Practical Insights into Atopic Dermatitis

Kwang Hoon Lee • Eung Ho Choi
Chang Ook Park
Editors

Practical Insights into Atopic Dermatitis

Springer

Editors
Kwang Hoon Lee
Department of Dermatology
Yonsei University College of Medicine
Seoul
Korea (Republic of)

Chang Ook Park
Department of Dermatology
Yonsei University College of Medicine
Seoul
Korea (Republic of)

Eung Ho Choi
Department of Dermatology
Yonsei University Wonju College
of Medicine
Wonju
Korea (Republic of)

ISBN 978-981-15-8158-8 ISBN 978-981-15-8159-5 (eBook)
https://doi.org/10.1007/978-981-15-8159-5

This Springer imprint is published by the registered company Springer Nature Singapore Pte Ltd.
The registered company address is: 152 Beach Road, #21-01/04 Gateway East, Singapore 189721, Singapore

Contents

Part I

Introduction

Introduction to Atopic Dermatitis

Kwang Hoon Lee

Atopic dermatitis is one of the most common chronic, recurrent eczematous disorders. It often begins in infancy or early adolescence, and is accompanied by severe itching and various skin symptoms. Moreover, there is an increasing number of atopic dermatitis patients worldwide [1].

Although atopic dermatitis has various epidemiological factors, such as region, age, gender, and sociocultural characteristics, the incidence of atopic dermatitis has been increasing all over the world due to environmental changes, such as the changes in eating habits, clothing, residential environment, and urbanization. In case of children under 6 years old, the incidence rate of atopic dermatitis has been reported to be about 3%. Furthermore, its incidence rate has been estimated to be over 20% in children, and 1–3% in adults for the last 20–30 years [2]. The symptoms usually improve in around the first birthday, kindergarten age, or just before puberty; however, they may persist until adulthood. According to recent clinical studies, there is a steadily increasing number of adults with acute atopic dermatitis even after their twenties. Since an increasing number of adults who experience the development of atopic dermatitis for the first time in their life, it is likely to be a serious social issue [3, 4].

K. H. Lee (✉)
Department of Dermatology, Cutaneous Biology Research Institute, Yonsei University College of Medicine, Seoul, Korea (Republic of)
e-mail: kwanglee@yuhs.ac

Patients with chronic and intractable itching, especially on their faces or hands, would be difficult to keep social relationships with others. Atopic dermatitis not only significantly damages quality of life by causing sleep deprivation, fatigue, or decrease in a sense of achievement, but also put burden on patients themselves and their families. Clinically, its symptoms vary depending on the age of patients. The progression of atopic dermatitis is classified into three phases based on the patient's age: infancy, childhood, adolescence and adulthood [1, 5, 6]. Infancy is a period that refers to babies from 2 or 3 months to 2 years. During childhood, from 3 years to before adolescence, patients experience redness around joint areas of legs, necks, ankles, and other flexural areas. On these parts of the skin, atopic dermatitis first develops as a form of acute eczema, which makes skin red, rugged, flaky, hard. At the same time, skin around the forehead and eyes becomes red, dark, hard, and flaky. Atopic dermatitis during adolescence and adulthood display symptoms like skin redness around the upper part of the body, such as face, neck, head. Then, as in the earlier phases, the affected skin gets dark, swollen, and hard. Various types of acute or chronic eczema develop around trunk, hands, feet, arms, legs, and other parts.

It is not difficult for most physicians to diagnose atopic dermatitis; however, it gets sometimes confusing to diagnose because atopic dermatitis is accompanied by various

K. H. Lee et al. (eds.), *Practical Insights into Atopic Dermatitis*,
https://doi.org/10.1007/978-981-15-8159-5_1

clinical symptoms and signs [4]. Thus, it becomes complicated to define characteristic clinical symptoms of atopic dermatitis. For example, since skin diseases like psoriasis, lichen planus, or herpes are distinguishable by inspection of primary skin lesions, they are easy to be diagnosed by doctors, especially by dermatologists. On the other hand, atopic dermatitis does not provoke prototypical eczematous skin lesions in most cases. While the patients scratch their skins, the skin lesions are aggravated and resulted in a number of secondary changes. Furthermore, even experts have some difficulties in diagnosing atopic dermatitis due to a lack of definitive examinations to decide upon. Many physicians also do not regard this disease as to be curable completely. Unfortunately, since there are not many appropriate treatments available for atopic dermatitis, it is liable to abuse alternative therapies, resulting in the economic damage to the atopic dermatitis patients. Recently, numerous adverse reactions have been reported to occur because of prevalent inaccurate and unverified information based on personal experiences throughout the Internet.

Even though there were not many basic or clinical studies about atopic dermatitis going on actively about 40 years ago, as atopic dermatitis prevalence rates have been rapidly increasing for the past 10 years, now there is a great number of both qualitatively and quantitatively excellent researches about atopic dermatitis due to a splendid development in genetics and immunology [7–11].

History and Definition of Atopic Dermatitis Terms

The description of atopic eczema is thought to have started when Robert Willan wrote the term, "eczema," in 1808. Indeed, the term 'eczema' itself began to be used by the Greek scholar Aetios, who used the term as the meaning of boiling and bubbling (eczeo or ekzein = to bubble up) in the sixth century AD [6].

Later, Wilson depicted the disease with similar skin symptoms as infantile eczema. Hebra also named prurigo, which is considered to be a subtype of atopic dermatitis nowadays, as "constitutional prurigo." Hebra further explained that the major symptom of prurigo is itching, and prurigo is characterized by frequent outbreaks in infants, erythematous lesions, papule and lichenoid lesions increase with age, chronic progressive course, seasonal fluctuations, and association with hay fever and asthma. The concept of constitution that prurigo begins during early childhood and continues to the rest of the life has become a critical part of dermatology. Brocq later invented the concept of "neurodermatitis" [6, 12].

With advancement of immunology and allergology in the early 1900s, a condition of hypersensitivity associated with asthma began to be referred as 'atopy'. In 1923, Coca and Cook [13] defined atopy as a tendency to run in families like hay fever or asthma, and to display hypersensitive reactions to foreign antigens. The word, atopy, means "not located in the right place and not in order" in Greek. In 1933, Wise and Sulzberger [5] included development of skin symptoms with atopic tendency as a characteristic of atopic dermatitis and named it atopic dermatitis or atopic eczema. Since it has been proved that IgE is a mediator of immediate-type hypersensitivity by Ishizaka [14], atopy has been equated with various IgE-mediated diseases by many people. However, it is controversial to simplify atopic dermatitis as an IgE-mediated disease, because IgE-mediated penicillin hypersensitivity or hypersensitive reactions to insect bites do not often run in families. Bruynzeel-Koomen et al. [15] first identified that IgE is attached to Langerhans cells, which are antigen-presenting cells, in skin lesions of atopic dermatitis patients, and this attachment has been further verified by other researchers since then. Klubal et al. [16] also observed that these IgE molecules described above adhere to Fc epsilon RI, a high-affinity receptor for IgE, on the surface of Langerhans cells in active skin lesions of atopic dermatitis patients. Consequently, these results demonstrated that inhalant allergens, such as house dust mites, might be able to penetrate directly into the skin and cause Th2 immune responses.

In 1983, Wuthrich [17] proposed the classification of extrinsic and intrinsic atopy by analogy with respiratory atopy. However, this classification system evoked controversy about nomenclature in around 2000, so it was discussed by the Task Force Teams of the European Academy of Allergology and Clinical Immunology (EAACI) and the World Allergy Organization (WAO) [18].

Those teams initially described that "atopy has an individual or familial tendency, and begins in infancy or adolescence mainly after being exposed to protein antigens, which are then sensitized to produce IgE antibodies. As a result, these patients show typical symptoms such as asthma, rhinitis, or eczema." Based on the above definition, if patients have asthma, rhinitis, or eczema, which do not have IgE detected, they can be determined to have no "atopic diseases." For that reason, the WAO Task Force Team redefined "eczema." Since then, they have confirmed the adjective, atopy, only when IgE antigens are found in patient's serum. Unfortunately, this classification also led to the division of atopic diseases into atopic and non-atopic eczema [6]. Up until 50 years ago, many researchers believed that allergies would not be involved in the pathogenesis of atopic dermatitis, but rather that dry skin and psychological factors were the main causes. Nevertheless, according to the research results and achievements of all pathophysiological mechanisms or responses to treatments today, atopic dermatitis and allergy are absolutely relevant and inseparable from each other.

The controversies surrounding this terminology have started with the motivation to understand the etiology of atopic dermatitis. Earlier terms were based on the clinical studies and symptoms of the disease, whereas the presence of IgE antibodies has become more important when defining the term nowadays. According to the definition made by WAO, WAO initially focused on IgE which is measured in patients, rather than on visible symptoms. They subsequently included the clinical symptoms when defining atopic dermatitis [6]. In the light of research and clinical experiences to date, atopic dermatitis is a disease that belongs to IgE-mediated diseases from one angle of perspectives. On the other hand, it covers a broader scope. With the above definition, we can understand atopic diseases present at both ends of spectrum, which refer to two phenomena, IgE antibody production, and nonspecific immune responses. It is likely to suspect that there is atopy disease where the two phenomena overlap. However, it may still cause some confusion because there exists a condition that does not have "latent atopy (IgE is detected in blood but does not display clinical symptoms)" or "intrinsic atopy (IgE is not detected but shows clinical symptoms)" on the margins of the spectrum.

Terms of Eczema and Atopic Dermatitis

Being a synonym for various types of dermatitis as well as atopic dermatitis, the term "eczema" has been used historically in numerous regions worldwide by many medical specialties. Eczema means "boiling" in Greek and was introduced in the medical literature to refer to a small group of skin diseases that show vesicular or bullous lesions by Robert Wilan [6].

As mentioned previously, Atopic dermatitis was initially called "porrigo larvalis," "lichen agrius," and "prurigo Besnier." The term "atopy" itself was introduced by Coca and Cooke [13] in 1923, establishing a new definition of hypersensitivity, one of the abnormal immunological reactions. In 1933, Sulzberger and Wise [5] first documented atopic dermatitis in a footnote of "1933 Year Book of Dermatology and Syphilogy." Since then, dermatitis and eczema have actually been used as synonyms to describe a subset of distinct clinical symptoms of patients. Some doctors also refer general eczema as atopic dermatitis.

There have been repeated and active discussions for centuries about the accurate meaning of eczema to determine whether eczema accompanies itching or not, whether it includes acute lesions with oozing and chronic ones like lichenification, and whether the cause is extrinsic or intrinsic. The word 'eczema' has not only been used continuously, but has also remained to be a demanding challenge for the American dermatology literatures. Since it is vague to determine what other diseases are included in eczema or to grasp an accurate definition of eczema, increasing number of people have desired to eliminate the term entirely [19]. Although some authors have agreed with this claim, many dermatologists have been opposed to the argument. Bear [20] said, "Rational doctors still use these irrational and incorrect terms because those terms are already well known and helpful. Even if it is possible to assign better names, misleading old words are not always discarded. This is because there still remain some purposes to use the term, and besides it is difficult to learn new terms quickly throughout the world."

According to the recent meta-analysis and review papers, "atopic dermatitis" and "eczema" are the most common nomenclatures for atopic dermatitis [21]. It is not easy to describe the characteristics of atopic dermatitis due to its broad spectrum. "Eczema" is the most universal term preferred by the public rather than physicians. Many clinicians often select the word "eczema" to explain some morphological changes. Other clinicians may consider "eczema" and atopic dermatitis as synonyms according to nomenclature methods specified by the World Allergy Society. Thus, heterogeneous use of these terms can be confusing for patients to understand their diseases.

Diagnosis of Atopic Dermatitis

Georg Rajka and Jon Hanifin [22] brought the most significant change in the words of atopic dermatitis by proposing diagnostic criteria for atopic dermatitis in 1979. Simultaneously, Scoring System for Atopic Dermatitis (SCORAD) was first introduced to assess a degree of atopic dermatitis severity and it led to the development of objective tools for evaluating conditions of patients with atopic dermatitis. In other words, this is when the concept of atopic dermatitis has begun to take shape and numerous new diagnostic criteria have been proposed. Nonetheless, atopic dermatitis still lacks accurate biomarkers and displays a variety of clinical presentations. Thus, it is difficult to make 100% satisfactory diagnostic criteria or definitions for atopic dermatitis.

Treatment of Atopic Dermatitis

Prior to the introduction of antibiotics and steroids, atopic dermatitis was mainly treated with internal medications, dietary habit change and topical therapies. Sulzberger recommended tar ointment as the most effective drug for treating eczema on the face of infants when there were no steroids out in the medical fields [5]. Current debate on atopic dermatitis has shifted from harmful fluids discussed in the past to inflammatory cytokines and disorder of hereditary barrier disruptions. When looking at from the outside-in (corneocentric) and inside-out (immunocentric) perspectives, there are new treatments for repairing skin barriers and some magical biologics for terminating persistent inflammation [10]. Besides, Arsenic was replaced by cyclosporine, tar by topical steroids and topical calcineurin inhibitors, and roentgen therapy by narrowband ultraviolet (UV) UVB and UVA1.

References

1. Bieber T. Atopic dermatitis. N Engl J Med. 2008;358:1483–94.
2. Nutten S. Atopic dermatitis: global epidemiology and risk factors. Ann Nutr Metab. 2015;66(Suppl 1):8–16.
3. Kim J, Chao LX, Simpson EL, Silverberg JI. Persistence of atopic dermatitis (AD): a systematic review and meta-analysis. J Am Acad Dermatol. 2016;75(4):681–7.
4. Chu H, Shin JU, Park CO, Lee H, Lee J, Lee KH. Clinical diversity of atopic dermatitis: a review of 5,000 patients at a single institute. Allergy Asthma Immunol Res. 2017;9(2):158–68.
5. Wise F, Sulzberger MB. Editor's remarks. In: Yearbook of dermatology and syphilology. Chicago: Year Book Medical; 1933.

6. Ring J. Atopic dermatitis: eczema. Switzerland: Springer; 2016.
7. Novak N, Leung DY. Advances in atopic dermatitis. Curr Opin Immunol. 2011;23:778–83.
8. Kim HJ, Shin JU, Lee KH. Atopic dermatitis and skin barrier dysfunction. Allergy Asthma Respir Dis. 2013;1(1):20–8.
9. Park CO, Noh S, Jin S, Lee NR, Lee YS, Lee H, Lee J, Lee KH. Insight into newly discovered innate immune modulation in atopic dermatitis. Exp Dermatol. 2013;22(1):6–9.
10. Paller AS, Kabashima K, Bieber T. Therapeutic pipeline for atopic dermatitis: end of the drought? J Allergy Clin Immunol. 2017;140(3):633–43.
11. Weidinger S, Beck LA, Bieber T, Kabashima K, Irvine AD. Atopic dermatitis. Nat Rev Dis Primers. 2018;4(1):1.
12. Rudikoff D, Cohen SR, Scheinfeld N. Atopic dermatitis and eczematous disorders. Boca Raton, FL: Taylor & Francis Group; 2014.
13. Coca AF, Cooke RA. On the classification of the phenomena of hypersensitiveness. J Immunol. 1923;8:163–82.
14. Ishizaka K, Ishizaka T. Identification of gE antibodies as carrier of reaginic activity. J Immunol. 1967;99:1187–98.
15. Bruynzeel-Koomen C, van Wichen DF, Toonstra J, Berrens L, Bruynzeel PL. The presence of IgE molecules on epidermal Langerhans cells in patients with atopic dermatitis. Arch Dermatol Res. 1986;278:199–205.
16. Klubal R, Osterhoff B, Wang B, Kinet JP, Maurer D, Stingl G. The high-affinity receptor for IgE is the predominant IgE-binding structure in lesional skin of atopic dermatitis patients. J Invest Dermatol. 1997;108:336–42.
17. Wuthrich B, Schmid-Grendelmeier P. The atopic eczema/dermatitis syndrome. Epidemiology, natural course, and immunology of the IgE-associated ("extrinsic") and the nonallergic 8 ("intrinsic") AEDS. J Invest Allergol Clin Immunol. 2003;13:1–5.
18. Johansson SGO, Bieber T, Dahl R, Friedmann PS, Lanier BQ, Lockey RF, et al. Revised nomenclature for allergy for global use. Allergy Clin Immunol Int J World Allergy Org. 2004;17:4–8.
19. Ackerman AB, Ragaz A. A plea to expunge the word 'eczema' from the lexicon of dermatology and dermatology and dermatopathology. Arch Dermatol Res. 1982;272:407–20.
20. Baer RL. No-the word 'eczema' should not be expunged but be retained for the time being. Am J Dermtopathol. 1982;4(4):327–8.
21. Siverberg JI, Thyssen JP, Paller AS, Drucker AM, Wollenberg A, Lee KH, Kabsshima K, Todd G, Schmid-Grenelmeier P, Bieber T. What's in a name? Atopic dermatitis or atopic eczema, but not eczema alone. Allergy. 2017;72(12):2026–30.
22. Hanifin IM, Rajka G. Diagnostic features of atopic dermatitis. Acta Derm Venereol. 1980;92(suppl):44–7.

Part II

Epidemiology

Epidemiology of Atopic Dermatitis

Jaeyong Shin

Epidemiology of Atopic Dermatitis at a Glance

- The prevalence of atopic dermatitis is on the rise, 10–20 percent of children and 1–3 percent of adults around the world.
- It is assumed that environmental factors may be associated with the difference in prevalence around the world.
- In the industrialized world, atopic dermatitis as a cause of increased hygiene hypothesis (Hygiene hypothesis), indoor and outdoor environments, increasing pollution, Westernized eating habits, etc. can be mentioned as the cause of everything.
- Atopic dermatitis not only puts an economic burden on the patient, but also social costs.

Atopic dermatitis (AD) is one of the most common skin diseases and is on the rise worldwide [1–6]. Especially in industrialized countries, 10–20% of children and 1–3% of adults suffered from atopic dermatitis [4, 6]. One of five children have symptoms of atopic dermatitis during certain times of life. Half of the AD patients initially show symptoms within the first 12 months [7]. Even though most of them experience spontaneous relief of symptoms during the school-age or adolescence, eczema lesions can be accompanied by itching often deteriorate intermittently. In addition, 25% of children's atopic dermatitis is thought to continue atopic dermatitis in the form of dry skin and eczema in their hands even after the symptoms of severe dermatitis have disappeared. Adult-onset AD has also been increasing. In this chapter, we look at the differences between the prevalence rate AD at home and abroad and its geographical location, the factors of the increase in AD, and the social cost of the skin disease.

Epidemiology of Atopic Dermatitis in Korea

Research on the prevalence rate of atopic dermatitis can be largely divided into methods by dermatologist's skin examination, methods of using questionnaire, and methods of using big data such as data requested by the Health Insurance Review and Assessment (HIRA) (Table 1). First, the dermatologist's skin examination method is the most accurate way to check the prevalence rate of atopic dermatitis in a specific population. However, skin screening requires a lot of effort and cost. Also, it takes a lot of time and resources that it is unrealistic to study on a large popula-

J. Shin (✉)
Department of Preventive Medicine,
Yonsei University College of Medicine, Seoul,
Korea (Republic of)
e-mail: drshin@yuhs.ac

K. H. Lee et al. (eds.), *Practical Insights into Atopic Dermatitis*,
https://doi.org/10.1007/978-981-15-8159-5_2

Table 1 The prevalence rate of atopic dermatitis in Korea

Author	Year	Age (year)	*n*	Prevalence rate	
1. Epidemiology based on the skin examination by dermatologists					
Kim et al.	1978	≤6	516	11.2%	Modified Hanifin's criteria
Lee et al.	1992	7–8	4018	3.78%	Modified Hanifin's criteria
Kim et al.	1994–1995	6–18	6070	6.0%	Hanifin and Rajka Criteria
		6–8	1926	10.0%	
		10–12	2362	5.4%	
		16–18	1782	2.5%	
Kim et al.	2009	≥19	2032	2.6%	Hanifin and Rajka Criteria
Kim et al.	2009	3–6	733	7.9%	Korean diagnostic criteria
		3–6	733	8.0%	Japanese diagnostic criteria
		3–6	733	11.2%	Hanifin and Rajka Criteria
Bae et al.	2010	19–24	1321	5.1%	Korean diagnostic criteria
Lee et al.	2012	7–12	1320	11.3%	Hanifin and Rajka Criteria
2. Epidemiology based on a survey					
Lee et al.	1995	6–12	25,361	7.3%	ISAAC questionnaire
		12–15	15,068	3.9%	
Oh et al.	2000	6–12	27,425	10.7%	ISAAC questionnaire
		12–15	14,777	6.1%	
Seo et al.	2006	8–11	30,893	15.3%	ISAAC questionnaire
Kim et al.	2009	>19	3563	7.1%	Questionnaire based on Hanifin and Rajka Criteria
Baek et al.	2009	0–12	8750	14.4%	ISAAC questionnaire
		0–6	1136	18.0%	
		7–12	7614	13.9%	
Ahn et al.	2010	6–7	3953	17.9%	ISAAC questionnaire
		13–14	4010	11.2%	
Lee et al.	2011	13–18	75,643	23.1%	The 7th Korea Youth Risk Behavior Web-based Survey
3. Epidemiology based on the Korean National Health Insurance Claims database					
Yu et al.	2008	All age groups	48,606,787	2.2%	
		≤18	11,119,894	6.9%	
		>18	37,486,893	0.9%	
Kim et al.	2014	All age groups	All residents in Korea	1.9%	
		<10		9.5%	
		≥10		1.2%	

tion. Second, the method of using questionnaires can be for the entire population. It also has an advantage to capture time trends across geographic areas. However, it is necessary to verify the validity and reliability of the survey tool. The diagnosis of atopic dermatitis depends on the subjective judgment of the respondents, and there is a risk for a recall bias. The most widely used questionnaire for epidemiological studies of atopic diseases is the ISAAC questionnaire produced by the International Study of Asthma and Allergy in Childhood Program [8–10]. ISAAC questionnaire consists of survey questions to confirm the occurrence of major atopic diseases over the past year, such as asthma, allergic rhinitis, atopic dermatitis, allergic conjunctivitis, food allergy, and drug allergy. The ISAAC questionnaire has been adopted to investigate the prevalence of atopic diseases internationally and has been conducted several times in Korea. Lastly, claim-based big national data by the HIRA is one of the important sources of epidemiological research. However, visits to hospitals are selective depending on individual characteristics, severity of the disease, and accompanying medical conditions. Since medical records are not designed for research, they may be medically inaccurate or incomplete. They may also include nonmedical content, especially according to salary recognition criteria.

Diagnosis of atopic dermatitis requires accurate medical history and skin examination [11–13]. Therefore, it is difficult to make an accurate diagnosis without examining patients in person. Therefore, it suggests that epidemiological studies by skin screening suggest the most accurate prevalence of atopic dermatitis. However, epidemiological surveys using questionnaires and big data-based research can provide new information that cannot be obtained from small-scale studies.

Epidemiology of Atopic Dermatitis by Skin Examination

Kim et al., in Jincheon County, North Chungcheong Province (Table 1), conducted the first epidemiological study of atopic dermatitis reported to the Korean Dermatological Society in 1978 [14]. They visited all families with infants in the area and conducted skin checkups of 516 children under the age of 6 and reported 11.2% (58 people) of the prevalence rate. According to this study, 67.3% of the patients had a family history of atopic diseases. Atopic dermatitis began after 2 months of birth, with the highest frequency between 18 and 24 months. It decreased after the age of 5 years.

Lee et al. [15] visited 10 elementary schools in Bucheon in 1992 and conducted skin checkups for 4018 students at the age of 7 years old. They reported a 3.78% (152/4018) prevalence of atopic dermatitis. The most common eczematous lesions are flexural areas (83.6%). It is also frequently accompanied by pityriasis alba (59.8%), perifollicular accentuation (57.8%), keratosis pilaris (56.5%), hyperlinear palms, (55.2%), and Dennie-Morgan folds (26.3%).

In 1994–1995, Kim et al. [16], conducted skin checkups on 6070 children and teenagers aged between 6 and 18 years in Seoul, Ulsan, and Chuncheon. They found that the prevalence rate of atopic dermatitis was 6.0% for all participants, 10.0% for the aged between 6 and 8 years, 5.4% for the aged 10–12 years old, and 2.5% for the aged 16–18 years old, respectively. Especially for those aged 6–8 years of the most common frequency, the prevalence of AD was 17.5% in Seoul and 9.6% in Chuncheon. It shows that the prevalence rate of atopic dermatitis was higher in large cities than in provincial cities.

Kim et al. [16] visited four kindergartens in Daegu to conduct skin examinations of 733 children aged between 3 and 6 years. They described that the prevalence of AD was 7.9% of the Korean atopic dermatitis diagnosis standards, 8.0% of the Japanese atopic dermatitis diagnosis standards, and 11.2% of Hanifin and Rajka diagnosis standards.

In 2012, Lee et al. [17] conducted skin checkups on a total of 1320 students (7–12 years old) at five elementary schools in Gwangju, with 11.3% (149/1320 years old) having atopic dermatitis.

Kim et al. [18] conducted skin checkups on healthy adults aged 19 years or older (n = 2032) who visited skin examination centers at six general hospitals in Seoul and Gyeonggi Province in 2009. They reported that the prevalence rate of adult atopic dermatitis was 2.6%. Adult patients had the highest atopic dermatitis at 4.5% in their 30s, decreasing with 1.2% in their 50s and 0.4% in their 60s or older. It also shows significantly higher prevalence rates in men (4.2%), compared to women (1.3%).

Bae et al. [19], visited a military unit in northern Gyeonggi Province in 2010 and conducted skin checkups of 1321 soldiers (19–24 years old). According to the study, atopic dermatitis (5.1%) was the third most common skin disease after acne (35.6%) and athlete's foot (15.2%). However, AD had the greatest impact on soldiers' quality of life in all three aspects: symptoms, function, and emotion.

Epidemiology of Atopic Dermatitis by Questionnaire

In 1995, Lee et al. [20] surveyed 40,429 children aged between 6 and 15 years. They found that 7.3% of elementary school students (6–12 years old) and 3.9% of middle school students (12–15 years old) had atopic dermatitis. It shows higher rate in Seoul (elementary school students: 8.8%; middle school: 4.9%) compared to provincial cities (elementary school students: 6.6%; middle school: 3.5%). The study was conducted again in 2000 under the same condition [21]. It shows a higher prevalence than in 1995, with 10.7% in elementary school and 6.1% in middle school. In 2010, Ahn et al., conducted a survey on the prevalence of atopic dermatitis nationwide in the same way in the same age group [22]. It also confirmed that atopic dermatitis has been steadily increasing in Korea, with 17.9% of elementary school students and 11.2% of middle school students.

In addition, many researchers studied the dynamics of atopic dermatitis under various conditions using different questionnaires. According to a survey of 30,893 children aged 8–11 years using ISAAC questionnaire in 2006 [23], Seo et al. found that atopic dermatitis had a prevalence rate of 15.3% (girls: 16.5%, boys: 13.7%). In particular, the number of cases of atopic dermatitis was high in industrialized cities (15.9% for boys and 18.7% for girls), large cities (15.4% for boys and 17.5% for girls), provincial cities (13.6% for boys and 17.0% for girls), and island areas (11.4% for boys and 14.2% for girls), respectively. According to a study conducted by Kim et al. on healthy adults who visited the skin examination centers in 2009, the prevalence of atopic dermatitis in adults was 2.6% of skin checkups and 7.1% of the ISAAC questionnaire, respectively. In 2009, Paik et al. [24] used ISAAC questionnaire for 8750 children (0–12 years old), and the prevalence rate of atopic dermatitis was 14.4% for all participants, 18.0% for preschool children (0–6 years old), and 13.9% for elementary school students (7–12 years old). According to the 7th Korea Centers for Disease Control and Prevention's online survey of youth health behaviors ($n = 75{,}643$) in 2011 [25], the prevalence of atopic dermatitis was 23.1% in adolescents (13–18 years old). The high risk for AD is associated with the higher the income of their families and the higher the educational background of their mothers.

Epidemiological Investigation of Atopic Dermatitis Based on Claims Data from the Health Insurance Review and Assessment Service

According to a survey of patients who visited hospitals more than once with the main diagnosis of atopic dermatitis (ICD-10 code: L20) using data requested by the Health Insurance Review and Assessment Service [26], the prevalence rate of atopic dermatitis nationwide was 2.2% (male 2.1%, female 2.4%) in 2008. The prevalence rate of atopic dermatitis by age group was decreasing with the increasing age group, 21.1% by 12 months of age, 26.5% by 12 months of age, 7.6% by 6 years of age, 3.4% by 12 years of age, 2.4% by 18 years of age, and 0.9% by 19 years of age, respectively. Kim et al. [27] reported that the prevalence rate of atopic dermatitis was 1.9%, 9.5% under the age of 10, and 1.2% over the age of 10 in 2014, under the same conditions.

Geographical Location According to Different Prevalence of Atopic Dermatitis

A representative study comparing prevalence rates of atopic diseases by country is the "International Study on the Epidemiological Survey of Pediatric Asthma and Allergy Diseases (ISAAC)" project. The ISAAC study was planned in three stages, with the aim of comparing prevalence rates among countries in Phase I, the risk factors for allergic diseases in Phase II, and the objective of repeating the first stage of investigation in Phase III to see changes in prevalence rates over time.

The first-stage ISAAC study was conducted by 155 organizations from 56 countries in 1992–1997 [28], covering a total of 715,033 children, while the third-stage ISAAC study was conducted by 233 institutions from 98 countries between 1999 and 2004 [29]. This is the largest epidemiological study ever conducted on a global scale to investigate the prevalence of atopic dermatitis, and the prevalence rate of atopic dermatitis can be compared according to geographical location. The global prevalence of atopic dermatitis in children (6–7 years old) was 6.1% in the first phase of ISAAC study (1992–1997), up 7.9% in the third phase (1999–2004), and showed a range of 0.9% (India) to 22.5% (Equator) depending on the country and institution. Even within one continent, the prevalence of atopic dermatitis showed a large deviation, generally high prevalence in Oceania, and low prevalence rates in India, the eastern Mediterranean, northern Europe, and Eastern Europe. Areas with particularly high prevalence rates of 15% or more were located in Asia-Pacific, Central and South America, Europe, and Oceania. In this study, the prevalence of atopic dermatitis in children in Korea was 11.3%, the 22nd highest among 56 countries.

The global prevalence of atopic dermatitis in adolescence (13–14 years old) increased from 7.3% in 1992–1997 to 8.8% in 1999–2004, with a range of 0.2% (China) to 24.6% (Colombia) [30]. This also has large regional deviations with generally high prevalence rates in Africa and Oceania, and with low prevalence rates in India, northern Europe, and Eastern Europe. In this study, the prevalence rate of atopic dermatitis in adolescence in Korea was 5.7%, the 65th among 98 countries.

In summary, the prevalence of atopic dermatitis was on the rise worldwide in both children and adolescence, and there was a huge difference of 60 times for each country. These large differences between regions suggest that environmental factors play an important role in the occurrence of atopic dermatitis.

Factors to Increase Atopic Dermatitis

In the ISAAC study, the global prevalence of atopic dermatitis shows an overall upward trend between 1992 and 1997 and 1999 and 2004. The change was observed in most countries except Western Europe, especially among countries in Africa, the Asia-Pacific region, South America, South Europe, and Eastern Europe. In a study using ISAAC questionnaire conducted in Korea, the prevalence rate of atopic dermatitis among elementary school students increased to 7.3% in 1995, 10.7% in 2000, 17.9% in 2010, 3.9% in 1995, 6.1% in 2000, and 11.2% in 2010. Deckers et al. [30] systematically examined literatures that reported the prevalence of atopic dermatitis between 1990 and 2010. They reported the increasing prevalence of atopic dermatitis in Africa, East Asia, Western Europe, and Northern Europe.

The prevalence rate of atopic diseases can fluctuate in a short period, depending on political and social changes. According to a study in Germany on the prevalence of atopic dermatitis in pre-unification children (5–6 years old) before and after unification, there was no significant change in West Germany [31], while East Germany saw a significant increase from 16.0% in 1991 to 23.4% in 1997. A similar phenomenon has been confirmed again in studies of other regions or immigrant groups where rapid urbanization has progressed.

Even within a country, there is a higher risk of atopic dermatitis in cities than in rural areas.

Table 2 Hypothesis of the rise in atopic dermatitis

Hypothesis of the rise in atopic dermatitis
1. Hygiene hypothesis
2. Indoor air pollution
3. Environmental pollution: Nitrogen dioxide with, the carbon monoxide, volatile compounds; and organic, fine dust
4. Climate : The Latitude the high, the low temperature, the low humidity, the low sunshine
5. Westernized food: Processed grains, the Red preserved meat, and saturated FAT
6. Others: Discontinuation of breastfeeding, early life exposure to antibiotics

According to a systematic review [32], 19 out of 26 studies comparing regional differences in atopic dermatitis show significantly higher prevalence than rural areas in cities.

Genetic predisposition and environmental factors work in the development of atopic dermatitis. The reason for the surge in atopic diseases such as asthma, allergic rhinitis, and atopic dermatitis can be explained as environmental factors stemming from industrialization. Changes in personal hygiene due to transformation to nuclear family and improvements in residential environment, the expansion of the use of hazardous chemicals, the increase in environmental pollutants resulting from industrialization, and Westernized eating habits are cited as factors for the occurrence and deterioration of atopic dermatitis (Table 2) [33].

Hygiene Hypothesis

In the late 1980s, Strachan raised the Hygiene Hypothesis to explain the high incidence of atopic dermatitis in families with few siblings [34]. Hygiene hypothesis is that Th1 immune response is not mature while the Th2 immune system prevails, in an industrialized society because of the decrease in family members, improvement in residential environment, and personal hygiene [35, 36]. They reduce the chance of exposure to viruses and germs in infancy or to endotoxins, increasing the prevalence of atopic diseases. The hypothesis suggests that external requirements in infancy can affect the determination of future immune responses, which is able to serve as a new opportunity to understand post-birth immune responses. However, the prevalence of atopic diseases in underdeveloped countries is often high, and atopic diseases occur frequently in population groups with low socioeconomic levels. This makes it difficult to explain the increase in atopic diseases only through the hygiene hypothesis. There is another analysis that hygiene hypothesis shows a stronger link in asthma and allergic rhinitis, while atopic dermatitis is relatively less persuasive.

Indoor Air Pollution

Indoor air pollution is regarded that it is a potential cause of increased atopic dermatitis. Many environmental factors, such as house dust mites, pollen, and exposure to air pollutants, are associated with the deterioration of atopic dermatitis as well as they increase the risk of atopic dermatitis [37]. There is a high risk of atopic dermatitis if the house was remodeled or new furniture purchased within 12 months of birth, and exposure to cigarette smoke before and after childbirth [38].

Environmental Pollution

Several studies suggest that the increase in environmental pollutants due to industrialization are direct factors in the increase in atopic dermatitis. The occurrence of atopic dermatitis is associated with residences closer to the side of the road, with high nitrogen dioxide (NO_2) and carbon monoxide (CO), which are harmful gases from automobiles [39]. Volatile organic compounds can also affect both the development and deterioration of atopic dermatitis, and recently, the relationship between Korea's spring fine dust and atopic dermatitis has been proven [40].

Climate

Climate is also closely related to triggering atopic dermatitis. Weiland et al. analyzed the first stage of ISAAC study conducted in 56 countries for a total of 715,033 children and adjusted income of each country, latitude, altitude, average annual temperature, and average relative humidity [41]. According to the study, it shows that the higher the latitude, the lower the annual average temperature is associated with the increased prevalence rate of atopic dermatitis. Low temperatures and low humidity are directly related to atopic dermatitis, and it has been proven that high humidity and adequate exposure to ultraviolet rays can reduce the occurrence of atopic dermatitis. As shown in these series of studies, climatic factors such as temperature, humidity, and exposure to ultraviolet rays are thought to have a direct impact on the development of atopic dermatitis [42]. However, climate factors are thought to work in combination with many other factors, as excessive sweating may worsen atopic dermatitis.

Diet

Westernized diet, characterized by processed grains, preserved red meats, and saturated fats, is one of the reasons for the increase in atopic dermatitis. The three-stage ISAAC study shows that atopic dermatitis is less common in children who frequently consume fresh fruits [43]. According to the study, the risk of atopic dermatitis also increases when eating fast food frequently. A similar result was also found in an ecological study comparing calories per capita by country, meat, and vegetable consumption with the prevalence of atopic dermatitis [44].

Westernized diet lacks ω-3 unsaturated fatty acids, which act as anti-inflammatory molecule, while it contains rich ω-6 unsaturated fatty acids, which act as an inflammatory agent. Frequent intake of fish rich in ω-3 unsaturated fatty acids during pregnancy reduced the incidence of atopic dermatitis. In contrast, mother's increased intake of ω-6 unsaturated fatty acids is also associated with the increased incidence of atopic dermatitis in fetus [45]. According to a prospective cohort study conducted in Germany, the risk of atopic dermatitis among children who usually consume margarine, was 2.1 times higher than that of children who usually consume butter. Margarine has 10–30 times higher linoleic acid, which is one of ω-6 unsaturated fatty acids, than butter [46]. As such, Westernization of eating habits is believed to affect the increase in atopic dermatitis.

Other Risk Factors

There has been a hypothesis that a cesarean section can change certain microbial strains of newborns [47]. According to the hypothesis, it may increase the risk of atopic dermatitis in infants. Based on the results of the meta-analysis of 26 observational studies [48], a cesarean section can increase the risk of food allergies, allergic rhinitis, and asthma in infants. However, it has not been confirmed to have a significant association with atopic dermatitis. It is also widely argued that breastfeeding can prevent the development of atopic dermatitis. However, according to the second phase of the ISAAC study (n = 51,119) [49], breastfeeding shows no preventive effect of atopic dermatitis. According to a systematic literature review of 27 prospective cohort studies on breastfeeding, Yang et al. [50] cannot describe any significant preventive effect of breastfeeding.

There was also much controversy over the impact of the use of antibiotics in infants on the development of atopic dermatitis. Tsukok et al. [51] conducted systematic literature studies and reviewed 20 observational studies (n = 289,384) and found that the use of antibiotics in mothers did not show any link to atopic dermatitis in the fetus, but the incidence of atopic dermatitis increased to 40% in the future if antibiotics were administered to infants within 12 months of age. However, 13 of the 20 studies included in the systematic literature review have the potential for recall biases due to a retrospective survey [52], and it is difficult to interpret this as a cause and result relationship because the infection in children with atopic dermatitis may increase and the use of antibiotics may be high.

Costs of Atopic Dermatitis

Kim et al. [53] analyzed the claims of the Health Insurance Review and Assessment Service in order to understand the cost of atopic dermatitis in Korea, and the annual medical cost of atopic dermatitis patients was 1.29 million won. In addition, as a result of prospective follow-up of actual atopic dermatitis-related costs of patients with atopic dermatitis ($n = 32$), direct medical expenses such as medical expenses and pharmaceutical expenses averaged 2.62 million won per year, When we consider all related indirect costs such as herbal treatment, transportation and purchasing moisturizer, it is estimated annually at 26.4 million Korean won.

The social cost includes visits of medical treatment and OTC purchases, emergency room visits, cost of hospitalization direct costs such as work and study in the book, such as the reduction of productivity indirect costs are included with all. Bickers et al. [54] estimated that skin disease due to consuming all the results of estimating the costs directly caused by atopic dermatitis of costs total $10 billion (psoriasis was 12 was $100 million), indirectly of the total, including the cost. The cost was $4.2 billion (psoriasis, $3.6 billion). According to a large-scale survey in the US adults with dermatitis [55], 32% of patients with atopic dermatitis said that atopic dermatitis affects their academic and work life, and 14% said that atopic dermatitis has a deteriorating career.

Conclusion

Atopic dermatitis is one of the most common skin diseases, which is not only economically burdensome for patients, but also socially expensive. Atopic dermatitis is increasing globally, especially in developing countries, and several recent epidemiological studies show that various environmental factors are involved in the increase in atopic dermatitis. However, there is still insufficient direct evidence to explain the causal relationship between individual factors and atopic dermatitis, and there is a great lack of discussion on how to suppress the increase in atopic dermatitis. In addition to the development of effective treatments, efforts to reduce the incidence of atopic dermatitis will also be needed.

References

1. Drucker AM, Wang AR, Li WQ, Sevetson E, Block JK, Qureshi AA. The burden of atopic dermatitis: summary of a report for the national eczema association. J Investig Dermatol. 2017;137:26–30.
2. Kaufman BP, Guttman-Yassky E, Alexis AF. Atopic dermatitis in diverse racial and ethnic groups-variations in epidemiology, genetics, clinical presentation and treatment. Exp Dermatol. 2018;27:340–57.
3. Nutten S. Atopic dermatitis: global epidemiology and risk factors. Ann Nutr Metab. 2015;66(Suppl 1):8–16.
4. Sacotte R, Silverberg JI. Epidemiology of adult atopic dermatitis. Clin Dermatol. 2018;36:595–605.
5. Silverberg JI. Public health burden and epidemiology of atopic dermatitis. Dermatol Clin. 2017;35:283–9.
6. Silvestre Salvador JF, Romero-Pérez D, Encabo-Durán B. Atopic dermatitis in adults: a diagnostic challenge. J Investig Allergol Clin Immunol. 2017;27:78–88.
7. Silverberg NB. Typical and atypical clinical appearance of atopic dermatitis. Clin Dermatol. 2017;35:354–9.
8. Brenninkmeijer EE, Schram ME, Leeflang MM, Bos JD, Spuls PI. Diagnostic criteria for atopic dermatitis: a systematic review. Br J Dermatol. 2008;158: 754–65.
9. Eichenfield LF, Tom WL, Chamlin SL, Feldman SR, Hanifin JM, Simpson EL, Berger TG, Bergman JN, Cohen DE, Cooper KD, Cordoro KM, Davis DM, Krol A, Margolis DJ, Paller AS, Schwarzenberger K, Silverman RA, Williams HC, Elmets CA, Block J, Harrod CG, Smith Begolka W, Sidbury R. Guidelines of care for the management of atopic dermatitis: section 1. Diagnosis and assessment of atopic dermatitis. J Am Acad Dermatol. 2014;70:338–51.
10. Pols DH, Wartna JB, Moed H, van Alphen EI, Bohnen AM, Bindels PJ. Atopic dermatitis, asthma and allergic rhinitis in general practice and the open population: a systematic review. Scand J Prim Health Care. 2016;34:143–50.
11. Avena-Woods C. Overview of atopic dermatitis. Am J Manag Care. 2017;23:S115–s23.
12. Barrett M, Luu M. Differential diagnosis of atopic dermatitis. Immunol Allergy Clin N Am. 2017;37:11–34.

13. Sidbury R, Kodama S. Atopic dermatitis guidelines: diagnosis, systemic therapy, and adjunctive care. Clin Dermatol. 2018;36:648–52.
14. Kim YH, Kim JW, Houh W. A study on incidence and genetic background of atopic dermatitis. Korean J Dermatol. 1979;17:105.
15. Lee SC, Byun DG, Lee WC, Kim JW. The prevalence and some minor clinical features of atopic dermatitis. Korean J Dermatol. 1995;33:1.
16. Kim C, Park C, Kim J, Koo D, Kim K, Kim T. Prevalence of atopic dermatitis in Korea. Acta Derm Venereol. 2000;80:353–6.
17. Lee S-C, Bae JM, Lee H-J, Kim HJ, Kim B-S, Li K, Cho J-W, Park CO, Cho SH, Lee KH. Introduction of the reliable estimation of atopic dermatitis in ChildHood: novel, diagnostic criteria for childhood atopic dermatitis. Allergy, Asthma Immunol Res. 2016;8:230–8.
18. Kim MJ, Kang TW, Cho EA, Kim HS, Min JA, Park H, Kim JW, Cha SH, Lee YB, Cho SH. Prevalence of atopic dermatitis among Korean adults visiting health service center of the Catholic Medical Center in Seoul Metropolitan Area, Korea. J Korean Med Sci. 2010;25:1828–30.
19. Bae JM, Ha B, Lee H, Park CK, Kim HJ, Park YM. Prevalence of common skin diseases and their associated factors among military personnel in Korea: a cross-sectional study. J Korean Med Sci. 2012;27:1248–54.
20. Lee SI, Shin MH, Lee HB, Lee JS, Son BK, Koh YY, Kim KE, Ahn YO. Prevalences of symptoms of asthma and other allergic diseases in Korean children: a nationwide questionnaire survey. J Korean Med Sci. 2001;16(2):155–64.
21. Oh J-W, Pyun B-Y, Choung J-T, Ahn K-M, Kim C-H, Song S-W, Son J-A, Lee S-Y, Lee S-I. Epidemiological change of atopic dermatitis and food allergy in school-aged children in Korea between 1995 and 2000. J Korean Med Sci. 2004;19:716–23.
22. Ahn K, Kim J, Kwon H-J, Chae Y, Hahm M-I, Lee K-J, Park YM, Lee S-Y, Han M, Kim WK. The prevalence of symptoms of asthma, allergic rhinoconjunctivitis, and eczema in Korean children: nationwide cross-sectional survey using complex sampling design. J Korean Med Assoc/Taehan Uisa Hyophoe Chi. 2011;54:769–78.
23. Suh M, Kim H-H, Sohn MH, Kim K-E, Kim C, Shin DC. Prevalence of allergic diseases among Korean school-age children: a nationwide cross-sectional questionnaire study. J Korean Med Sci. 2011;26:332–8.
24. Baek J-O, Hong S, Son D-K, Lee J-R, Roh J-Y, Kwon H-J. Analysis of the prevalence of and risk factors for atopic dermatitis using an ISAAC questionnaire in 8,750 Korean children. Int Arch Allergy Immunol. 2013;162:79–85.
25. Lee K-S, Rha Y-H, Oh I-H, Choi Y-S, Choi S-H. Socioeconomic and sociodemographic factors related to allergic diseases in Korean adolescents based on the Seventh Korea Youth Risk Behavior Web-based Survey: a cross-sectional study. BMC Pediatr. 2016;16:19.
26. Yu J-S, Lee C-J, Lee H-S, Kim J, Han Y, Ahn K, Lee S-I. Prevalence of atopic dermatitis in Korea: analysis by using national statistics. J Korean Med Sci. 2012;27:681–5.
27. Kim B-K, Kim J-Y, Kang M-K, Yang M-S, Park H-W, Min K-U, Cho S-H, Kang H-R. Allergies are still on the rise? A 6-year nationwide population-based study in Korea. Allergol Int. 2016;65:186–91.
28. Williams H, Robertson C, Stewart A, Aït-Khaled N, Anabwani G, Anderson R, Asher I, Beasley R, Björkstén B, Burr M. Worldwide variations in the prevalence of symptoms of atopic eczema in the International Study of Asthma and Allergies in Childhood. J Allergy Clin Immunol. 1999;103:125–38.
29. Mallol J, Crane J, von Mutius E, Odhiambo J, Keil U, Stewart A, ISAAC Phase Three Study Group. The International Study of Asthma and Allergies in Childhood (ISAAC) phase three: a global synthesis. Allergol Immunopathol. 2013;41:73–85.
30. Deckers IA, McLean S, Linssen S, Mommers M, Van Schayck C, Sheikh A. Investigating international time trends in the incidence and prevalence of atopic eczema 1990–2010: a systematic review of epidemiological studies. PLoS One. 2012;7:e39803.
31. Krämer U, Schmitz R, Ring J, Behrendt H. What can reunification of East and West Germany tell us about the cause of the allergy epidemic? Clin Exp Allergy. 2015;45:94–107.
32. Schram M, Tedja A, Spijker R, Bos J, Williams H, Spuls PI. Is there a rural/urban gradient in the prevalence of eczema? A systematic review. Br J Dermatol. 2010;162:964–73.
33. Cramer C, Link E, Koletzko S, Lehmann I, Heinrich J, Wichmann H-E, Bauer C-P, Berg AV, Berdel D, Herbarth O. The hygiene hypothesis does not apply to atopic eczema in childhood. In: New trends in allergy and atopic eczema. Basel: Karger; 2012. p. 15–23.
34. Strachan DP. Hay fever, hygiene, and household size. Br Med J. 1989;299:1259.
35. Yazdanbakhsh M, Kremsner PG, Van Ree R. Allergy, parasites, and the hygiene hypothesis. Science. 2002;296:490–4.
36. Wills-Karp M, Santeliz J, Karp CL. The germless theory of allergic disease: revisiting the hygiene hypothesis. Nat Rev Immunol. 2001;1:69–75.
37. Tupker RA, De Monchy JG, Coenraads PJ, Homanb A, van der Meer JB. Induction of atopic dermatitis by inhalation of house dust mite. J Allergy Clin Immunol. 1996;97:1064–70.
38. Herbarth O, Fritz GJ, Rehwagen M, Richter M, Röder S, Schlink U. Association between indoor renovation activities and eczema in early childhood. Int J Hyg Environ Health. 2006;209:241–7.
39. Wen HJ, Chen PC, Chiang TL, Lin SJ, Chuang YL, Guo YL. Predicting risk for early infantile atopic dermatitis by hereditary and environmental factors. Br J Dermatol. 2009;161:1166–72.

40. Ahn K. The role of air pollutants in atopic dermatitis. J Allergy Clin Immunol. 2014;134:993–9.
41. Weiland S, Hüsing A, Strachan D, Rzehak P, Pearce N. Climate and the prevalence of symptoms of asthma, allergic rhinitis, and atopic eczema in children. Occup Environ Med. 2004;61:609–15.
42. Silverberg JI, Hanifin J, Simpson EL. Climatic factors are associated with childhood eczema prevalence in the United States. J Investig Dermatol. 2013;133:1752–9.
43. Ellwood P, Asher MI, García-Marcos L, Williams H, Keil U, Robertson C, Nagel G, Group IPIS. Do fast foods cause asthma, rhinoconjunctivitis and eczema? Global findings from the International Study of Asthma and Allergies in Childhood (ISAAC) phase three. Thorax. 2013;68:351–60.
44. Ellwood P, Asher M, Björkstén B, Burr M, Pearce N, Robertson C. Diet and asthma, allergic rhinoconjunctivitis and atopic eczema symptom prevalence: an ecological analysis of the International Study of Asthma and Allergies in Childhood (ISAAC) data. Eur Respir J. 2001;17:436–43.
45. Willers S, Devereux G, Craig L, McNeill G, Wijga A, El-Magd WA, Turner S, Helms P, Seaton A. Maternal food consumption during pregnancy and asthma, respiratory and atopic symptoms in 5-year-old children. Thorax. 2007;62:773–9.
46. Sausenthaler S, Kompauer I, Borte M, Herbarth O, Schaaf B, von Berg A, Zutavern A, Heinrich J, Group LS. Margarine and butter consumption, eczema and allergic sensitization in children. The LISA birth cohort study. Pediatr Allergy Immunol. 2006;17:85–93.
47. Yu M, Han K, Kim DH, Nam GE. Atopic dermatitis is associated with Caesarean sections in Korean adolescents, but asthma is not. Acta Paediatr. 2015;104:1253–8.
48. Bager P, Wohlfahrt J, Westergaard T. Caesarean delivery and risk of atopy and allergic disease: meta-analyses. Clin Exp Allergy. 2008;38:634–42.
49. Flohr C, Nagel G, Weinmayr G, Kleiner A, Strachan DP, Williams HC. Lack of evidence for a protective effect of prolonged breastfeeding on childhood eczema: lessons from the International Study of Asthma and Allergies in Childhood (ISAAC) Phase Two. Br J Dermatol. 2011;165:1280–9.
50. Yang YW, Tsai CL, Lu CY. Exclusive breastfeeding and incident atopic dermatitis in childhood: a systematic review and meta-analysis of prospective cohort studies. Br J Dermatol. 2009;161:373–83.
51. Tsakok T, McKeever TM, Yeo L, Flohr C. Does early life exposure to antibiotics increase the risk of eczema? A systematic review. Br J Dermatol. 2013;169:983–91.
52. Madhok V, Futamura M, Thomas KS, Barbarot S. What's new in atopic eczema? An analysis of systematic reviews published in 2012 and 2013. Part 1. Epidemiology, mechanisms of disease and methodological issues. Clin Exp Dermatol. 2015;40:238–42.
53. Kim C, Park KY, Ahn S, Kim DH, Li K, Kim DW, Kim MB, Jo SJ, Yim HW, Seo SJ. Economic impact of atopic dermatitis in Korean patients. Ann Dermatol. 2015;27:298–305.
54. Bickers DR, Lim HW, Margolis D, Weinstock MA, Goodman C, Faulkner E, Gould C, Gemmen E, Dall T. The burden of skin diseases: 2004. A joint project of the American Academy of Dermatology Association and the Society for Investigative Dermatology. J Am Acad Dermatol. 2006;55:490–500.
55. Silverberg JI. Health care utilization, patient costs, and access to care in us adults with eczema: a population-based study. JAMA Dermatol. 2015;151:743–52.

Part III

Clinical Manifestations

Clinical Manifestations

Howard Chu, Chang Ook Park,
and Kwang Hoon Lee

Atopic dermatitis (AD) is a chronically relapsing skin disorder that usually occurs during infancy and early childhood [1]. Due to the chronicity of the disease, differentiating from other skin diseases and making the correct diagnosis is crucial. However, there is not a diagnostic laboratory test or a single characteristic feature of AD, thus the recognition of the overall clinical manifestation is the key in the diagnosis. The set of major and minor clinical features of AD is listed in Table 1, in which the diagnosis is made when three of the four major features and three of 28 minor features are fulfilled [2].

Intense pruritus is the main clinical feature seen in patients with AD, which often aggravates in the nighttime, causing significant sleep disturbances and thus lowering the quality of life of the patients [3, 4]. The cutaneous symptoms of AD can be described according to acute, subacute, or chronic status of the lesions. In acute stages, extensive erythematous patches can be observed that may be accompanied by exudative papules and vesicles. For subacute lesions, erythematous papules and plaques with excoriations and dry scales are prominent. When the lesions become chronic, as a result of prolonged scratching, lichenification is commonly observed with severe erythematous scaly plaques. During such a condition, lesions of different stages may be seen simultaneously [5].

Patients with AD generally share such similar cutaneous symptoms, yet some characteristic features can be distinguished among different age groups of early infancy, childhood, and adulthood.

Clinical Features According to Age

Early Infancy (<2 Years Old)

In infants, AD may develop as early as 2–3 months after birth. Non-discrete confluent erythematous exudative patches arise that typically involve the cheeks and face. The scalp, forehead, ears, and the extensor surfaces of the limbs are also commonly affected [6, 7]. Drooling is an important factor to consider, as saliva can further cause irritations to the skin. Due to the pruritus and inability to restrain from scratching, symptoms can easily exacerbate and can be susceptible to bacterial infections, leading to secondary impetiginization.

Childhood (2~12 Years Old)

Several distinct features can be seen in childhood AD, that is, after the age of two, and before becoming an adolescent. During this period, the

H. Chu (✉) · C. O. Park (✉) · K. H. Lee
Department of Dermatology, Cutaneous Biology Research Institute, Yonsei University College of Medicine, Seoul, Korea (Republic of)
e-mail: yuanhao@naver.com; copark@yuhs.ac

K. H. Lee et al. (eds.), *Practical Insights into Atopic Dermatitis*,
https://doi.org/10.1007/978-981-15-8159-5_3

Table 1 The Hanifin and Rajka diagnostic criteria for atopic dermatitis [2]

Major criteria
1. Pruritus
2. Typical morphology and distribution – Facial and extensor involvement in infants – Flexural lichenification and linearity in children and adults
3. Chronic or chronically relapsing dermatitis
4. Personal or family history of atopy
Minor criteria
1. Xerosis
2. Ichthyosis/palmar hyperlinearity/keratosis pilaris
3. Immediate (type 1) skin test reactivity
4. Elevated serum IgE
5. Early age of onset
6. Tendency toward cutaneous infections
7. Tendency toward nonspecific hand or foot dermatitis
8. Nipple eczema
9. Cheilitis
10. Recurrent conjunctivitis
11. Dennie-Morgan infraorbital fold
12. Keratoconus
13. Anterior subcapsular cataracts
14. Orbital darkening
15. Facial pallor/facial erythema
16. Pityriasis alba
17. Anterior neck folds
18. Itch when sweating
19. Intolerance to wool and lipid solvents
20. Perifollicular accentuation
21. Food intolerance
22. Course influenced by environmental/emotional factors
23. White dermographism/delayed blanch

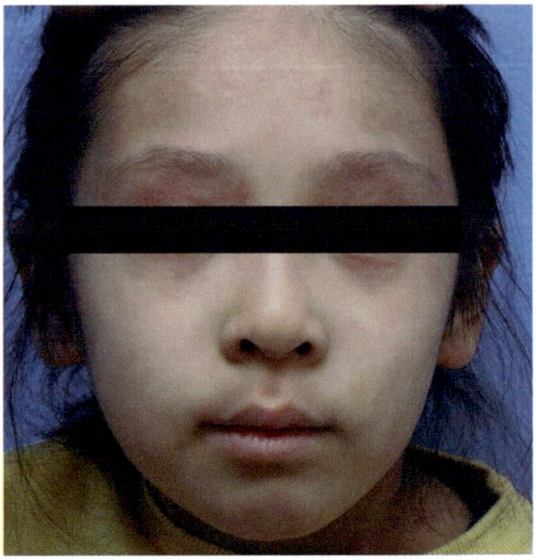

Fig. 1 Perioral, periorbital eczematous lesion of childhood AD

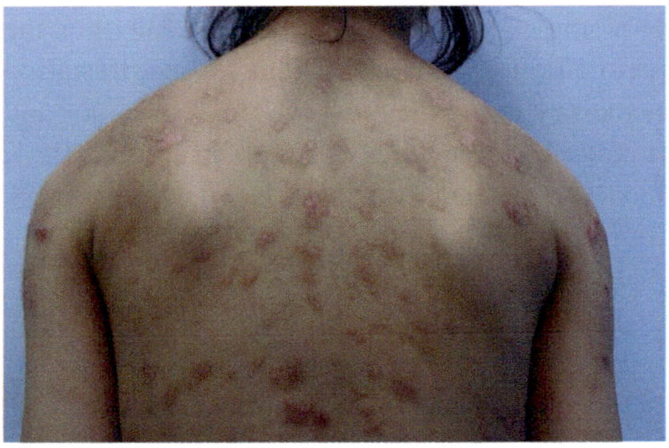

Fig. 2 Diffusely scattered erythematous, lichenified papules, and plaques on the back of childhood AD patient

facial skin is less involved, whereas more lesions develop on the areas of antecubital and popliteal fossa of the arms and legs, the typical features of flexural eczemas seen in AD [6, 7]. Also, more involvements of the buttocks, wrists, and ankles can be observed. When symptoms develop on the face, eczemas of the eyelids, perioral area, and periauricular fissures are the characteristic features (Fig. 1). Cheilitis is also commonly seen, in which the upper lip is more typically involved. Sometimes the soles and toes can be affected, which can be difficult to distinguish from fungal infections, and may require a fungus study for the correct diagnosis.

Compared to the symptoms during infancy, as the disease becomes more chronic, subacute lesions can be more frequently observed, which may be more localized with more xerosis and exfoliation than exudative lesions. Also, hyperpigmentation and lichenification can develop more frequently in the lesions (Fig. 2).

Adolescent (>12 Years Old)

Symptoms of AD during adolescence resemble many features seen in childhood AD [6, 7]. Likewise, erythematous patches, papulation, and hyperpigmentation of the periorificial area, periocular regions, neck, flexural areas are the typically observed symptoms (Figs. 3 and 4). Also, eczemas tend to develop more commonly on the upper trunk during this age period (Fig. 5). In addition to cheilitis and periocular eczemas of the facial areas, a widespread facial erythema can be frequently observed, especially in severe patients. Lichenification and xerosis are also commonly seen features, as in childhood AD, as the disease becomes more chronic.

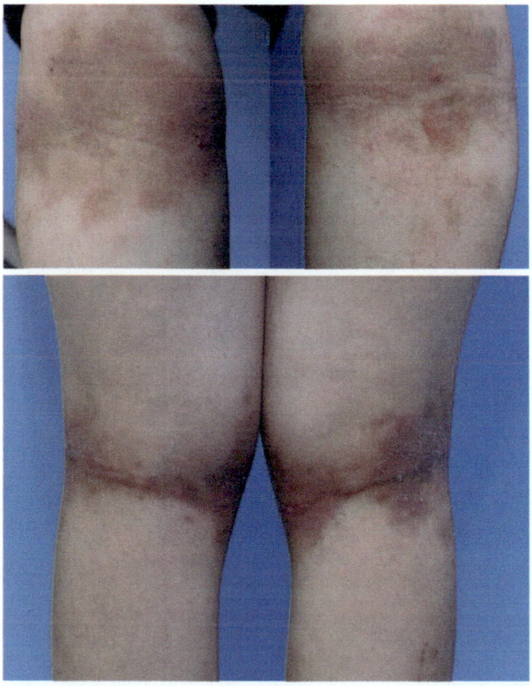

Fig. 3 The typical eczemas observed in AD patients on the flexural areas of the arms and legs

Adulthood (>18 Years Old)

In adult AD patients, the symptoms are nearly an extension of that of adolescent AD [8, 9]. Eczemas involve the flexural areas of arms and legs, neck, and the face, and chronic lesions with xerosis and lichenification can be commonly observed (Fig. 6). As the child ages and enters adulthood, the lesions become relatively more defined on the flexural areas, as well as a more distinctive facial erythema (Fig. 7). In females, nipple eczemas can recurrently develop (Fig. 8). Also, chronic hand eczema frequently occurs (Fig. 9), and it may be the only symptom that remains in a portion of the patients throughout adulthood.

Dermatologic Conditions that May Accompany AD

In addition to the typical symptoms of AD mentioned above, various distinct subtypes and conditions develop frequently in patients with AD.

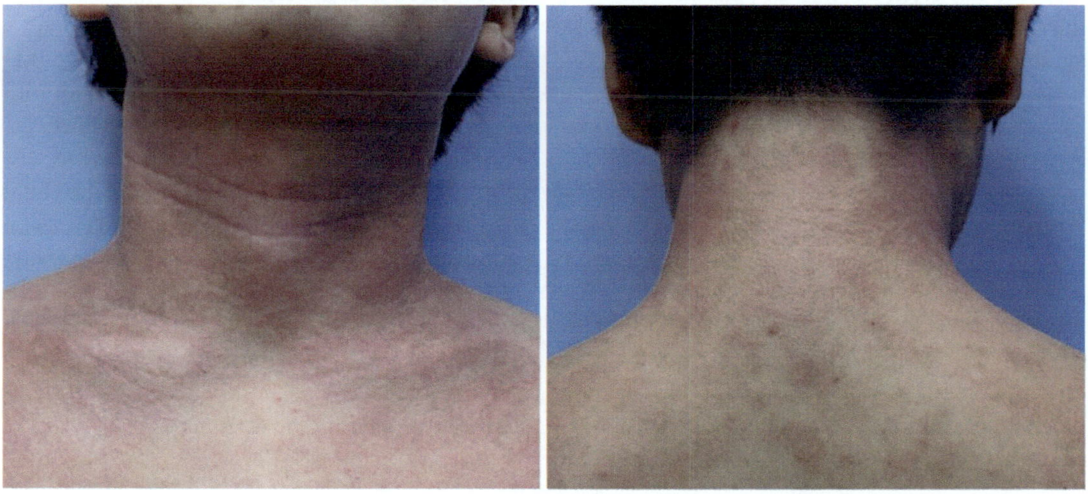

Fig. 4 Erythematous, lichenified eczematous lesion affects anterior and posterior neck in adolescent AD patient

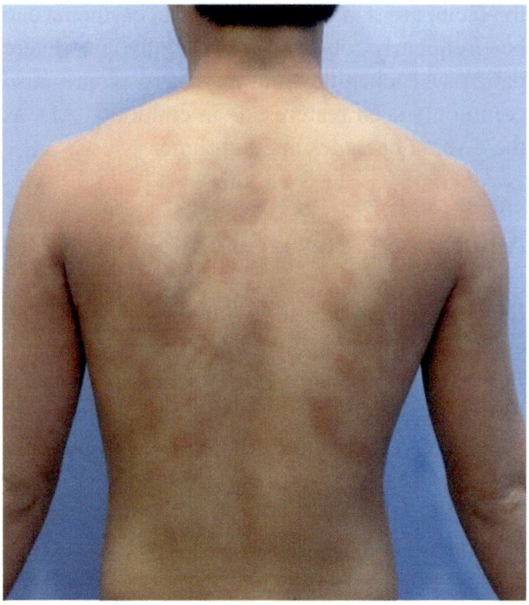

Fig. 5 Eczemas tend to develop more commonly on the upper trunk during the adolescent period

Nummular Eczema

Nummular eczema is defined as relatively well-demarcated round coin-sized exudative erythematous patches (Fig. 10) and is a subtype that is more often seen in children and adults. It develops most commonly on the extremities, while the trunk is also commonly affected. Although nummular eczema is not always associated with atopy, it can often develop in patients with AD, thus the evaluation of the patient's past history is significant [4, 10].

Prurigo Nodularis

Prurigo nodularis consists of 0.5~3 cm-sized papules or nodules often with central erosion or crusts and is usually extremely pruritic (Figs. 11 and 12). Prurigo nodularis usually develops in adults with chronic severe AD. It is known to develop in 2–3% of the patients and may be recalcitrant to various treatment methods [4, 5].

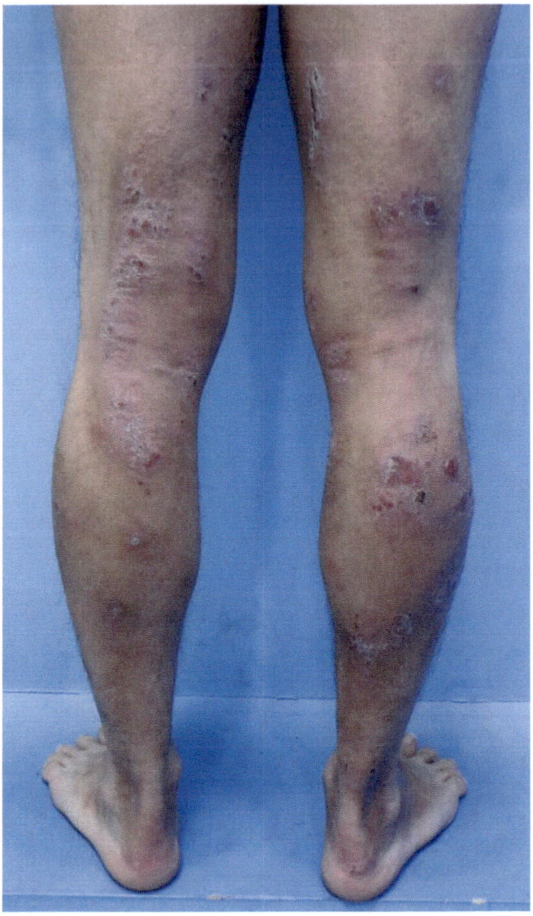

Fig. 6 Severe eczemas with scales, crusts, and lichenification can be seen on a chronic adult AD patient

Exfoliative Dermatitis

Exfoliative dermatitis may occur in severe AD patients, presenting as generalized erythema with scales accompanied by extensive oozing crusts, which may also involve lymphadenopathy [5, 10] (Fig. 13). Complications are rare but may be fatal when left untreated. Exfoliative dermatitis can be caused by *Staphylococcus aureus* (*S. aureus*) infection and/or coinfection of herpes simplex virus or by inappropriate therapies [11]. It can also be induced by rebound effect in severe AD patients after the cessation of systemic corticosteroid while during the treatment.

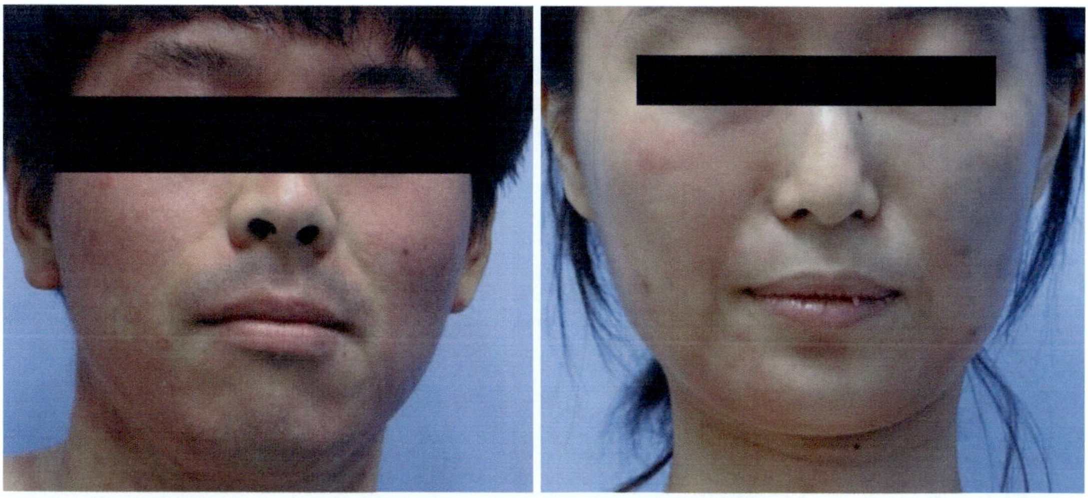

Fig. 7 Chronic diffuse confluent erythema on the face of an adult patient

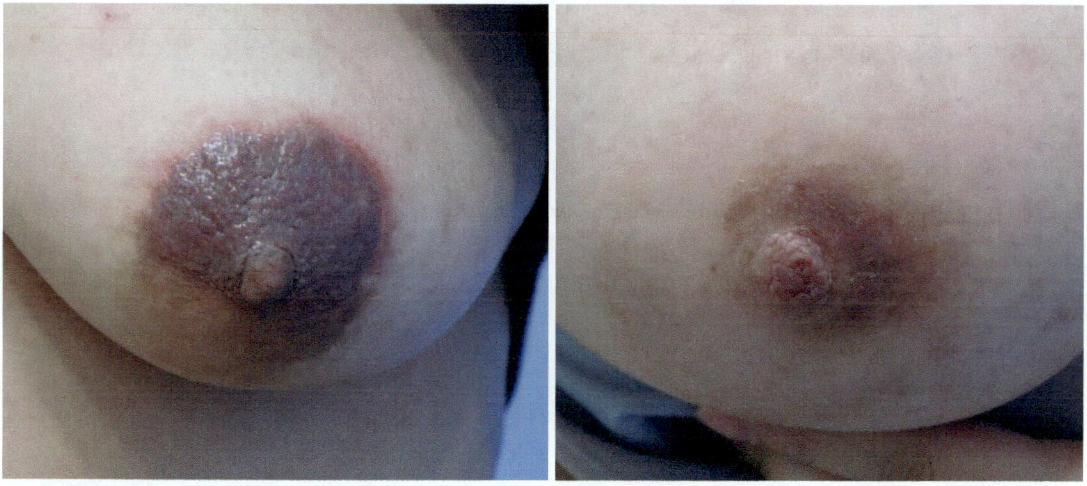

Fig. 8 Erythematous lichenified eczematous plaque with scales on the nipples

Infections

Due to the defective skin barriers in AD patients, the incidences of cutaneous infections in AD patients are higher than that of non-AD subjects [12, 13]. Various pathogens may be associated including viruses, fungi, bacteria, and more, and because the therapeutic methods are different for each, differentiating the infected pathogen is important.

Viral Infection

The most commonly acquired viral infection is from herpes simplex virus [11, 12]. Herpes simplex virus infection presents as multiple tiny vesiculations. Because of the skin barrier defect in AD, patients are more susceptible to viral infections. It is known to occur in approximately 3% of AD patients, and when left untreated, severe complications, such as keratoconjunctivitis, meningitis, and virema, can occur in rare

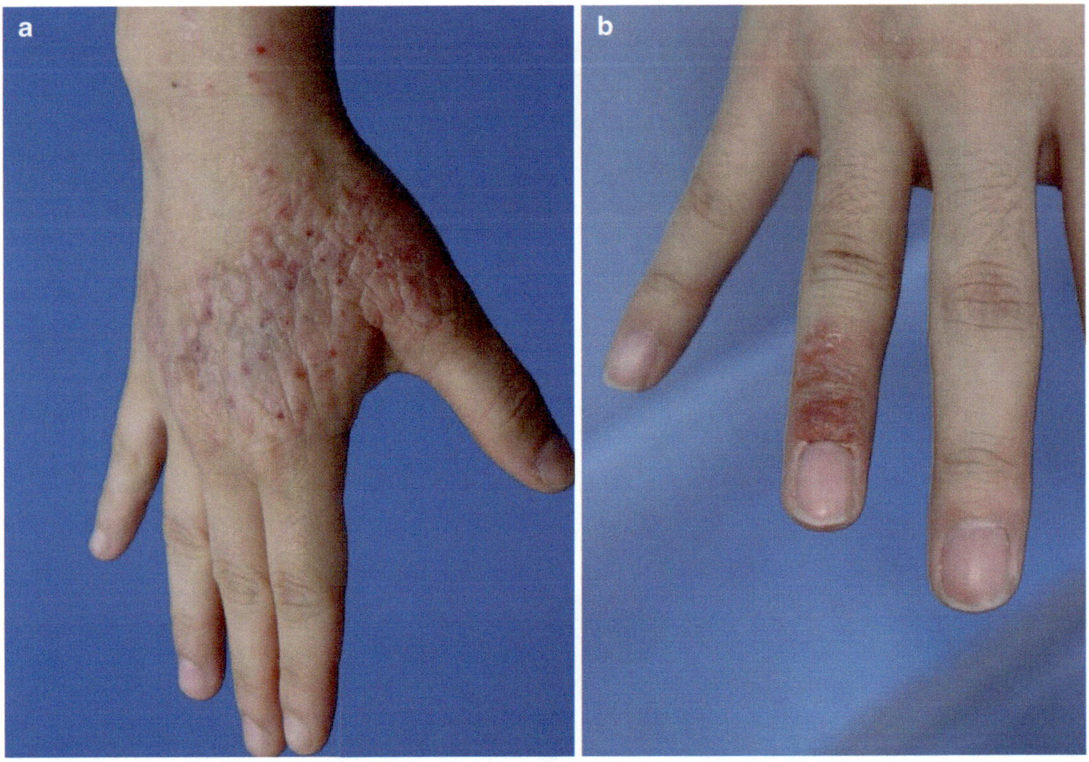

Fig. 9 (**a**) Eczema with marked lichenification on the hand of an AD patient, (**b**) Focal eczematous lesion on the finger of an AD patient

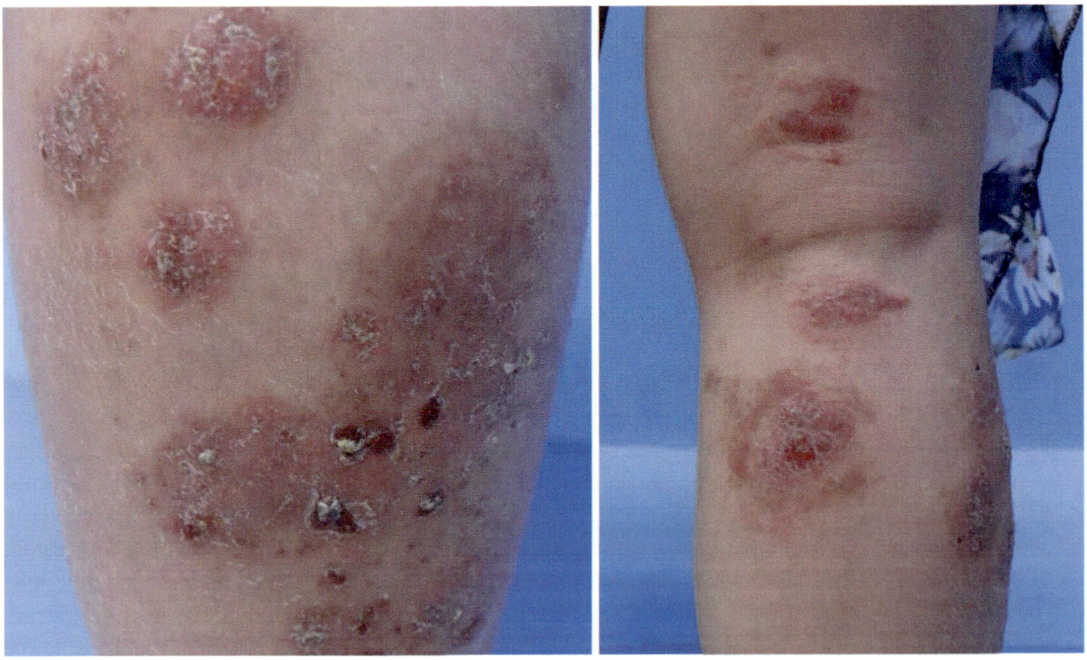

Fig. 10 Round shaped, erythematous lichenified plaques on both the posterior legs

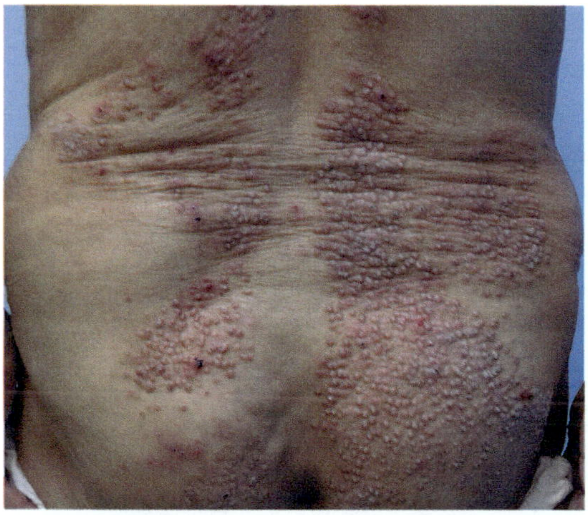

Fig. 11 Multiple lesions of prurigo nodularis that developed on the trunk of a chronic AD patient

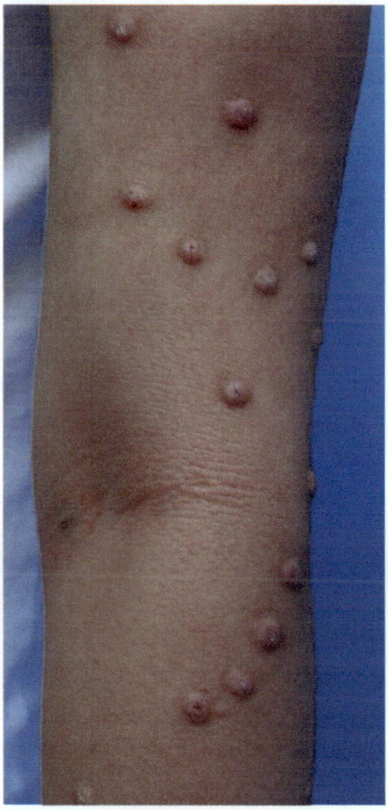

Fig. 12 Multiple skin colored, crusted nodules on the arm: Typical morphology and distribution of prurigo nodularis

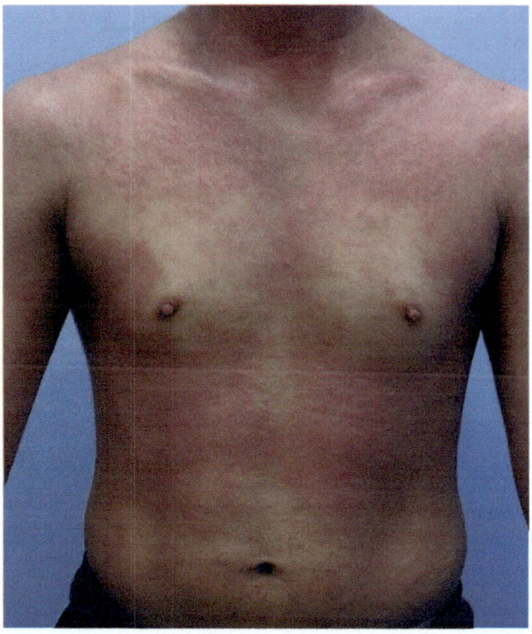

Fig. 13 Exfoliative dermatitis: generalized erythema with scales, oozing crusts on whole body

cases. Herpes can be infected in all ages, and it may develop into Kaposi's varicelliform eruption or eczema herpeticum, which consists of multiple vesicles and pustules that disseminate around the lesions and may be pruritic. The vesicles show central umbilication and tend to coalesce, in which hemorrhagic crusts often develop. If left untreated, these lesions may spread and become generalized (Fig. 14).

Fungal Infection

Superficial fungal infections commonly occur in AD patients and may aggravate the patients' symptoms [12]. The incidence of *Trichophyton rubrum* infection has been found to be higher in AD patients than that of non-AD individuals. Tinea pedis can be easily mistaken for foot eczemas in AD patients, thus a fungus study may be necessary, especially when the symptoms are not well managed with the conventional treatments. *Malassezia furfur* (*Pityrosporum ovale*) is a lipophilic fungus that is commonly detected in sebor-

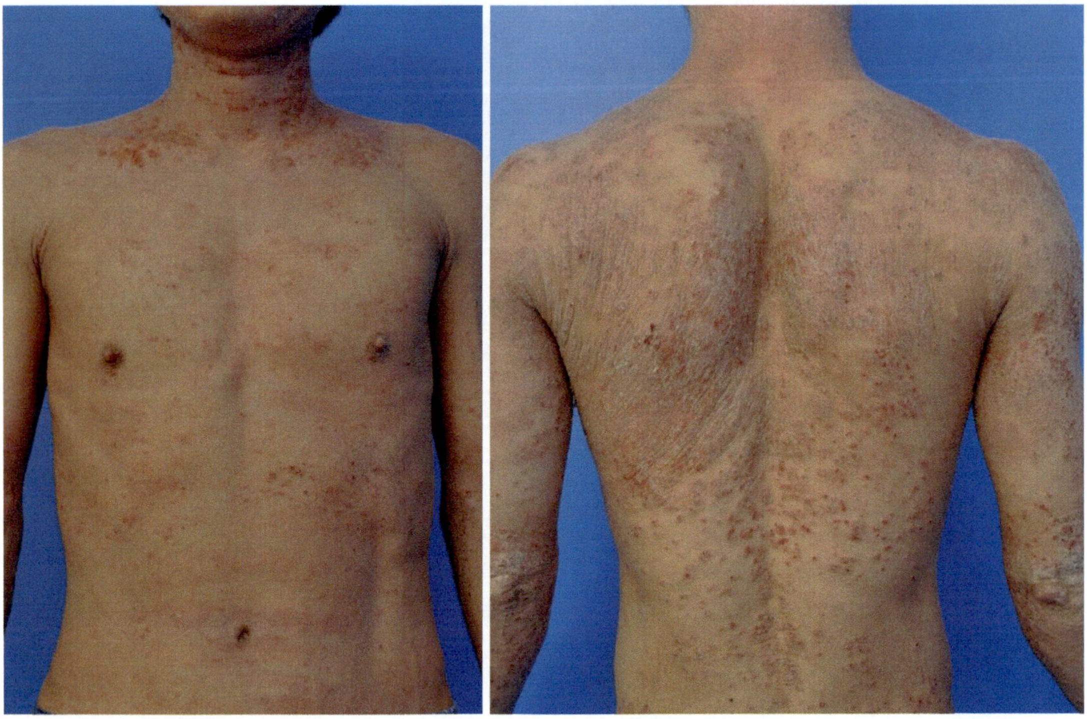

Fig. 14 Multiple crusted papules and vesicles with oozing, crusting; suggestive of viral infections on underlying AD, which is called "Eczema herpeticum"

rheic skin. In AD patients, especially those with head and neck dermatitis, specific IgE levels to *M. furfur* have been found to be elevated [27]. Antifungal agents may be effective in these patients, suggesting the deleterious role of fungus in AD patients.

Bacterial Infection

S. aureus can be detected as high as 90% in the lesions of AD patients, and in more than 70% of the uninvolved skin [11]. Once infected, yellowish exudate and crusts form on the lesions, occasionally with pustules, which are signs to infer secondary infections by *S. aureus* (Fig. 15). *S. aureus* infection is well-known to be an aggravating factor of AD; thus, an appropriate management is important. Topical antibiotics can be used to easily manage the condition, but systemic antibiotics may be required in severe cases. Recurrent *S. aureus* infections may occur, especially in severe AD patients, but evolvement into severe deep infections are rare, in which syndromes with immunodeficiency should be suspected.

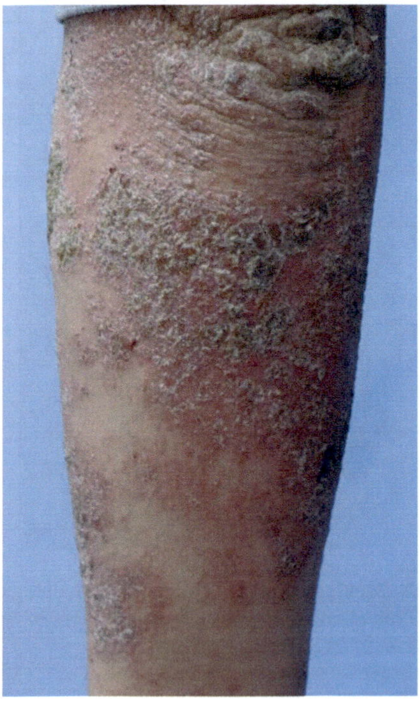

Fig. 15 Lesions with yellowish oozing crusts showing signs of *S. aureus* infection on the arm of an AD patient

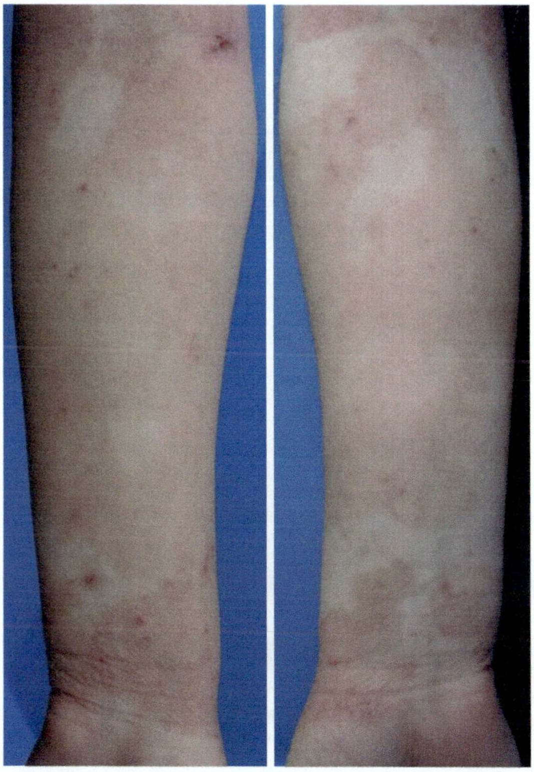

Fig. 16 Vitiligo associated with atopic dermatitis

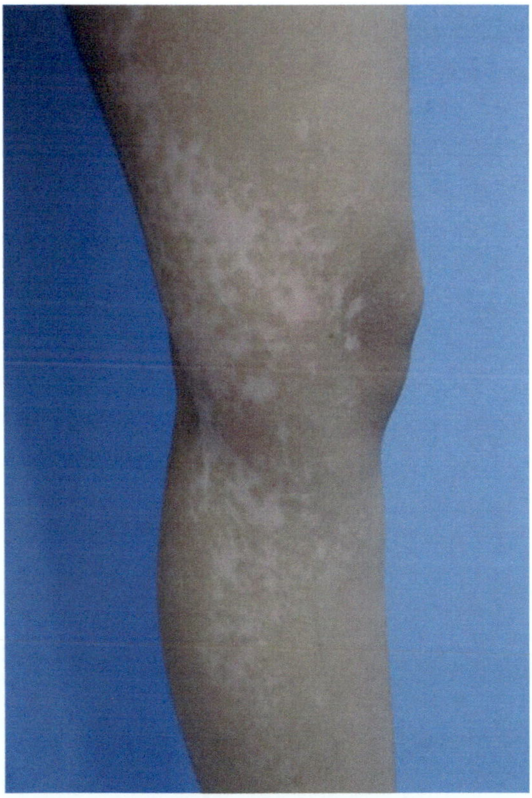

Fig. 17 Vitiligo associated with atopic dermatitis

Others

Most of the dermatologic conditions that develop in association with AD are related to the defect in the skin barrier, while some may be associated with the immunologic aspects, as AD is characterized by abnormal T cells with augmented Th2 response [4, 13]. In addition to the conditions described previously, allergic contact dermatitis, irritant contact dermatitis, alopecia areata, vitiligo (Figs. 16 and 17), cutaneous amyloidosis, and urticaria have been known to be associated. Congenital diseases including ichthyosis vulgaris, Netherton syndrome, Wiskott-Aldrich syndrome, hyper-IgE syndrome, and anhidrotic ectodermal dysplasia can also show features of AD.

Other conditions, such as keratosis pilaris, lichen amyloidosis, and pityriasis alba, may develop regardless of the presence of AD, but develop more frequently in AD patients [4, 5]. Keratosis pilaris is keratotic papules of the follicles that usually affects the extensor aspects of the arms, anterior thighs, and lateral aspects of the face. Lichen amyloidosis is a form of cutaneous amyloidosis that appears as multiple brownish papules, which has been suggested to develop secondary to persistent scratching (Fig. 18). Pityriasis alba is described as hypopigmented patches that may have fine scales that usually appear on the face and upper arms (Fig. 19).

Systemic Conditions that May Accompany AD

Atopic March

Although AD may present with cutaneous manifestations only, a significant portion of the patients has concomitant systemic allergic conditions that are frequently termed by "atopic march." In general, atopic march begins with

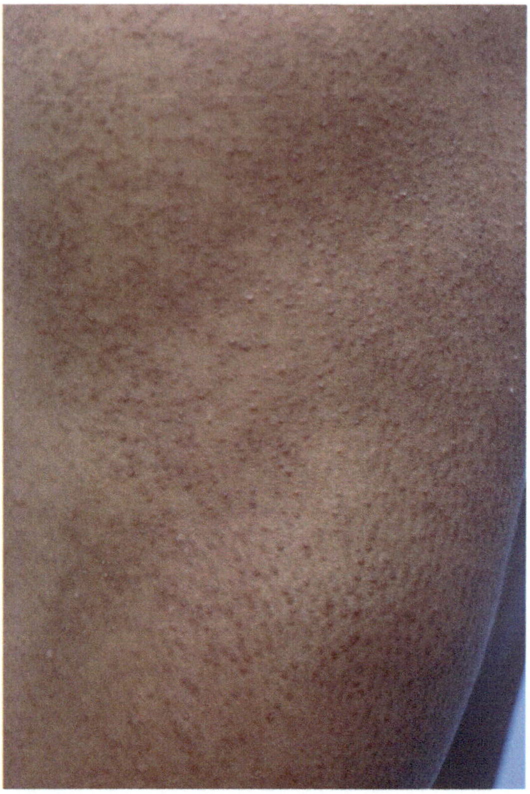

Fig. 18 Lesions of lichen amyloidosis that developed on the arms of a chronic AD patient

the development of AD in infancy, with the peak incidence at the first year of life and declines afterward, followed by allergic asthma and allergic rhinitis that slowly arises during childhood [14]. Children with higher severity of AD were more likely to develop allergic asthma and/or allergic rhinitis. AD and these other atopic diseases share a common genetic background and immunologic pathogenesis, with elevated IgE levels, peripheral and lesional eosinophilia, augmented Th2 cytokines, epithelial barrier dysfunction, and sensitization to aeroallergens [15].

Ocular Symptoms

Many ocular symptoms may accompany AD, including blepharitis, conjunctivitis, keratoconus, cataract, uveitis, and retinal detachment

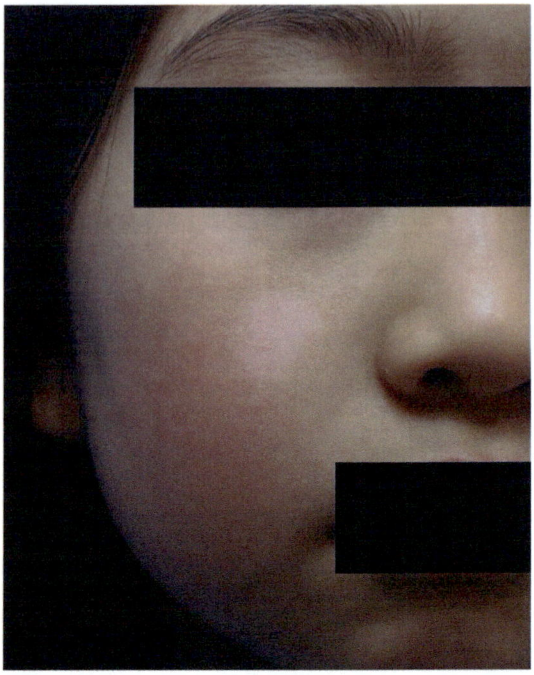

Fig. 19 A small white patch of pityriasis alba that appeared on the right cheek of a girl with AD

[16]. The incidence of these conditions in AD patients varies between 2.5 and 67%. These symptoms are usually associated with the allergic response, and often aggravates by the patients rubbing their eyes due to the itching. Topical steroid ointment is often used for the management of the symptoms, but it should only be used for a short period of time, as the risk of cataract arises. Patients with a family history of glaucoma should be refrained from using topical steroids and instead, topical calcineurin inhibitors should be used.

Autoimmune Diseases

The association between AD and autoimmune diseases has been suggested [15, 17, 18]. Children diagnosed with autoimmune thyroid diseases have been found to have a higher risk of developing AD. Meanwhile, rheumatic arthritis, multiple sclerosis, and type I diabetes mellitus, which are Th1-mediated autoimmune diseases, have been reported to have a protective role in the development of AD, and on the other hand, atopy may lower the severity of these diseases.

Metabolic Syndrome

Recent studies have shown the relationship between obesity and allergic diseases [19, 20]. These evidence have been first suggested in allergic asthma, and the association to AD is being added lately. Obese subjects have been suggested to have higher risk of developing atopy and higher disease severity than nonobese subjects. Adipose tissue is known to produce inflammatory cytokines, which may contribute to the increased severity. There have been studies that suggest the associations between metabolic syndrome, hypertension, and central obesity with AD.

Psychiatric Disorders

AD, especially in severe cases, the patients' quality of lives are seriously affected, resulting in psychological stress. This stress has been found in studies to provoke and exacerbate AD [21]. The most common psychiatric disorders observed in AD are anxiety and depressive disorders. Patients with concomitant allergic rhinitis and/or allergic asthma were found to have a higher risk of developing anxiety disorders. In addition to ADHD, children with AD were susceptible to distress, anxiety, poor self-esteem, and low self-confidence [22]. Due to the intense itching, sleep disturbances are common, with difficulty in falling asleep, frequent waking during sleep, and reduced amount of sleep, resulting in low functional capacity and a poor social relationship. Also, recent studies have demonstrated the relationship between atopic diseases and schizophrenia, in which the two disease entities share a common immunological mechanism. Psychological stress has been known to induce systemic inflammation and may affect the homeostasis of the epidermal barrier, thus an appropriate management of psychological stress is also crucial in the management of AD.

Differential Diagnosis

Several dermatologic disorders may resemble the clinical features of AD and may be difficult to distinguish sometimes [5]. Because the treatment methods and the natural course of the diseases are different, accurate diagnosis is significant.

Seborrheic Dermatitis

The clinical features of seborrheic dermatitis are characterized by ill-defined erythematous patches with scales that present on the seborrheic areas which area nasolabial folds, glabella, retroauricular areas, and the scalp [23]. It usually develops before 3 months of age and during adulthood. The findings are relatively distinct in adults, yet when it develops in infants, the features may highly resemble that of AD [5]. However, seborrheic dermatitis presents with greasy rather than dry scales on salmon red-colored erythema, involvement of the scalp, and often with the absence of pruritus, which are several features that may aid in differentiating from AD.

Contact Dermatitis

Although contact dermatitis localizes on areas where certain allergens or irritants have come in contact and thus, may not be difficult to distinguish from AD [3]. However, when it develops on areas where symptoms of AD typically present or if the distribution is atypical, it may be easily mistaken for AD [24]. A thorough review of the history is necessary for the correct diagnosis and may require a patch test when ambiguous.

Scabies

Infestation with *Sarcoptes scabiei* results in erythematous papules with an intense pruritus, which can be mistaken with AD, especially in those with a history of AD [25]. The lesions develop in areas such as the finger web, axilla, and genital areas in adults, which usually differ from the presentation of AD. But in infants, the lesions may appear on the whole body including the face, scalp, palms and soles, and when secondary changes of eczema and impetigo develop, the diagnosis maybe even more difficult. However, the development of the symptoms among the family members and the history of contact with a patient with scabies would highly suggest the infestation. The diagnosis can be made by the isolation of the mite found in burrows located on the fingers, wrists, and genital areas.

Malignancy

Cutaneous T-cell lymphomas may present as eczematous lesions, especially in the early stages, and can be misdiagnosed as AD [26]. Mycosis fungoides is the most common, which usually develops between 55 and 60 years of age, but approximately 5–10% develop in pediatrics. When the symptoms are severe, irresponsive to the conventional treatments of AD, and show distribution that varies from typical symptoms of AD, a biopsy should be performed.

Prognosis

The natural course of AD is not exactly known and varies among studies. However, it has been generally understood to show improvements during childhood as the patient ages, with possibly some aggravations during adolescence, and disappearance of the symptoms usually before the age of 30 years [7]. Statistically, AD disappears in 40% of the patients before adolescence, and 60% of the remaining before the age of 30 years. Filaggrin mutation has been known to be associated with the persistence of the disease [8]. Also, high disease severity during childhood, past history of allergic rhinitis and/or allergic asthma, family history of AD, early onset, and high IgE levels are some of the well-known poor prognostic factors.

References

1. Bieber T. Atopic dermatitis. N Engl J Med. 2008;358(14):1483–94. https://doi.org/10.1056/NEJMra074081.
2. Hanifin JM. Diagnostic features of atopic dermatitis. Acta Derm Venereol Suppl. 1980;92:44–7.
3. Thestrup-Pedersen K. Clinical aspects of atopic dermatitis. Clin Exp Dermatol. 2000;25(7):535–43. https://doi.org/10.1046/j.1365-2230.2000.00696.x.
4. Chu H, Shin JU, Park CO, Lee H, Lee J, Lee KH. Clinical diversity of atopic dermatitis: a review of 5,000 patients at a single institute. Allergy, Asthma Immunol Res. 2017;9(2):158–68. https://doi.org/10.4168/aair.2017.9.2.158.
5. Deleuran M, Vestergaard C. Clinical heterogeneity and differential diagnosis of atopic dermatitis. Br J Dermatol. 2014;170(Suppl 1):2–6. https://doi.org/10.1111/bjd.12933.
6. Lyons JJ, Milner JD, Stone KD. Atopic dermatitis in children: clinical features, pathophysiology, and treatment. Immunol Allergy Clin N Am. 2015;35(1):161–83. https://doi.org/10.1016/j.iac.2014.09.008.
7. Pyun BY. Natural history and risk factors of atopic dermatitis in children. Allergy, Asthma Immunol Res. 2015;7(2):101–5.
8. Kim JP, Chao LX, Simpson EL, Silverberg JI. Persistence of atopic dermatitis (AD): a systematic review and meta-analysis. J Am Acad Dermatol. 2016;75(4):681–7. e11.
9. Silvestre Salvador JF, Romero-Perez D, Encabo-Duran B. Atopic dermatitis in adults: a diagnostic challenge. J Investig Allergol Clin Immunol. 2017;27(2):78–88. https://doi.org/10.18176/jiaci.0138.
10. Silverberg NB. Typical and atypical clinical appearance of atopic dermatitis. Clin Dermatol. 2017;35(4):354–9. https://doi.org/10.1016/j.clindermatol.2017.03.007.
11. Ong PY, Leung DY. Bacterial and viral infections in atopic dermatitis: a comprehensive review. Clin Rev Allergy Immunol. 2016;51(3):329–37. https://doi.org/10.1007/s12016-016-8548-5.
12. Sun D, Ong PY. Infectious complications in atopic dermatitis. Immunol Allergy Clin N Am. 2017;37(1):75–93. https://doi.org/10.1016/j.iac.2016.08.015.
13. Paller A, Jaworski JC, Simpson EL, Boguniewicz M, Russell JJ, Block JK, et al. Major comorbidities of atopic dermatitis: beyond allergic disorders. Am J Clin Dermatol. 2018;19(6):821–38. https://doi.org/10.1007/s40257-018-0383-4.
14. Paller AS, Spergel JM, Mina-Osorio P, Irvine AD. The atopic march and atopic multimorbidity: many trajectories, many pathways. J Allergy Clin Immunol. 2019;143(1):46–55. https://doi.org/10.1016/j.jaci.2018.11.006.
15. Silverberg JI, Gelfand JM, Margolis DJ, Boguniewicz M, Fonacier L, Grayson MH, et al. Association of

atopic dermatitis with allergic, autoimmune, and cardiovascular comorbidities in US adults. Ann Allergy Asthma Immunol. 2018;121(5):604–12.e3. https://doi.org/10.1016/j.anai.2018.07.042.
16. Carmi E, Defossez-Tribout C, Ganry O, Cene S, Tramier B, Milazzo S, et al. Ocular complications of atopic dermatitis in children. Acta Derm Venereol. 2006;86(6):515–7.
17. Mittermann I, Aichberger KJ, Bünder R, Mothes N, Renz H, Valenta R. Autoimmunity and atopic dermatitis. Curr Opin Allergy Clin Immunol. 2004;4(5):367–71.
18. Rabin R, Levinson A. The nexus between atopic disease and autoimmunity: a review of the epidemiological and mechanistic literature. Clin Exp Immunol. 2008;153(1):19–30.
19. Ali Z, Ulrik CS, Agner T, Thomsen SF. Association between atopic dermatitis and the metabolic syndrome: a systematic review. Dermatology. 2018;234(3–4):79–85. https://doi.org/10.1159/000491593.
20. Brunner PM, Silverberg JI, Guttman-Yassky E, Paller AS, Kabashima K, Amagai M, et al. Increasing comorbidities suggest that atopic dermatitis is a systemic disorder. J Investig Dermatol. 2017;137(1):18–25. https://doi.org/10.1016/j.jid.2016.08.022.
21. Oh SH, Bae BG, Park CO, Noh JY, Park IH, Wu WH, et al. Association of stress with symptoms of atopic dermatitis. Acta Derm Venereol. 2010;90(6):582–8. https://doi.org/10.2340/00015555-0933.
22. Slattery MJ, Essex MJ, Paletz EM, Vanness ER, Infante M, Rogers GM, et al. Depression, anxiety, and dermatologic quality of life in adolescents with atopic dermatitis. J Allergy Clin Immunol. 2011;128(3):668.
23. Borda LJ, Wikramanayake TC. Seborrheic dermatitis and dandruff: a comprehensive review. J Clin Investig Dermatol. 2015;3(2):10. https://doi.org/10.13188/2373-1044.1000019.
24. Aquino M, Fonacier L. The role of contact dermatitis in patients with atopic dermatitis. J Allergy Clin Immunol Pract. 2014;2(4):382–7. https://doi.org/10.1016/j.jaip.2014.05.004.
25. Boralevi F, Diallo A, Miquel J, Guerin-Moreau M, Bessis D, Chiaverini C, et al. Clinical phenotype of scabies by age. Pediatrics. 2014;133(4):e910–6. https://doi.org/10.1542/peds.2013-2880.
26. Boulos S, Vaid R, Aladily TN, Ivan DS, Talpur R, Duvic M. Clinical presentation, immunopathology, and treatment of juvenile-onset mycosis fungoides: a case series of 34 patients. J Am Acad Dermatol. 2014;71(6):1117–26. https://doi.org/10.1016/j.jaad.2014.07.049.
27. Bayrou O, Pecquet C, Flahault A, Artigou C, Abuaf N, Leynadier F. Head and neck atopic dermatitis and malassezia-furfur-specific IgE antibodies. Dermatology. 2005;211(2):107–13.

Pruritus

Hye One Kim

Introduction

Pruritus, also called itching, is an unpleasant sensation of the skin that causes the urge to scratch or rub the skin [1]. Pruritus is a relatively common symptom that anyone can experience at any point in their life. A large cross-sectional study in Germany reported chronic pruritus in about 16% of the population [2]. Pruritus can occur not only from skin diseases but also from systemic diseases throughout the body. Pruritus accompanying chronic inflammatory skin diseases markedly lowers the quality of life of patients. Particularly, atopic dermatitis is a typical disease in which severe itching occurs among many skin diseases. In patients with atopic dermatitis, the threshold for itch and alloknesis is markedly reduced, and infections can promote exacerbation and thereby increase the itch.

Pruritus is a very subjective sensation that varies widely from person to person, and even the same stimulus in the same person can cause differences in pruritus at different times. It can be aggravated by physical and mental stress, fatigue, and anxiety. Moreover, pruritus often happens during night sleep. In severe cases, pruritus can cause difficulty in falling asleep, and the pruritus itself may cause severe stress, resulting in such as irritability and depression. Pruritus induces repetitive scratching that causes skin irritation, lichenification, and damage to the peripheral nerves, which can make the pruritus worse.

Classification and Causes of Pruritus

The most common cause of chronic pruritus is senile pruritus due to dry skin without a specific disease. In addition, it may be secondary to skin diseases and systemic diseases. Many mammals use neurophysiological reflexes, such as scratching, to remove harmful environmental stimuli, such as invading pathogens and insects. Clinically, pruritus can be divided into six types: pruritus caused by systemic diseases, pruritus caused by skin diseases, neuropathic pruritus, psychogenic pruritus, pruritus with multiple factors, and from unknown causes [3].

Pruritic skin diseases mainly include eczematous dermatitis, hives, food allergies, insect bites, and scabies. The degree of itching varies depending on the affected area and how sensitive the patient is. Severe scratching or rubbing to eliminate the pruritus without proper treatment of causal diseases may result in scratches, abrasions, erythema, lichenification, ulcers, hives, and pigmentation of the skin.

If pruritus occurs on the skin due to systemic diseases, then kidney disease, liver disease, gas-

H. O. Kim (✉)
Department of Dermatology, Hallym University Kangnam Sacred Heart Hospital, College of Medicine, Hallym University, Seoul, Korea (Republic of)
e-mail: hyeonekim@gmail.com

K. H. Lee et al. (eds.), *Practical Insights into Atopic Dermatitis*,
https://doi.org/10.1007/978-981-15-8159-5_4

trointestinal disease, or cancer could be the problem. Moreover, allergic reactions caused by medication may cause pruritus accompanied by skin rashes. In chronic renal failure and in patients with long-term kidney failure, pruritus tends to become more pronounced when hemodialysis occurs later than when early. It may appear months earlier than other systemic symptoms in those with Hodgkin's disease, a type of malignant hematological tumor. Pruritus may also accompany various obstructive biliary diseases (primary biliary sclerosis, cirrhosis, cirrhosis, etc.) in which bile ducts are blocked, or in which bile ducts are characteristic. Malignant hematological tumors other than Hodgkin's disease, intestinal parasites, hyperthyroidism, and pruritus may also occur in association with hypofunction, diabetes, and acquired immunodeficiency. If it is suspected that pruritus is caused by systemic diseases, patients should be asked to provide their detailed medical history and medications. Renal function and blood sugar tests should be performed and patients checked for the presence of causative disease, and if present, the causative disease should be treated properly. In general, patients with chronic pruritus report several characteristics, which include such as idiopathic pruritus, pruritus after mechanical stimulation, aquagenic pruritus, pain, tingling sensations, and mixed symptoms. Some disorders may exhibit characteristic clinical features [4] (Table 1).

Pathophysiology of Pruritus (Fig. 1) [5]

Mediator of Pruritus

Itching is mediated by unmyelinated C-fiber afferents and thinly myelinated Aδ fiber afferents. Nerves can be stimulated by various neuronal mediators [6]. Mediators found to be involved in pruritus include histamine, substance P, prostaglandins, proteases, opioids, and platelet activators [4, 6].

Histamine, a representative itch mediator, was proposed by Lewis in 1927 to cause pruritus in inflammatory skin diseases [7]. Injection of histamine into the skin causes pruritus. In addition to pruritus, histamine causes erythema and edema through direct action on blood vessels and by the release of neuropeptides from the sensory nerves [7]. The major source of histamine in the skin is mast cells. Histamine is synthesized and stored in the mast cells, from which it can be secreted in response to stimulation. Histamine causes pruritus through the H1 receptor, and H1 receptor antihistamines are effective in relieving pruritus in many inflammatory skin diseases, including almost all types of hives [8]. Mast cells are present throughout the skin, and in skin diseases that cause pruritus, such as atopic dermatitis, many mast cells are infiltrated by skin lesions [7]. Mediators of mast cells include histamine, proteases (e.g., tryptase), proteoglycans (e.g., heparin and chondroitin sulfate), eicosanoids (e.g., prostaglandin D2, leukotriene B4, and C4), and a number of cytokines (interleukin-3, -4, -6, -9, -10). Mast cells can induce pruritus through the release of mediators. To date, agents that selectively inhibit mast cell activation have not been developed and no inhibitor exists. Instead, there are drugs that affect the mediator after its release [7]. These include corticosteroid, cyclosporine, H1 antihistamines, and β-adrenergic receptor antagonists.

Substance P is a neuropeptide synthesized in dorsal root ganglia that acts as a neurotransmitter of Group C nerve fibers. It is a strong vasodilator and causes erythema and pruritus, as well as promoting the release of histamine by other mediators [9].

Prostaglandin E is involved in inflammatory skin diseases although it does not directly cause pruritus. However, it has the property of increasing pruritus through other mediators [10].

Opioids, when injected into the dermis, cause histamine secretion and pruritus. Opioid receptors are expressed not only in the central nervous system but also in the skin and can be used therapeutically by the administration of individual antagonists or agents [7]. The role of skin opioid receptors is not yet fully studied and could be an interesting topic.

Platelet activators are secreted from inflammatory cells and are potent inflammation inducers. They have been reported to cause pruritus

Table 1 Typical pruritus of various diseases

	Diagnosis	Characteristics
Dermatological disorders	Atopic dermatitis	With flare-ups or in the interval Scratching exacerbates pruritus Accompanied with allokinesis, stinging, burning sensation
	Psoriasis	Usually limited to the lesional skin
	Urticaria	Accompanied with wheal and flare Can be mechanically induced such as scratching, pressure
Internal medical disorders	Chronic kidney disease	2–3 months after dialysis Accompanied with xerosis or prurigo Generalized or localized
	Cholestatic liver disease	Not diminished by scratching Generalized
	Polycythemia vera	After contact with water With stinging sensation and pain Generalized or localized
	Lymphoproliferative disease	Such as Hodgkin's disease Premonitory onset Area of affected lymph nodes such as anterior chest
Neurological disorders	Brachioradial pruritus	Aggravated with sunlight Intractable pruritus to topical steroid etc. Brachioradialis muscle (C6 dermatome) Unilateral or bilateral
	Notalgia paraesthetica	Hyperpigmented lesions Between the scapula or back
Psychiatric disorders	Somatoform disorder	Sometimes severe lesions With other sensations such as burning, stinging, prickling Generalized or localized
	Delusional parasitosis	Symptoms like bugs moving up or down Particles are collected as evidence by patients
	Adjustment disorder	Accompanied with depression or other psychosomatic symptoms

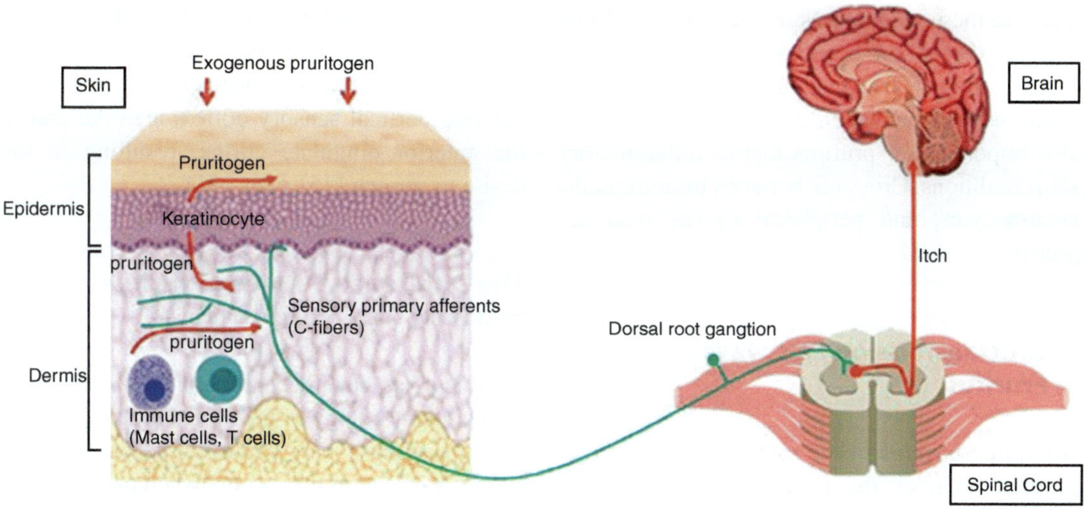

Fig. 1 Pathway of itch (From Atsuko Kamo, et al., J Clin Cosmet Dermatol 1(3) according to the Creative Commons license Journal of Clinical and Cosmetic Dermatology)

directly in animals, but in humans, the pruritus is indirectly induced by histamine release from mast cells [11].

Mechanism of Pruritus: Signaling at Neuronal Terminals

A variety of stimuli activates the receptors in nerve fibers and eventually initiates the potential when the ion channel is opened to trigger the pruritus. There are various calcium ion channels related to pruritus in the nerve fibers, and TRPV1 (transient receptor potential vanilloid 1) and TRPA1 (transient receptor potential ankyrin 1) are the representative channels. A heat-sensitive channel, TRPV1, was found to be necessary for the induction of histamine-mediated itch [12]. Many histaminergic and non-histaminergic pruritoceptors require TRPA1 and TRPV1 for itch signaling to the spinal cord. In addition to heat stimulation, TRPV1 can be activated by capsaicin application and various inflammatory mediators [7].

In addition to histamine receptors and TRPV1 at the nerve endings, TSLP/IL-7Ra is responsible for refractory itch. When TSLP (thymic stromal lymphopoietin) is bound to the TSLP/IL-7Ra receptor, TRPA1 is activated and extracellular calcium floods into the cell. Increasing calcium levels in these cells serves as the first signal that initiates the action potential and transmits the pruritus signal. This channel is also expressed in keratinocytes, dendrites, and mast cells and is also important for pruritus due to inflammatory skin conditions. Crosstalk between immune cells, keratinocytes, and peripheral nerves mediates pruritus.

Neurotransmission Pathways in Pruritus

A brief description of the route of occurrence of pruritus includes the epidermis and near the dermo-epidermal junction, and it is optionally transmitted to non-myelinated C nerve fibers and thinly myelinated Aδ afferent fibers. These afferent fibers are found in the epidermis, upper dermis, and around skin appendages, which express many sensory receptors [7]. The neural pathways that cause pruritus are not fully understood but are involved in the transmission of signals along histamine sensitive and non-histamine sensitive peripheral C nerve fibers. These account for 5% of the C nerve fibers in the body. Itch-specific peripheral neurons are positive for Mas-related G-protein-coupled receptor (GPCR) A3 (MargprA3) because the genetic ablation of MargprA3 positive neurons reduced scratching behavior in response to chloroquine and histamine, without affecting the pain responses in a mouse model [13]. Some of these fibers are sensitive to histamine, but some are not. Histamine-responsive (histaminergic) and non-histaminergic pruritoceptors use largely distinct receptors and distinct cutaneous nerve fibers that follow separate spinothalamic tracts to connect with different neural pathways in the central nervous system (CNS). In general, the non-histaminergic pathway is more important than histaminergic pathway in pruritus of atopic dermatitis.

Complex interactions between T cells, mast cells, neutrophils, eosinophils, keratinocytes, and neurons involving increased release of cytokines, proteases, and neuropeptides exacerbate pruritus [14]. The primary afferent C nerve fibers carry the signal to synapses with secondary delivery neurons and pass through the dorsal horn of the spine and into the thalamus via the opposite spinal thalamic pathway. Pruritus then passes to the cerebral cortical sensory cortex, area 3a, and to the anterior cingulate cortex, resulting in the desire to scratch [15].

The Difference Between Pruritus and Pain Transmission [16, 17]

Many studies have been conducted to determine the pathophysiology of how pruritus and pain differ. It was previously claimed that pruritus was simply a sensation that occurs when pain stimulation is weak, and that other patterns of action-potential transmission in nerves might differ. A relatively recent theory is called the spatial contrast

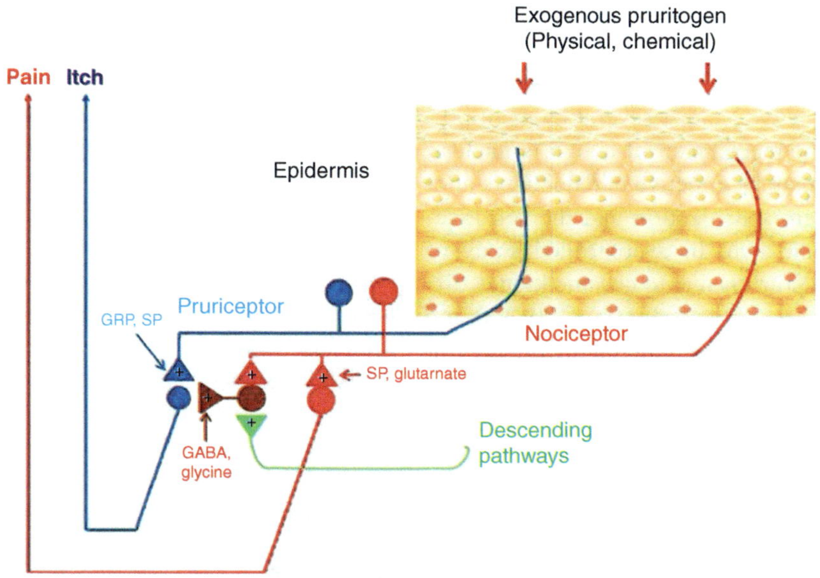

Fig. 2 Neurotransmission pathways of pain and itch (From Tasuku Akiyama, et al., i. PLoS ONE 6(7): e22665 according to the Creative Commons license of Akiyama et al.)

theory (Fig. 2) [18]. That is, even within C nerve fibers, many nociceptors and channels that deliver pruritus and pain are mixed, and each may exist independently or form an intersection. When some of the nociceptors are stimulated, pruritus occurs and this stimulation tends to inhibit other nociceptors of the surrounding nerve fibers and vice versa. This is considered pain in the case of stimuli in which several nociceptors are activated. Therefore, when a human feels pruritus, he or she scratches that causes vigorous irritation. Then the person feels only pain and no pruritus. However, the theory of pathophysiology of pruritus remains a subject that needs further study.

Treatment of Pruritus

Systemic Therapy

Antihistamines

Oral H1 antihistamines act by blocking the H1 receptor on afferent C nerve fibers. They can also inhibit the release of pruritic pruritus mediators from mast cells when administered at high doses [4]. H1 antihistamines are systemic drugs that are used as primary treatment in patients with pruritus due to the relative safety, wide availability, and economic efficiency of these drugs [19]. However, the data on the efficacy of systemic antihistamines on pruritus are limited [20]. To date, the data from randomized clinical trials do not support the efficacy of antihistamines in diseases other than urticaria [14].

Antihistamines include classic first-generation antihistamines and new second-generation antihistamines. First-generation antihistamines include diphenhydramine, chlorpheniramine, and hydroxyzine. First-generation antihistamines easily cross the blood–brain barrier, leading to sedation and anticholinergic side effects [21]. Anticholinergic side effects include dry mouth, diplopia, visual field disorders, urinary obstruction, and vaginal dryness. In addition, the first-generation antihistamines are suitable for night therapy because they show central sedation by attaching not only to H1 receptors but also to muscarinic, α-adrenergic, dopamine, and serotonin receptors. Now, the new second-generation antihistamines are recommended as first-line therapy [22]. These drugs produce less sedation, little anticholinergic effect, less drug-drug interactions, and need lower doses compared to the first generation. Second-generation antihistamines include fexofenadine, cetirizine, levocetirizine, loratadine, rupatadine, and ebastine.

Neurological Drugs

The structural analogs of the neurotransmitter γ-aminobutyric acid (i.e., gabapentin and pregabalin) are effective against several kinds of pruritus [14]. The mechanism of action is unclear, but these seem to be effective in reducing central nervous system sensitization and the sensitization of chronic itch. In a controlled study of patients with pruritus due to chronic kidney disease, low doses of gabapentin (100–300 mg three times a week) were much more effective at reducing pruritus than placebo was [23]. Although there are no controlled studies, the use of these drugs to reduce neuropathic pruritus, such as pruritus and brachioradial pruritus, has been reported in a case [14].

Antidepressants

Selective serotonin reuptake inhibitors (paroxetine, sertraline, fluvoxamine, and fluoxetine) have been reported to reduce various types of general itch in addition to psychogenic itch [24]. Tricyclic antidepressants, such as amitriptyline, are also sometimes used to treat chronic pruritus but are the subject of no randomized studies [25].

Opiate Agonists and Antagonists

Opiate agonists and antagonists are effective in cholestasis, chronic urticaria, atopic dermatitis, and chronic kidney disease. Randomized controlled trials showed antipruritic effects of mu-opioid antagonists (naltrexone, nalmefene, naloxone) in patients with chronic urticaria, atopic dermatitis, eczema, and cholestatics [14]. There may be side effects such as nausea, loss of appetite, abdominal cramps, and diarrhea. In addition, randomized, placebo-controlled clinical trials showed that kappa-opioid agonist nalfurafine hydrochloride significantly reduced pruritus in patients with chronic kidney disease [26]. It has been reported that kappa-opioid analog and mu-opioid antagonists (butorphanol) reduce pruritus associated with non-Hodgkin's lymphoma, cholestasis, and other refractory pruritus [27].

Immunomodulators [28]

Cyclosporine and azathioprine are effective drugs for inflammatory skin diseases such as atopic dermatitis and chronic urticaria, which are hardly affected by antihistamines. However, caution should be exercised in cases with high blood pressure, infection, elevated BUN/creatinine, and risk of nephrotoxicity. Nephrotoxicity is often asymptomatic and requires careful monitoring. Mycophenolate mofetil has an immunosuppressive effect by specifically blocking lymphocyte proliferation and antibody production, and has been reported in severe atopic dermatitis, chronic idiopathic urticaria, and autoimmune diseases in adults. In terms of safety, it is known that its frequency of toxicity is lower than that of cyclosporine.

Mycophenolate mofetil has the anti-inflammatory action of methotrexate on lymphocytes and neutrophils and is thought to be effective for treating pruritus. It has been proven effective for the treatment of atopic dermatitis and chronic urticaria. Although dapsone has been reported to be effective in various types of chronic urticaria and angioedema, monitoring has been reported due to rare but serious side effects such as dose-dependent anemia, skin rashes, peripheral neuropathy, gastrointestinal side effects, hepatotoxicity, methemoglobulinosis, and hematological abnormalities.

Biologics and Small Molecules (Fig. 3)

Dupilumab, a fully human monoclonal antibody that blocks Interleukin-4 and Interleukin-13 in patients with atopic dermatitis (a representative skin disease that can cause pruritus) has been shown to be effective in patients with severe atopic dermatitis and pruritus [29].

In addition, atopic dermatitis is characterized by a TH2-mediated immune response. Activated TH2 cells in patients have higher IL-31 levels and higher levels of IL-31 in skin. Nemolizumab, which blocks IL-31, markedly diminished pruritus within the first 2 weeks in patients with atopic dermatitis [30]. Omalizumab, a recombinant human monoclonal IgG antibody, attaches to the free IgE and degrades mast cell function. Recognizing the clinical efficacy and stability of chronic urticaria, the European urticaria treatment guidelines recommend that it be used preferen-

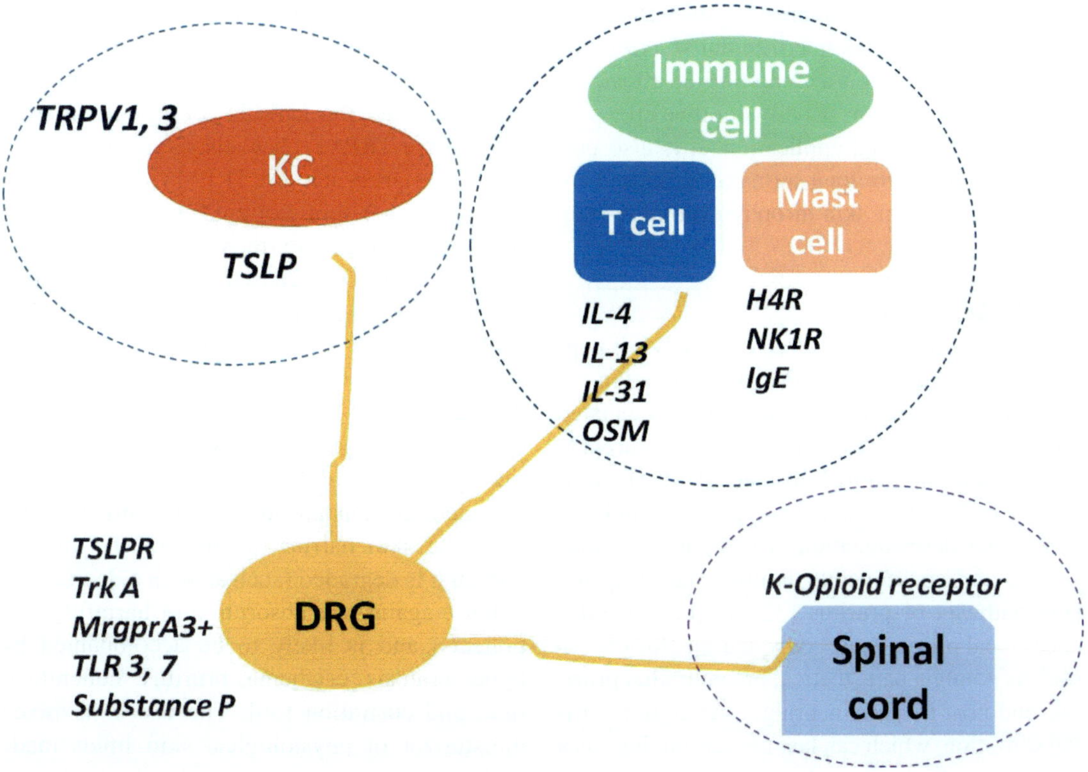

Fig. 3 Mediators that may be targets of treatment for pruritus

tially over cyclosporine if the urticaria does not respond to antihistamine doses. In chronic urticaria, as with other treatments, symptoms may slowly reappear 4–10 weeks after discontinuation of omalizumab [28]. Apremilast (PDE4 inhibitor) modulates the pruritus of psoriasis by controlling the production of inflammatory/non-inflammatory cytokines [28].

UV Treatment

Treatment with UV-B alone, or in combination with UV-A, reduces the itch caused by chronic kidney disease and improves the itch of skin diseases such as psoriasis, atopic dermatitis, and other kinds of eczema. In addition, it can be safely used in patients and pregnant women with the underlying disease, in which cases it is difficult to use systemic drugs because there are few side effects except a temporary reaction during which the skin looks like it is sunburned [31].

Topical Drugs

Topical Steroids

Topical steroid preparations are effective in the treatment of various inflammatory skin diseases, and reduction of the inflammation improves the pruritus associated with it. However, because it does not directly suppress pruritus, the effect may be of limited use for pruritus that is not associated with inflammatory skin diseases. In addition, long-term use may weaken the skin barrier function.

Topical Calcineurin Inhibitors

Topical calcineurin inhibitors are mainly used for inflammatory skin diseases such as atopic dermatitis. In addition to their anti-inflammatory effect, they are thought to have the effect of relieving pruritus by activation of TRPV1 in peripheral C nerve fibers with subsequent desensitization [19]. Pruritus improves within 48 h of the first application, and the effect of suppressing the itch lasts if the application is continued. Initial stinging due to TRPV1 activation is a common side effect, but the stinging symptoms usually improve after several days of repeated application. It is also preferred to steroids for long-term use because there is no side effect of skin atrophy even after long use [19].

TRPV1 Activator

Capsaicin is a substance derived from chili peppers, which activates TRPV1. Activation of TRPV1 stimulates peripheral nerves associated with pruritus or pain, releasing certain neuroprotein peptides, including Substance P, which eventually leads to deficiency. It also induces continuous desensitization of neurons to various stimuli and consequently inhibits the transmission pathway of pruritus [32]. Capsaicin influences local pruritus caused by neuropathic causes such as notalgia paresthetica, brachioradial pruritus, and post-herpetic neuralgia. An initial burning sensation, which can last for several days, is a major side effect, so applying topical anesthesia first and then applying capsaicin for 2 weeks at the beginning of the treatment may help reduce the burning sensation.

TRPV 1 Inhibitor

Local itch caused by neuropathic issues such as notalgia paresthetica, brachioradial pruritus, and post-herpetic neuralgia may be helped by capsaicin creams that activate TRPV1 and then desensitize the skin. However, many patients suffer from burning sensations after application. Recently, topical agents that antagonize and relieve pruritus instead of activating TRPV1 are currently in clinical trials in patients with atopic dermatitis (PAC-14028, AMOREPACIFIC).

TRPM8 Activator

TRPM8 is a major receptor for temperature-sensitive nerve fibers associated with the detection of cooling on body surfaces such as skin [31].

Activation of TRPM8 acts to relieve pruritus through several pathways [33]. First, it activates antipruritic kappa-opioid receptors [34]. The influx of calcium associated with TRPM8 in neurons increases the threshold for pruritus [35]. Lotions containing calamine or menthol give the skin a sensation that relieves pruritus symptoms and act through the activation of the cold receptor (TRPM8 or TRPA1) channels. Cryosim-1, a synthetic substance, acts as a TRPM8 selective agent and makes the skin feel cold without changing the tissue temperature, thereby suppressing discomfort such as that caused by pruritus. Cooling is felt within 1 min, and unlike natural substances such as menthol, it lasts 2–4 h.

Moisturizer

Dry skin is caused by changes in the composition of epidermal lipids and the increase of transdermal moisture loss. In patients with dry skin, the skin barrier function of the stratum corneum is degraded (such as with a decrease in defense against the absorption of harmful components) and is likely to be accompanied by hyperkeratosis, erythema, pruritus, lichenification, and custration [36]. The use of a mixed moisturizer of physiological skin lipids made with a composition similar to the skin's physiological lipid (ceramides, cholesterol, fatty acids, etc.) is the most basic in the treatment of pruritus because it softens the stratum corneum and restores the barrier function, relieving pruritus [37]. However, preservatives should be tested before use, because preservatives and scents in the moisturizers can cause allergic dermatitis in some patients, after which the pruritus could become more severe.

Conclusions

Pruritus is a common symptom that occurs not only in skin diseases but also under a variety of other circumstances, such as secondary to systemic or psychotic illnesses. Without general treatment, the patient suffers from extreme pain and poor quality of life. The factor stimulating the itch and the extent of the symptoms affect the treatment. Although a variety of therapies are used to relieve pruritus, data for direct comparison of a number of studies on the efficacy of those treatments is limited. Numerous new medications are being developed in response to pruritus, which could be helpful if used properly according to the individual's condition.

References

1. Ikoma A, Steinhoff M, Stander S, Yosipovitch G, Schmelz M. The neurobiology of itch. Nat Rev Neurosci. 2006;7(7):535–47. https://doi.org/10.1038/nrn1950.
2. Stander S, Schafer I, Phan NQ, Blome C, Herberger K, Heigel H, et al. Prevalence of chronic pruritus in Germany: results of a cross-sectional study in a sample working population of 11,730. Dermatology. 2010;221(3):229–35. https://doi.org/10.1159/000319862.
3. Stander S, Weisshaar E, Mettang T, Szepietowski JC, Carstens E, Ikoma A, et al. Clinical classification of itch: a position paper of the International Forum for the Study of Itch. Acta Derm Venereol. 2007;87(4):291–4. https://doi.org/10.2340/00015555-0305.
4. Metz M, Stander S. Chronic pruritus—pathogenesis, clinical aspects and treatment. J Eur Acad Dermatol Venereol. 2010;24(11):1249–60. https://doi.org/10.1111/j.1468-3083.2010.03850.x.
5. Moniaga CS, Tominaga M, Takamori K. Mechanisms and management of itch in dry skin. Acta Derm Venereol. 2020;100(2):adv00024. https://doi.org/10.2340/00015555-3344.
6. Yosipovitch G. The pruritus receptor unit: a target for novel therapies. J Invest Dermatol. 2007;127(8):1857–9. https://doi.org/10.1038/sj.jid.5700818.
7. Stander S, Raap U, Weisshaar E, Schmelz M, Mettang T, Handwerker H, et al. Pathogenesis of pruritus. J Dtsch Dermatol Ges. 2011;9(6):456–63. https://doi.org/10.1111/j.1610-0387.2011.07585.x.
8. Greaves MW, Wall PD. Pathophysiology of itching. Lancet. 1996;348(9032):938–40. https://doi.org/10.1016/s0140-6736(96)04328-0.
9. Harrison S, Geppetti P. Substance p. Int J Biochem Cell Biol. 2001;33(6):555–76. https://doi.org/10.1016/s1357-2725(01)00031-0.
10. Lovell CR, Burton PA, Duncan EH, Burton JL. Prostaglandins and pruritus. Br J Dermatol. 1976;94(3):273–5. https://doi.org/10.1111/j.1365-2133.1976.tb04383.x.
11. Fjellner B, Hagermark O. Experimental pruritus evoked by platelet activating factor (PAF-acether) in human skin. Acta Derm Venereol. 1985;65(5):409–12.
12. Imamachi N, Park GH, Lee H, Anderson DJ, Simon MI, Basbaum AI, et al. TRPV1-expressing primary afferents generate behavioral responses to pruritogens via multiple mechanisms. Proc Natl Acad Sci U S A. 2009;106(27):11330–5. https://doi.org/10.1073/pnas.0905605106.
13. Han L, Ma C, Liu Q, Weng HJ, Cui Y, Tang Z, et al. A subpopulation of nociceptors specifically linked to itch. Nat Neurosci. 2013;16(2):174–82. https://doi.org/10.1038/nn.3289.
14. Lumpkin EA, Caterina MJ. Mechanisms of sensory transduction in the skin. Nature. 2007;445(7130):858–65. https://doi.org/10.1038/nature05662.
15. Davidson S, Giesler GJ. The multiple pathways for itch and their interactions with pain. Trends Neurosci. 2010;33(12):550–8. https://doi.org/10.1016/j.tins.2010.09.002.
16. Akiyama T, Iodi Carstens M, Carstens E. Transmitters and pathways mediating inhibition of spinal itch-signaling neurons by scratching and other counter-stimuli. PLoS One. 2011;6(7):e22665. https://doi.org/10.1371/journal.pone.0022665.
17. Namer B, Reeh P. Scratching an itch. Nat Neurosci. 2013;16(2):117–8. https://doi.org/10.1038/nn.3316.
18. Akiyama T, Carstens E. Neural processing of itch. Neuroscience. 2013;250:697–714. https://doi.org/10.1016/j.neuroscience.2013.07.035.
19. Pereira U, Boulais N, Lebonvallet N, Pennec JP, Dorange G, Misery L. Mechanisms of the sensory effects of tacrolimus on the skin. Br J Dermatol. 2010;163(1):70–7. https://doi.org/10.1111/j.1365-2133.2010.09757.x.
20. O'Donoghue M, Tharp MD. Antihistamines and their role as antipruritics. Dermatol Ther. 2005;18(4):333–40. https://doi.org/10.1111/j.1529-8019.2005.00034.x.
21. Adelsberg BR. Sedation and performance issues in the treatment of allergic conditions. Arch Intern Med. 1997;157(5):494–500.
22. Grattan C, Powell S, Humphreys F. Management and diagnostic guidelines for urticaria and angio-oedema. Br J Dermatol. 2001;144(4):708–14. https://doi.org/10.1046/j.1365-2133.2001.04175.x.
23. Gunal AI, Ozalp G, Yoldas TK, Gunal SY, Kirciman E, Celiker H. Gabapentin therapy for pruritus in haemodialysis patients: a randomized, placebo-controlled, double-blind trial. Nephrol Dial Transplant. 2004;19(12):3137–9. https://doi.org/10.1093/ndt/gfh496.
24. Stander S, Bockenholt B, Schurmeyer-Horst F, Weishaupt C, Heuft G, Luger TA, et al. Treatment of chronic pruritus with the selective serotonin re-uptake inhibitors paroxetine and fluvoxamine: results of an open-labelled, two-arm proof-of-concept study. Acta Derm Venereol. 2009;89(1):45–51. https://doi.org/10.2340/00015555-0553.
25. Yosipovitch G, Samuel LS. Neuropathic and psychogenic itch. Dermatol Ther. 2008;21(1):32–41. https://doi.org/10.1111/j.1529-8019.2008.00167.x.
26. Kumagai H, Ebata T, Takamori K, Muramatsu T, Nakamoto H, Suzuki H. Effect of a novel kappa-receptor agonist, nalfurafine hydrochloride, on severe itch in 337 haemodialysis patients: a Phase III, randomized, double-blind, placebo-controlled study. Nephrol Dial Transplant. 2010;25(4):1251–7. https://doi.org/10.1093/ndt/gfp588.
27. Dawn AG, Yosipovitch G. Butorphanol for treatment of intractable pruritus. J Am Acad Dermatol.

2006;54(3):527–31. https://doi.org/10.1016/j.jaad.2005.12.010.
28. Leslie TA, Greaves MW, Yosipovitch G. Current topical and systemic therapies for itch. Handb Exp Pharmacol. 2015;226:337–56. https://doi.org/10.1007/978-3-662-44605-8_18.
29. Beck LA, Thaci D, Hamilton JD, Graham NM, Bieber T, Rocklin R, et al. Dupilumab treatment in adults with moderate-to-severe atopic dermatitis. N Engl J Med. 2014;371(2):130–9. https://doi.org/10.1056/NEJMoa1314768.
30. Ruzicka T, Hanifin JM, Furue M, Pulka G, Mlynarczyk I, Wollenberg A, et al. Anti-interleukin-31 receptor A antibody for atopic dermatitis. N Engl J Med. 2017;376(9):826–35. https://doi.org/10.1056/NEJMoa1606490.
31. Rivard J, Lim HW. Ultraviolet phototherapy for pruritus. Dermatol Ther. 2005;18(4):344–54. https://doi.org/10.1111/j.1529-8019.2005.00032.x.
32. Knotkova H, Pappagallo M, Szallasi A. Capsaicin (TRPV1 Agonist) therapy for pain relief: farewell or revival? Clin J Pain. 2008;24(2):142–54. https://doi.org/10.1097/AJP.0b013e318158ed9e.
33. Knowlton WM, Palkar R, Lippoldt EK, McCoy DD, Baluch F, Chen J, et al. A sensory-labeled line for cold: TRPM8-expressing sensory neurons define the cellular basis for cold, cold pain, and cooling-mediated analgesia. J Neurosci. 2013;33(7):2837–48. https://doi.org/10.1523/jneurosci.1943-12.2013.
34. Galeotti N, Di Cesare Mannelli L, Mazzanti G, Bartolini A, Ghelardini C. Menthol: a natural analgesic compound. Neurosci Lett. 2002;322(3):145–8. https://doi.org/10.1016/s0304-3940(01)02527-7.
35. Linte RM, Ciobanu C, Reid G, Babes A. Desensitization of cold- and menthol-sensitive rat dorsal root ganglion neurones by inflammatory mediators. Exp Brain Res. 2007;178(1):89–98. https://doi.org/10.1007/s00221-006-0712-3.
36. Lee DH, Seo ES, Hong JT, Lee GT, You YK, Lee KK, et al. The efficacy and safety of a proposed herbal moisturising cream for dry skin and itch relief: a randomised, double-blind, placebo-controlled trial—study protocol. BMC Complement Altern Med. 2013;13:330. https://doi.org/10.1186/1472-6882-13-330.
37. Park CS. The skin barrier and moisturizer. J Skin Barrier Res. 2007;9(1):11–7.

Part IV

Diagnosis

Diagnosis and Severity Assessment of Atopic Dermatitis (Korean Guideline Included)

Jung Eun Kim and Sang Wook Son

Diagnosis of Atopic Dermatitis

Diagnostic Criteria for AD

Gold Standard Criteria for AD Diagnosis

The diagnosis of Atopic Dermatitis (AD) is clinically made and is based on the morphology and distribution of the lesion, and the associated signs and symptoms. The first comprehensive diagnostic criteria for AD are made by Hanifin and Rajka and it was developed empirically on "clinical experience" and consensus between experts. It was minimally validated but, most widely used for diagnosis for AD [1]. Hanfin-Rajka criteria consist of 4 major criteria and 23 minor criteria consisting of associated signs and symptoms (Table 1). Patients need to fulfill at least three major criteria and three minor features. It is not easy to use these comprehensive criteria in real clinical practice, but it remains as gold standard criteria when a detailed examination is needed for diagnosis of atypical disease presentation [2].

There have been many attempts to refine and shorten the original criteria to make them clinically easy to be applicable. The UK Working Party Criteria were modified with core set of the Hanifin-Rajka criteria for epidemiological studies. The criteria was the most validated criteria that was proven in 19 studies [2]. It consists of one mandatory and five major criteria (Table 1) [3–5]. Both Hanfin-Rajka criteria and UK working party diagnostic criteria are the most commonly used worldwide [6, 7].

Several modified versions of the Hanifin-Rajka criteria, which reflects each racial characteristics and medical environment are developed and used in various countries. [8–11]. Korean diagnostic criteria for AD was based on the Hanifin-Rajka criteria, and established considering phenotype of AD in Korean populations. It consists of 4 major criteria and 13 minor criteria (Table 2). The major criteria of AD is similar to conventional diagnostic criteria, but three additional minor features (periauricular eczema, scalp scale, and skin prick test reactivity) were significant for the diagnosis of AD in Korean patients (11). This means that ethnic backgrounds influence the phenotype of AD and illustrate the need for development of diagnostic criteria in specific ethnic populations and in specific subgroups.

J. E. Kim
Department of Dermatology, Eunpyeong St.Mary's Hospital, The Catholic University of Korea, Seoul, Korea (Republic of)

S. W. Son (✉)
Department of Dermatology, Korea University Ansan Hospital, Ansan-si, Korea (Republic of)

Division of Brain Korea 21 Project for Biomedical Science, Department of Dermatology, Laboratory of Cell Signalling and Nanomedicine, Korea University College of Medicine, Seoul, Korea (Republic of)
e-mail: skin4u@korea.ac.kr

K. H. Lee et al. (eds.), *Practical Insights into Atopic Dermatitis*,
https://doi.org/10.1007/978-981-15-8159-5_5

Table 1 Gold standard criteria for AD diagnosis

Hanifin-Rajka criteria	UK working party diagnostic criteria
Major criteria (three or more) • Pruritus • Dermatitis affecting flexural surfaces in adults and the face and extensors in infants • Chronic or relapsing dermatitis • Personal or family history of cutaneous or respiratory atopy *Minor criteria (three or more)* • Facial pallor or erythema • Hypopigmented patches • Infraorbital darkening • Infraorbital folds or wrinkles • Cheilitis • Recurrent conjunctivitis • Anterior neck folds • Triggers of atopic dermatitis: foods, emotional factors, environmental factors, and skin irritants such as wool, solvents, and sweat • Susceptibility to cutaneous viral and bacterial infections • Impaired cell-mediated immunity • Immediate skin test reactivity • Raised serum IgE • Keratoconus • Anterior subcapsular cataracts • Early age of onset • Dry skin • Ichthyosis • Hyperlinear palms • Keratosis pilaris • Hand and foot dermatitis • Nipple eczema • White dermatographism • Perifollicular accentuation	*Major criteria (mandatory)* • Itchy skin condition *Minor criteria* (three or more) • Flexural involvement • Asthma/hay fever • Generalized dry skin • Onset of rash under the age of 2 years • Visible flexural dermatitis

We often encounter patients with adult-onset AD without any atopic background and some of them have atypical clinical features. It is not easy to diagnose AD in these cases, who do not match with the UK Working Party Criteria. We will discuss the reported diagnostic criteria or features in various age groups.

Diagnostic Criteria in Different Age Groups

Several expert groups have suggested modified diagnostic criteria in certain age groups due to their heterogeneity in clinical manifestation. Most diagnostic criteria that are used in different age groups were developed based on the Hanifin and Rajka criteria or Working Party criteria, and characteristic features that could be seen in a specific age group have been emphasized and others have been simplified.

Diagnostic Criteria for Pediatric AD

International Study for Asthma and Allergy in Childhood (ISAAC) criteria questionnaire to diagnosis of eczema were derived from the UK criteria and are widely used for epidemiological surveys, thus it may not be appropriate to use in diagnosing AD in individual setting [12, 13].

The experts group in the American Academy of Dermatology have suggested consensus diagnostic criteria for pediatric AD. Pruritus and eczema are essential features for pediatric AD and early age at onset, a personal and/or family history of atopy, IgE reactivity and xerosis are important features that support the diagnosis in children. Other associated features such as periorbital changes may be helpful to diagnosis, but considered as nonspecific in children [14].

Table 2 Diagnostic criteria for AD in Korean

Major features (two or more)
1. Pruritus
2. Typical morphology and distribution
(a) Under the age of 2 years: face, trunk, and extensor involvement
(b) Over the age of 2 years: face, neck, and flexural involvement
3. Personal or family history (atopic dermatitis, asthma, and allergic rhinitis)
Minor features (four or more)
1. Xerosis
2. Facial erythema/facial pallor
3. Periorbital eczema or orbital darkening
4. Periauricular eczema
5. Cheilitis
6. Tendency toward nonspecific hand or foot dermatitis
7. Scalp scale
8. Perifollicular accentuation
9. Itch when sweating
10. White dermographism
11. Skin prick test reactivity
12. Elevated serum IgE
13. Tendency toward cutaneous infections

In Korea, Reliable Estimation of Atopic Dermatitis of Child Hood (REACH) diagnostic criteria [15] were developed for AD children aged 4–12 years. The REACH consists of two major and nine minor criteria. Two major criteria are "recurrent eczema in the last 12 months" and "eczema on the antecubital or popliteal fossa." Nine minor criteria are atopy history, localized eczema involving the following six areas including eye, "recurrent eczema in the last 12 months" popliteal fossae is diagnosed if one fulfills the two major criteria. AD without eczema on the antecubital or popliteal fossae is diagnosed if one fulfills the one major criteria and four minor criteria or more [15]. REACH emphasize the importance of flexural dermatitis in children AD compared to pediatric criteria suggested by the American Academy of Dermatology.

Diagnostic Features of Adult-Onset AD

The proportion of adult-onset AD is known as about 25% in recent meta-analysis [16]. Since adult-onset AD presents different clinical phenotypes comparing persistent AD from childhood, there are diagnostic particularities in, which are getting important for physicians to consider. Diagnosis of AD in adults has remained a clinical challenge since to date there are no specific criteria for the adult population to date. Some clinical characteristics were identified for adult-onset AD. When compared to patients with pre-adult onset, those with adult-onset disease were related to higher female ratio, high altitude resident area, lower socioeconomic status, smoking in adulthood, and less history of familial history, asthma, filaggrin-null mutations, and allergen-specific IgE [17]. A study reported that flexural areas of arms are the most commonly involved area among adult-onset patients, followed by eyelid/periocular area, hands, and neck. Adult-onset AD tended to show less severity than persistent AD from childhood, but more severe in itching [18]. Another study reported that adult onset-AD patients often present a nonflexural distribution as well as flexural dermatitis [19].

Recently, Italian experts suggested diagnostic guidelines for adult AD. The criteria involve four major contents consisting of morphological features, localization, clinical history, and differential diagnosis [20]. Adult AD frequently presents atypical morphologic variants such as pruritic papules or nodules other than typical eczema, xerosis, and lichenification [19], They specify that characteristic localization of adult AD are hands, face and neck, and flexural areas [20]. The diagnostic criteria for adult-onset AD should be confirmed through larger studies with cumulative consistent evidence of clinical characteristics in the future.

Diagnostic Features of AD in Elderly

Recently, elderly-onset AD has been considered a distinct AD phenotype. AD developed in elderly without any previous allergic comorbidities is more difficult to diagnose. Skin manifestations in elderly AD are known to be basically similar to those of adult AD. Tanei et al. reported unique "reverse sign of lichenification" in elderly AD, which means lichenified eczema is shown around unaffected flexural areas instead of classic lichenification involving flexural areas [21].

Dezoteux et al. have characterized that elderly-onset AD (>45 years old) present less head and neck involvement compared to persistent AD since childhood [22, 23].

However, even elderly without AD go through impaired skin barrier, xerosis, and possible Th2 immune deviation as part of aging that is similar to disease condition of AD [22]. Besides, elderly patients usually have more comorbidities and take more medications that can cause itching and dry skin, complicating the diagnosis of AD in elderly [21, 22]. It is difficult to apply Hanfin-Rajka criteria and the UK working party diagnostic criteria to AD in elderly diagnosis. To date, AD in the elderly has not been well characterized and more knowledge about AD in the elderly is needed to establish diagnostic clues and work-up guidelines when evaluating elderly patients [24].

Differential Diagnosis

The diagnosis of AD is primarily clinical, additional workup such as serum total and specific IgE only contributes to identifying external aggravating factors. A diagnosis of AD is made after differential diagnosis of the following diseases: psoriasis, scabies infestation, and seborrheic dermatitis. Allergic or irritant contact dermatitis should also be excluded. Nummular dermatitis is an important four differential diagnosis of AD, but differential diagnosis is often vague from atypical form of adult AD [25].

If the lesions do not respond to topical anti-inflammatory treatment or have atypical in morphology or distribution, physicians should consider T-cell lymphoma, nutritional deficiencies, or metabolic syndromes. If an AD child had a history of recurrent respiratory tract infections, or skin infections, or failure to thrive, immunodeficiency syndromes should be suspected. To rule out the conditions above, laboratory tests such as serum immunoglobulins, potassium hydroxide (KOH), patch test, or skin biopsy can be performed [25].

In case of elderly patients, xerotic eczema, senile pruritus, and chronic prurigo should be additionally considered as essential differential diagnoses. Since elderly patients commonly have other underlying diseases such as hypertension, cerebrovascular diseases, and diabetes mellitus, which possibly cause pruritus or xerosis as a consequence of the conditions and/or side effects of medication [21].

Disease Severity Assessment of AD

Many different scoring systems to assess AD's severity have been developed and used for clinical practice and research purposes. There are about 62 different types of disease severity measures and 28 quality of life (QOL) assessment scales have been used [26]. Since most evaluation methods are evaluated according to the extent of lesions and subjective symptoms, the score values often show difference by interobserver and intraobserver. In addition, the severity may be assessed differently depending on which assessment method is used in a patient, since each evaluation method has different metrics that rate high weights. Scoring atopic dermatitis (SCORAD) assesses subjective symptoms such as itching and sleep disturbance, which is not included in the Eczema Area and Severity Index (EASI). In this chapter, we will review the most representative severity scoring systems of AD rated by physicians and patients.

Physicians' Measurement Tools

SCORAD

The SCORAD index is developed by the European Task Force of Atopic Dermatitis and validated to measure clinical signs and symptoms of AD and adequate interobserver reliability [27]. SCORAD index remained the most widely used instrument. SCORAD measures the extent and the intensity of disease, and the patient's subjective symptoms. The extent of involved lesional area is estimated by the rule of nines. Different ratios of body surface area are applied between adults and infants.

The intensity is scored from 0 to 3 (none to severe) regarding erythema, edema/papulation, oozing/crusting, excoriations, dryness, and lichenification. Lastly, for the subjective symptoms, itching and sleep loss are evaluated with a scale from 0 to 10 [25]. SCORAD has its three levels of severity as follows: mild: <25; moderate: 25–50; and severe: >50 [28].

EASI

EASI is a widely used objective evaluation tool of AD severity in various countries and well correlate to SCORAD. Unlike SCORAD, EASI only scores to measure patients' visible lesions only, but not their subjective symptoms. EASI assesses the degree of erythema, edema, excoriation, and lichenification signs in four body parts comprising of head and neck, trunk, upper extremities, and lower extremities. The EASI describes AD severity as follows: mild, EASI score < 16; moderate, 16 ≤ EASI score < 23; and severe, EASI score ≥ 23. EASI of 16 corresponds to SCORAD index of 25 and EASI of 23 corresponds to SCORAD index of 50. Corresponding scores between SCORAD and EASI have some variations according to study methods. Some studies define moderate to severe AD as follows: mild, EASI score 1–5; moderate, EASI score 6–22; and severe, EASI score 23–72 points.

Investigator's Global Assessment

An Investigator's Global Assessment (IGA) is a literally physician's global assessment that is based on the erythema, edema, papulation, and oozing. IGA score defines AD severity as follows: (1) almost clear, (2) mild disease, (3) moderate, (4) severe, and (5) very severe [29]. IGA is a commonly used tool in clinical trials, since it is relatively simple to perform, especially daily record keeping. To prove the efficacy of a drug, the Food and Drug Administration (FDA) requires that achieving an IGA score ≤ 1, indicating clear or nearly clear skin is obligatory for FDA approval. However, IGA is not a validated scale either does not provide clinical information about body surface area, and symptoms in detail as SCORAD or EASI. Silverberg et al. have reported that IGA does not correlate with other validated scales such as EASI, Dermatology Life Quality Index (DLQI), and Patient-Oriented Eczema Measure (POEM) in their clinical trials and IGA may not be proper as a clinical outcome measurement tool [30].

Patient-Reported Outcome Measures

Although majority of the subjective and objective symptoms are correlated, QoL of AD patients may not necessarily be proportional to the objective severities of AD. Besides, SCORAD and EASI may not be applicable to routine clinical practice because they are time consuming. Patient-Reported Outcome Measures (PROMs) have advantages in time saving and easy to use for patients without any specific education although they are less accurate than physician's assessment. The Self-administered-EASI (SA-EASI) and Patient-Oriented SCORAD (PO-SCORAD) index are patients' assessment version of EASI and SCORAD. They are also validated and correlate well with EASI and SCORAD, respectively [31]. Using patients' assessed scales, clinicians can save time and focus on the treatment outcome and the next treatment. Considering one's medical environment, clinicians may utilize patient-reported tools for routine practice [32].

In these respects, the score changes of PROM before and after treatment should be utilized to determine treatment responses together with the change of physicians' assessment. It brings the needs for the development of consensus on PROM. The consensus on the definition of AD severity measured by physicians such as SCORAD, and EASI has been made by various expert committee. A modified Delphi method is widely used to achieve a consensus based on expert opinions. Recently, there is a movement to establish consensus-based PROM by letting patients and care providers participate in voting similar to that of physicians' consensus-making process [33].

Patient-Oriented Eczema Measure

POEM is a validated instrument to measure the core outcome of subjective symptoms of AD and is widely used in clinical trials. It consists of seven questions regarding the frequency of a particular symptom over the past 1 week. It asks about itch, sleep disturbance, dryness, flaking, weeping or oozing, bleeding, and cracking. Likert five-point scale that gives a total maximum score of 28 [34]. POEM is easy and quick to use but has some limitations because it scores only the frequency of symptoms, not the intensity. And it does not assess the redness, key symptoms of AD [34, 35]. POEM is known to have moderate correlations with EASI and SCORAD since POEM does not assess QoL [28]. Comparing SA-EASI or PO-SCORAD to POEM, prior scales have a property to assess clinical signs rather than patient-reported symptoms. For those reasons, POEM was proposed as the preferred PROM in the latest HOME IV meeting and other clinical trials [35, 36]. The optimal severity grades for the POEM was suggested as following: mild AD, POEM 0–7; moderate AD, POEM 8–19; severe AD, POEM 20–28 [36].

Patient Global Assessment

Patient Global Assessment (PGA) asks overall severity of symptoms or global impact of the disease and widely used as in clinical trials. PGA is similar to that of IGA and uses a 5-point global assessment of disease severity (clear = 0, almost clear = 1, mild = 2, moderate = 3, severe = 4) [33]. It is suitable to follow up the treatment response compared to baseline due to its simplicity.

Pruritus Scales

Visual analog scale (VAS), numerical rating scale (NRS), language rating scale (VRS), and itching severity scale (ISS) were used as a measure of itching, but most scales have not been validated. Among them, VAS and NRS are the most commonly used due to its simplicity [26].

With the VAS, patients are asked to indicate a point corresponding to their pruritus on a horizontal 10-cm line. With the NRS, patients score the intensity of pruritus from 0 to 10 (0: no itch; mild pruritus: 1–3; moderate pruritus: 4–6; severe pruritus: 7–9; 10: worst imaginable itch) [37]. VRS indicates an intensity of pruritus as follows: 0, none; 1, mild; 2, moderate; 3, severe; and 4, very severe. ISS consists of several questionnaires regarding frequency, features of itch, extent of itch, itch intensity graded as "best, average, or worst," effect on mood, sexual desire/function, and sleep [38].

NRS is easy to perform, and the Korean and Italian guidelines recommend to use NRS to assess disease severity and if a patient with an EASI score less than 16, who experience daytime or night time itching NRS over 7 should be considered as at least moderated AD [39, 40]. A recent study validated pruritus scales and revealed that VAS, NRS, and VRS correlated well with each other, but have a low correlation with itch related QoL [41]. ISS is time consuming but correlated with Itchy QoL and reliable [33]. Serial assessment of pruritus is necessary before and after treatment to assess response to treatment.

Quality of Life Index

DLQI, Infant's Dermatology Quality of Life Index (IDQOL), and Children's Dermatology Life Quality Index (CDLQI) are the most commonly used instrument in clinical trials [26] The Dermatology Life Quality Index (DLQI) is a validated instrument to assess the QoL of patients with various skin disorders. DLQI consists of ten questionnaires regarding their symptoms and feelings, daily activities, leisure, work and school, personal relationships, and treatment. IDQOL and CDLQI consist of similar questionnaires to DLQI but the questionnaires are modified properly to the patients' age.

Each question is scored from 0 (no impact) to 3 (worst impact) and the maximum score is 30. QoL impairment shown in total DLQI corresponds as follows: no effect: 0–1, minimal effect: 2–5, moderate effect: 6–10, large effect: 11–20, and extremely large effect: 21–30. A population-based cohort study revealed that DLQI grades as mild = 0–5, moderate = 6–10, severe = 11–30 in adult AD patients [36]. Korean and Italian guidelines suggest that patients with DLQI over 10 should be considered as at least moderate severity of AD regardless of their EASI score [39, 40].

DLQI, CDLQI, and the IDQOL generally well reflect patients' QoL, but time consuming for routine use in clinical practice [8, 42, 43]. Generally, QoL assessment is not recommended for routine clinical practice, but is indicated for the patients who complain of severe pruritus or QoL impairment to provide an appropriate treatment [39]. To assess the treatment responses, it is recommended to perform baseline and at the time point to measure treatment responses.

To evaluate the daily impact on QoL of the patients and to reflect the clinical AD course, more simple tools are developed such as the Atopic Dermatitis Score 7 (ADS7), the Atopic Dermatitis Symptom Score (ADSS), and Atopic Dermatitis Control Tool (ADCT) [33, 44–46].

Core Outcome Sets to Measure Disease Severity

Various countries have their own treatment guidelines by assessing AD severity using SCORAD or EASI primarily (Table 3). AD is characterized by severe itching and chronic relapsing courses, which affect a profound impact on the patients' lives. So far, various instruments that reflect patients' subjective symptoms have been developed to assess treatment responses but, only a few countries adopt the tools to classify disease severity. For example, Korean and Italian experts recommend to use itching and QoL index in AD severity classification in addition to objective severity assessment tools such as EASI [39, 48]. This approach to reflect patients' subjective symptoms in AD severity is necessary, but clinicians should be careful not to be affected by patients' exaggerated complaints or insists. To avoid too many patients over-graded as moderate to severe AD, more precise and elaborate measurement tools should be established with consensus by clinicians and patients.

Table 3 Recommendation on severity assessment tools in various guidelines

	Objective assessment	Subjective assessment	References
USA	EASI, SCORAD		[47]
Europe	SCORAD		[28]
Italy	EASI, involved area	NRS, DLQI	[40, 48]
Korea	SCORAD, EASI	NRS, DLQI	[39]
Asia–Pacific	Not described	Not described	[49]
Japan	Severity index using BSA, SCORAD		[9]

The combination of physicians' objective assessment tools with patients' subjective symptom scores and other measures of QoL would reflect a more comprehensive disease severity and treatment responses of patients. Thus which combination of objective and subjective core outcome instrument sets would be useful should be further addressed to improve the quality of AD treatment in the future.

To evaluate AD severity, not only clinical signs and symptoms, but also long-term control of the disease and impairment of QoL should be considered together. The Harmonizing Outcome Measures for Eczema (HOME) initiative has defined clinical signs, symptoms, quality of life, and long-term control as the core outcome domains [27]. While EASI and SCORAD are concluded as the best tools in measuring the clinical sign of AD based on its validation, responsiveness, and inter-observer reliability, POEM and DLQI were the most recommended core outcome measurement tools among instruments on PROM [27].

Disease severity classification is important to provide proper management and treatment for AD. The severity of AD shows individual variation, but it also goes through various clinical courses within a patient depending on time and environment. It is important to assess the severity correctly and provide proper treatment at each stage. Thus, a single static assessment of disease severity has a limit in that it is easily affected by patients' recall bias and disease status depending on the time point of assessment. Regarding proper frequency of assessment or length of periods that can reflect long-term disease control status should be further addressed.

Definition of Moderate to Severe AD

Diagnosis and management of AD should not be considered separately. The severity is crucial factor to decide the treatment on AD. While

Table 4 Representative AD severity classifications according to clinicians' investigative instruments in various countries

	Mild AD	Moderate AD	Severe AD
US practical recommendation [47]	SCORAD < 25 Or EASI ≤ 7	SCORAD 25–50 Or 7 < EASI ≤ 21	SCORAD > 50 Or EASI > 21
European guideline [28]	SCORAD < 25 Or transient eczema	SCORAD 25–50 Or recurrent eczema	SCORAD > 50 Or persistent eczema
Italian guideline [48]	EASI < 6[a]	EASI 6–22[a]	EASI 23–72
Korean guideline [39]	EASI < 16[b]	EASI 16–22[b]	EASI ≥ 23
Japanese guideline [9]	Only mild rashes are observed irrespective of the area	Rashes with severe inflammation are observed in less than 10% of the BSA[c]	Rashes with severe inflammation are observed > 10% of the BSA[c]

[a]The severity can be upstaged if there are face, neck, hand, foot, or genitalia involvement, NRS is over 7 or quality of life impairment with DLQI
[b]The severity can be upstaged if NRS ≥ 7 or DLQI > 10
[c]*BSA* body surface area

mild AD is regulated by topical immunomodulatory drugs, moderate to severe AD patients are recommended to use systemic immunomodulatory drugs including biologics as mainstay of active treatment. Thus, which patients are indicated to moderate to severe AD patients is very important. For management of AD, measurement of disease severity before treatment and after proper duration of treatment depending on medications is recommended for routine clinical practice. Several severity classifications have been suggested using various objective and subjective disease severity assessment tools such as SCORAD, EASI, pruritus scale, and life quality indices. Table 4 shows the definition of mild, moderate, and severe AD which is being used in various guidelines in various countries.

2019 AD Diagnostic guidelines by KADA (Korean Atopic Dermatitis Association), it defines patients with 16 ≤ EASI < 23, as moderate AD and EASI ≥ 23 as severe AD, respectively. It could raise the severity of the disease if the patient's itching numerical rating scale is more than 7 or dermatology life quality index is over 10 [39]. This is because the patient's clinical signs alone may not be sufficient to assess exact severity. Patients can be much more painful than they look. In the recent European guidelines, not only adopting SCORAD index but also considering recurrence or persistent disease courses in assessing severity is notable. If one has treatment refractoriness, it is enough to diagnose as moderate to severe AD regardless of SCORAD index [28]. The definition of persistent or recurrent AD is not clearly established yet and differ between countries, but experts have a common idea about proactive therapy is indicated for persistent or recurrent AD and the use of systemic immunomodulatory drugs is recommended for severe AD patients. For non-responders to treatment, clinicians should consider changing the treatment modality. In this respect, correct and detailed definition of persistent or recurrent AD, and non-responder is very important.

Spanish AD experts adopted more realistic definition of severe AD who are in need of the administration of immunosuppressive drugs or biologics, and/or hospitalization due to an AD flare [50].

Other Objective Factors to Consider in Determining AD Severity

There have been attempts that the involvement of head and neck, hand or foot, or genitalia, psychological or physical comorbidities such as depression or ocular complications should also be reflected in the patient's severity classifications of AD.

Involved Area

Patients having persistent facial eczema after treatment tend to have low esteem and social difficulties, it may lead to psychological complications. The involvement of exposed or functionally important areas has huge impact on patients' QoL. It should be definitely considered to disease classification. The Italian guideline recommends that if a patient with an EASI score less than 16, has skin lesions in one's face, hands, genital area should be considered as at least moderate AD and the same rule apply to moderate AD patients with affected areas mentioned above, then they get to be categorized into severe AD [40]. However, face, neck, hands, foot, or genitalia are frequently affected in AD patients. So far, there is no proven assessment tool that can stratify disease severity in these areas. The time is not ripe yet to upstage the disease severity with the presence of AD lesions only in these locations. A rational and practical measurement tool should be developed to reflect the severity in these areas.

Comorbidities

Some experts insist that patients with several allergic comorbidities or non-allergic complications should be regarded as severe AD. AD patients with other allergic comorbidities such as food allergies, asthma and allergic rhinitis tend to suffer from more severe diseases than those without other atopic diseases.

Numerous studies reported that severe AD patients are more prone to emotional or psychological illnesses. A higher prevalence of attention-deficit hyperactivity disorder (ADHD), anxiety, conduct disorder, and autism in children with AD was proven compared with children without AD [51]. The risk of ADHD seems to increase in relation to night pruritus–induced sleep disturbance. The Singapore guidelines for AD recommends that AD patients with psychological dysfunction should be considered as severe AD [52]. Several guidelines recommend that patients with over moderate severity or treatment-refractoriness are recommended to receive psychosomatic counseling by experts [53, 54].

Eye complications associated with AD may be mild such as eyelid dermatitis and allergic rhinoconjunctivitis, but can lead to significant morbidity such as cataracts or blindness related to keratoconus [55].

Assessment of comorbidities or complications is quite complicated, and there is no consensus to determine which allergic or nonallergic comorbidities or what degree is severe. However, AD patients who have certain critical physical or mental illnesses such as cataracts, keratoconus, or depression should be considered as severe AD and actively treated to prevent further sequelae.

Treatment Responses

Treatment Refractoriness of AD

SCORAD, EASI, and IGA are the most commonly used tools to determine treatment responses by the score changes before and after treatment in clinical trials. The assessment of the response to a treatment can be made at different times depending on the type of treatment. The determination of the therapeutic effect of biological agents is made on the fourth month of treatment and EASI 50–74 is used as primary end points in a few clinical trials [56].

The definition of nonresponder in treating AD is not established as well as which primary outcome would be used in real clinical practice. Using SCORAD to define responder is not suitable in clinical practice due to its complexity, and IGA is too rough scale and not enough to reflect the improvement in patients' objective symptoms. Korean experts suggest that the determination of treatment refractoriness should reflect both physician's assessment and patients' subjective assessment such as the effects on relieving pruritus and QoL [39]. EASI 50 is used as a yardstick for measurement of treatment response. If there is no appropriate response after 3–4 months of treatment, a higher grade of treatment is needed [39]. If the Pruritus NRS scale does not reach below 4 NRS points or the DLQI score does not fall below 6 points after 3 months of appropriate treatment, it should be defined as treatment-refractory AD [39].

On the while, an expert group in the United Kingdom defined severe recalcitrant AD as history of inadequate clinical response to topical corticosteroids (potent strength on the body and moderate strength on the face) and an objective SCORAD ≥ 30 [57].

Minimal clinically meaningful difference (MCID) in SCORAD or EASI is an important concept to refer to treatment responsiveness. A study reported that the MCID for SCORAD was 8.7 points, 8.2 for the objective SCORAD, and 6.6 for the EASI [58].

MCID in patient-reported symptoms score in response to treatment is getting emphasized. There have been no validated subjective symptoms measurement tools as well as their minimal clinically meaningful change to define responders to treatment. POEM is the most widely studied outcome to assess treatment efficacy and certain studies reported that MCID for adult patients is ranged from 3.4 to 6 point reduction in POEM and MCID for children and adolescents is from 6 to 8 points [56, 58, 59]. Howells et al. recommend the following thresholds be used as clinically important changes in POEM scores ≥ 4 after treatment [59]. Each estimate in different studies were calculated by various manners [58], including anchor-based methods, ROC curve analysis, logistic regression models, and distribution-based methods but showed in similar range [59, 60].

So far, standards as to what extent of decreased QoL will be judged as moderate or severe AD, and how much improvement in QoL score be regarded as the appropriate level therapeutic effect is unclear. Korean experts committee made an agreement based on the expert opinion that DLQI over 10 should be considered as at least moderate AD regardless of objective symptoms and signs and that patients not maintaining adequate QoL (DLQI ≥ 6) after appropriate treatment are in need of treatment change [39]. DLQI and CDLQI are the most used tools to assess QoL as primary outcome in clinical trials. Within-person change of 6–8 points in CDLQI was suggested as a reasonable responder threshold in clinical trial with dupilumab [56]. Such standards for improvement in QoL should be established based on a large number of studies that address minimum QoL level in sustaining a healthy life.

Persistent or Recurrent AD

Some patients with AD respond well during the treatment period, but develops into AD lesions at least moderate level within 3 months of the discontinuation of the treatment. Korean guidelines suggest that this should be defined as a recurrent AD and physicians should make a change in the treatment [39]. Similarly, Italian guidelines described that treatment changes should be made when clinically significant increases in severity index within 1 month after the cessation of treatment, although they did not define the exact level of clinically significant recurrence of AD [40].

Until now, there is no definition of a clinically meaningful recurrence that has been universally accepted using objective and subjective assessment tools. Many physicians treating AD feel the need to develop these indicators in the real practice. The index, if developed, would be very helpful to physicians and patients who are treated.

Conclusion

AD severity classification is an essential element to choose the option of treatments and treatment responsiveness also provides an important contribution to the determination of treatment. Discussion and efforts to achieve a consensus regarding comprehensive tools to assess both objective and subjective symptoms of AD are being kept on for improvement of clinical practice. Technically, electronic platforms that collect PROM and integrate them into medical record systems will come true, and it will enable dermatologists to capture enough information to identify the individuals' overall disease status in a short time.

References

1. Hanifin JM, Rajka G. Diagnostic features of atopic dermatitis. Acta Derm Venereol Suppl. 1980;92(1):44–7.
2. Andersen RM, Thyssen JP, Maibach HI. Qualitative vs. quantitative atopic dermatitis criteria—in historical and present perspectives. J Eur Acad Dermatol Venereol. 2016;30(4):604–18.

3. Williams HC, Burney PG, Hay RJ, Archer CB, Shipley MJ, Hunter JJ, et al. The U.K. Working Party's Diagnostic Criteria for Atopic Dermatitis. I. Derivation of a minimum set of discriminators for atopic dermatitis. Br J Dermatol. 1994;131(3):383–96.
4. Williams HC, Burney PG, Pembroke AC, Hay RJ. The U.K. Working Party's Diagnostic Criteria for Atopic Dermatitis. III. Independent hospital validation. Br J Dermatol. 1994;131(3):406–16.
5. Williams HC, Burney PG, Pembroke AC, Hay RJ. Validation of the U.K. diagnostic criteria for atopic dermatitis in a population setting. U.K. Diagnostic Criteria for Atopic Dermatitis Working Party. Br J Dermatol. 1996;135(1):12–7.
6. Chalmers DA, Todd G, Saxe N, Milne JT, Tolosana S, Ngcelwane PN, et al. Validation of the U.K. Working Party diagnostic criteria for atopic eczema in a Xhosa-speaking African population. Br J Dermatol. 2007;156(1):111–6.
7. Wanitphakdeedecha R, Tuchinda P, Sivayathorn A, Kulthanan K. Validation of the diagnostic criteria for atopic dermatitis in the adult Thai population. Asian Pac J Allergy Immunol. 2007;25(2–3):133–8.
8. Eichenfield LF, Tom WL, Chamlin SL, Feldman SR, Hanifin JM, Simpson EL, et al. Guidelines of care for the management of atopic dermatitis: section 1. Diagnosis and assessment of atopic dermatitis. J Am Acad Dermatol. 2014;70(2):338–51.
9. Katayama I, Aihara M, Ohya Y, Saeki H, Shimojo N, Shoji S, et al. Japanese guidelines for atopic dermatitis 2017. Allergol Int. 2017;66(2):230–47.
10. Lopez Carrera YI, Al Hammadi A, Huang YH, Llamado LJ, Mahgoub E, Tallman AM. Epidemiology, diagnosis, and treatment of atopic dermatitis in the developing countries of Asia, Africa, Latin America, and the Middle East: a review. Dermatol Ther. 2019;9(4):685–705.
11. Park YL, Kim HD, Kim KH, Kim MN, Kim JW, Ro YS, et al. Report from ADRG: a study on the diagnostic CRITERIA of Korean atopic dermatitis. Korean J Dermatol. 2006;44(6):659–63.
12. Asher MI, Keil U, Anderson HR, Beasley R, Crane J, Martinez F, et al. International Study of Asthma and Allergies in Childhood (ISAAC): rationale and methods. Eur Respir J. 1995;8(3):483–91.
13. Worldwide variation in prevalence of symptoms of asthma, allergic rhinoconjunctivitis, and atopic eczema: ISAAC. The International Study of Asthma and Allergies in Childhood (ISAAC) Steering Committee. Lancet. 1998;351(9111):1225–1232.
14. Eichenfield LF, Hanifin JM, Luger TA, Stevens SR, Pride HB. Consensus conference on pediatric atopic dermatitis. J Am Acad Dermatol. 2003;49(6):1088–95.
15. Lee SC, Bae JM, Lee HJ, Kim HJ, Kim BS, Li K, et al. Introduction of the reliable estimation of atopic dermatitis in childhood: novel, diagnostic criteria for childhood atopic dermatitis. Allergy Asthma Immunol Res. 2016;8(3):230–8.
16. Lee HH, Patel KR, Singam V, Rastogi S, Silverberg JI. A systematic review and meta-analysis of the prevalence and phenotype of adult-onset atopic dermatitis. J Am Acad Dermatol. 2019;80(6):1526–32.e7.
17. Abuabara K, Ye M, McCulloch CE, Sullivan A, Margolis DJ, Strachan DP, et al. Clinical onset of atopic eczema: results from 2 nationally representative British birth cohorts followed through midlife. J Allergy Clin Immunol. 2019;144(3):710–9.
18. Megna M, Patruno C, Balato A, Rongioletti F, Stingeni L, Balato N. An Italian multicentre study on adult atopic dermatitis: persistent versus adult-onset disease. Arch Dermatol Res. 2017;309(6):443–52.
19. Napolitano M, Megna M, Patruno C, Gisondi P, Ayala F, Balato N. Adult atopic dermatitis: a review. G Ital Dermatol Venereol. 2016;151(4):403–11.
20. Patruno C, Amerio P, Chiricozzi A, Costanzo A, Cristaudo A, Cusano F, et al. Optimizing a clinical guidance for diagnosis of atopic dermatitis in adults: joint recommendations of the Italian Society of Dermatology and Venereology (SIDeMaST), Italian Association of Hospital Dermatologists (ADOI), and Italian Society of Allergological, Occupational and Environmental Dermatology (SIDAPA). G Ital Dermatol Venereol. 2019;155(1):1–7.
21. Tanei R, Hasegawa Y. Atopic dermatitis in older adults: a viewpoint from geriatric dermatology. Geriatr Gerontol Int. 2016;16(Suppl 1):75–86.
22. Williamson S, Merritt J, De Benedetto A. Atopic dermatitis in the elderly: a review of clinical and pathophysiological hallmarks. Br J Dermatol. 2020;182(1):47–54.
23. Dezoteux F, Astrid B, Chuffard M, Drumez E, Azib S, Staumont-Salle D. Atopic dermatitis in elderly adults. Eur J Dermatol. 2019;29(4):371–4.
24. Bieber T, D'Erme AM, Akdis CA, Traidl-Hoffmann C, Lauener R, Schappi G, et al. Clinical phenotypes and endophenotypes of atopic dermatitis: where are we, and where should we go? J Allergy Clin Immunol. 2017;139(4s):S58–s64.
25. Simpson EL, Leung DYM, Eichenfield LF, Boguniewicz M. Atopic dermatitis. In: Kang S, Amagai M, Bruckner A, Enk AH, Margolis DJ, McMichael AJ, Orringer JS, editors. Fitzpatrick's dermatology in general medicine. 9th ed. New York: McGraw Hill Education; 2019. p. 363–85.
26. Hill MK, Kheirandish Pishkenari A, Braunberger TL, Armstrong AW, Dunnick CA. Recent trends in disease severity and quality of life instruments for patients with atopic dermatitis: a systematic review. J Am Acad Dermatol. 2016;75(5):906–17.
27. Schmitt J, Spuls PI, Thomas KS, Simpson E, Furue M, Deckert S, et al. The Harmonising Outcome Measures for Eczema (HOME) statement to assess clinical signs of atopic eczema in trials. J Allergy Clin Immunol. 2014;134(4):800–7.
28. Wollenberg A, Barbarot S, Bieber T, Christen-Zaech S, Deleuran M, Fink-Wagner A, et al. Consensus-based European guidelines for treatment of atopic eczema (atopic dermatitis) in adults and children: part I. J Eur Acad Dermatol Venereol. 2018;32(5):657–82.

29. Anderson K, Putterman E, Rogers RS, Patel D, Treat JR, Castelo-Soccio L. Treatment of severe pediatric atopic dermatitis with methotrexate: a retrospective review. Pediatr Dermatol. 2019;36(3):298–302.
30. de Bruin-Weller M. Time to get rid of the Investigator's Global Assessment as the primary outcome for clinical trials in atopic dermatitis? Br J Dermatol. 2019;181(1):12–3.
31. Faye O, Meledie N'Djong AP, Diadie S, Coniquet S, Niamba PA, Atadokpede F, et al. Validation of the Patient-Oriented SCORing for Atopic Dermatitis tool for black skin. J Eur Acad Dermatol Venereol. 2019;34(4):795–9.
32. Fishbein AB, Silverberg JI, Wilson EJ, Ong PY. Update on atopic dermatitis: diagnosis, severity assessment, and treatment selection. J Allergy Clin Immunol Pract. 2019;8(1):91–101.
33. Perez-Chada L, Taliercio VL, Gottlieb A, Van Beek M, Duffin KC, Reeder M, et al. Achieving consensus on patient-reported outcome measures in clinical practice for inflammatory skin disorders: on behalf of International Dermatology Outcome Measures and the American Academy of Dermatology. J Am Acad Dermatol. 2019;S0190-9622(19):32745–8.
34. Charman CR, Venn AJ, Williams HC. The patient-oriented eczema measure: development and initial validation of a new tool for measuring atopic eczema severity from the patients' perspective. Arch Dermatol. 2004;140(12):1513–9.
35. Spuls PI, Gerbens LAA, Simpson E, Apfelbacher CJ, Chalmers JR, Thomas KS, et al. Patient-Oriented Eczema Measure (POEM), a core instrument to measure symptoms in clinical trials: a Harmonising Outcome Measures for Eczema (HOME) statement. Br J Dermatol. 2017;176(4):979–84.
36. Silverberg JI, Gelfand JM, Margolis DJ, Fonacier L, Boguniewicz M, Schwartz LB, et al. Severity strata for POEM, PO-SCORAD, and DLQI in US adults with atopic dermatitis. Ann Allerg Asthma Immunol. 2018;121(4):464–71.
37. Vakharia PP, Chopra R, Sacotte R, Patel N, Immaneni S, White T, et al. Severity strata for five patient-reported outcomes in adults with atopic dermatitis. Br J Dermatol. 2018;178(4):925–30.
38. Majeski CJ, Johnson JA, Davison SN, Lauzon CJ. Itch Severity Scale: a self-report instrument for the measurement of pruritus severity. Br J Dermatol. 2007;156(4):667–73.
39. Kim JE, Shin MK, Park GH, Lee UH, Lee JH, Han TY, et al. 2019 consensus Korean diagnostic guidelines to define severity classification and treatment refractoriness for atopic dermatitis: objective and subjective assessment of severity. Ann Dermatol. 2019;31(6):654–61.
40. Calzavara Pinton P, Cristaudo A, Foti C, Canonica GW, Balato N, Costanzo A, et al. Diagnosis and management of moderate to severe adult atopic dermatitis: a Consensus by the Italian Society of Dermatology and Venereology (SIDeMaST), the Italian Association of Hospital Dermatologists (ADOI), the Italian Society of Allergy, Asthma and Clinical Immunology (SIAAIC), and the Italian Society of Allergological, Environmental and Occupational Dermatology (SIDAPA). G Ital Dermatol Venereol. 2018;153(2):133–45.
41. Jang YH, Kim SM, Eun DH, Park KD, Park GH, Kim BS, et al. Validity and reliability of itch assessment scales for chronic pruritus in adults: a prospective multicenter study. J Am Acad Dermatol. 2020;82(1):80–6.
42. Beattie PE, Lewis-Jones MS. An audit of the impact of a consultation with a paediatric dermatology team on quality of life in infants with atopic eczema and their families: further validation of the Infants' Dermatitis Quality of Life Index and Dermatitis Family Impact score. Br J Dermatol. 2006;155(6):1249–55.
43. Rehal B, Armstrong AW. Health outcome measures in atopic dermatitis: a systematic review of trends in disease severity and quality-of-life instruments 1985–2010. PLoS One. 2011;6(4):e17520.
44. Darrigade AS, Colmant C, de Montjoye L, Herman A, Bugli C, Tromme I, et al. Atopic dermatitis score 7 (ADS7): a promising tool for daily clinical assessment of atopic dermatitis. Allergy. 2019;75(5):1264–6.
45. Lee JY, Kim M, Yang HK, Kim HM, Cho J, Kim YM, et al. Reliability and validity of the Atopic Dermatitis Symptom Score (ADSS). Pediatr Allergy Immunol. 2018;29(3):290–5.
46. Pariser DM, Simpson EL, Gadkari A, Bieber T, Margolis DJ, Brown M, et al. Evaluating patient-perceived control of atopic dermatitis: design, validation, and scoring of the Atopic Dermatitis Control Tool (ADCT). Curr Med Res Opin. 2019;36:1–10.
47. Boguniewicz M, Fonacier L, Guttman-Yassky E, Ong PY, Silverberg J, Farrar JR. Atopic dermatitis yardstick: practical recommendations for an evolving therapeutic landscape. Ann Allergy Asthma Immunol. 2018;120(1):10–22.e2.
48. Damiani G, Calzavara-Pinton P, Stingeni L, Hansel K, Cusano F, Pigatto PDM. Italian guidelines for therapy of atopic dermatitis-Adapted from consensus-based European guidelines for treatment of atopic eczema (atopic dermatitis). Dermatol Ther. 2019;32(6):e13121.
49. Rubel D, Thirumoorthy T, Soebaryo RW, Weng SC, Gabriel TM, Villafuerte LL, et al. Consensus guidelines for the management of atopic dermatitis: an Asia-Pacific perspective. J Dermatol. 2013;40(3):160–71.
50. Sicras-Mainar A, Navarro-Artieda R, Armario-Hita JC. severe atopic dermatitis in Spain: a real-life observational study. Ther Clin Risk Manag. 2019;15:1393–401.
51. Paller A, Jaworski JC, Simpson EL, Boguniewicz M, Russell JJ, Block JK, et al. Major comorbidities of atopic dermatitis: beyond allergic disorders. Am J Clin Dermatol. 2018;19(6):821–38.
52. Tay YK, Chan YC, Chandran NS, Ho MS, Koh MJ, Lim YL, et al. Guidelines for the management of atopic dermatitis in singapore. Ann Acad Med Singap. 2016;45(10):439–50.

53. Wollenberg A, Barbarot S, Bieber T, Christen-Zaech S, Deleuran M, Fink-Wagner A, et al. Consensus-based European guidelines for treatment of atopic eczema (atopic dermatitis) in adults and children: part II. J Eur Acad Dermatol Venereol. 2018;32(6):850–78.
54. Kim JE, Kim HJ, Lew BL, Lee KH, Hong SP, Jang YH, et al. Consensus guidelines for the treatment of atopic dermatitis in Korea (part II): systemic treatment. Ann Dermatol. 2015;27(5):578–92.
55. Beck KM, Seitzman GD, Yang EJ, Sanchez IM, Liao W. Ocular co-morbidities of atopic dermatitis. Part I: associated ocular diseases. Am J Clin Dermatol. 2019;20(6):797–805.
56. Simpson EL, de Bruin-Weller M, Eckert L, Whalley D, Guillemin I, Reaney M, et al. Responder threshold for Patient-Oriented Eczema Measure (POEM) and Children's Dermatology Life Quality Index (CDLQI) in adolescents with atopic dermatitis. Dermatol Ther. 2019;9(4):799–805.
57. Irvine AD, Jones AP, Beattie P, Baron S, Browne F, Ashoor F, et al. A randomized controlled trial protocol assessing the effectiveness, safety and cost-effectiveness of methotrexate vs. ciclosporin in the treatment of severe atopic eczema in children: the TREatment of severe Atopic eczema Trial (TREAT). Br J Dermatol. 2018;179(6):1297–306.
58. Schram ME, Spuls PI, Leeflang MM, Lindeboom R, Bos JD, Schmitt J. EASI, (objective) SCORAD and POEM for atopic eczema: responsiveness and minimal clinically important difference. Allergy. 2012;67(1):99–106.
59. Howells L, Ratib S, Chalmers JR, Bradshaw L, Thomas KS. How should minimally important change scores for the Patient-Oriented Eczema Measure be interpreted? A validation using varied methods. Br J Dermatol. 2018;178(5):1135–42.
60. Gaunt DM, Metcalfe C, Ridd M. The Patient-Oriented Eczema Measure in young children: responsiveness and minimal clinically important difference. Allergy. 2016;71(11):1620–5.

Part V

Pathophysiology

Genetics of Atopic Dermatitis

Eung Ho Choi

Introduction

Atopic dermatitis (AD) is one of the major chronic inflammatory skin diseases, with a prevalence of up to 20% in infants and children and up to 5% in adults. Most patients show an onset of the disease in early childhood and a spontaneous remission until adolescence, but there may be relapses and the disease can also begin or persist in adulthood [1]. The pathophysiology of AD is complex, with an altered epidermal barrier and abnormal immunological and inflammatory pathways that lead to a T_H2-dominated immune response with a T_H17 component in acute AD lesions and progressive conversion to a T_H1-dominated response in chronic AD lesions [2].

Atopic Dermatitis Is a Heritable Disease and a Complex Trait

In the family, atopic diseases tend to cluster, so the term *atopic diathesis* is used. Family, twin, and adoption studies have provided important evidence that genetic factors are important in determining individual differences in susceptibility to atopic disorders and that there is a range of phenotypic expressions for this genetic predisposition [3]. Twin studies found concordance rates of 72–86% in monozygotic twins and 21–23% in dizygotic twins, and segregation analyses suggested that genetic factors account for more than 70% of susceptibility changes to AD [4–6]. As with most conditions of medical relevance, AD does not follow simple Mendelian monogenic inheritance, but is considered a complex trait (polygenic and multifactorial). Complex traits are the result of a complex network of numerous susceptible loci, many of which have an additive or synergistic effect but only a small role when considered in isolation [7]. Among other reasons, failure to identify and replicate individual genetic risk factors for complex diseases is due to epistasis (gene-by-gene interactions), which obscures the effects of individual single loci [8]. In addition, disease-causing genes interact with nongenetic environmental factors to determine the final phenotype.

Methods for Identifying Atopic Dermatitis Risk Genes

Identifying the genetic factors of a complex disease is not an easy task, but recent developments in molecular biology have made great strides. It is still difficult to understand the complex network of genes, proteins, and metabolites that interact through biochemical and physical interactions to determine the

E. H. Choi (✉)
Department of Dermatology, Yonsei University Wonju College of Medicine, Wonju, Korea (Republic of)
e-mail: choieh@yonsei.ac.kr

K. H. Lee et al. (eds.), *Practical Insights into Atopic Dermatitis*,
https://doi.org/10.1007/978-981-15-8159-5_6

phenotype [9]. In general, there are three types of studies used to identify gene variants associated with susceptibility to AD: genome-wide linkage scans followed by fine mapping of a linked region, candidate gene association studies, and genome-wide association (GWA) studies. In addition, animal models are useful supplements for human-based genetic studies [10]. However, for AD there is no single comprehensive animal model so far, so in order to explore pathophysiological mechanisms, many disease components need to be modeled as characteristics (and combinations accordingly) isolated from animals [11].

Genome-Wide Studies

Genome-wide linkage analysis (GWLA) is a systematic and unbiased approach to identify genetic loci for human complex diseases and to search for evidence of major genetic effects. A genome-wide association study (GWAS), also known as a whole-genome association study, is an observational study of a genome-wide set of genetic variants in different individuals to see if any variant is associated with a trait.

GWLAs are hypothesis-free scans that compare the transmission of disease and genetic information within families. For this purpose, a relatively small set of polymorphic markers covering the entire genome is examined. Linkage studies have been very successful in mapping rare single gene disorders, but this technique has proven less powerful in mapping complex diseases involving multiple low-risk gene mutations. Moreover, the linkage regions generally extend to include hundreds of genes and require subsequent fine mapping analyses [12]. Until now, several GWLAs of AD have been conducted. The results of these genomic screens differ significantly from each other, and replication under thresholds where the distance between binding peaks is less than 10 centimorgans (cM) can only be considered for the locus of chromosome 3p24 [13, 14]. In independent studies, the lack of replication of binding peaks may be due to genetic heterogeneity or differences in identification schemes and phenotype definitions, sample sizes, marker panels, and analytical methods, but it is likely to reflect the limitations of linkage studies in the dissection of complex characteristics, especially when used for particularly small sample sizes [15]. Apart from filaggrin (*FLG*), which explains some of the important linkage signals on 1q21 [15], the underlying disease genes for all other susceptibility loci identified by that approach remain difficult to find. Interestingly, the regions linked to AD show very little overlap with those of asthma, suggesting that susceptibility to asthma and eczema is mediated by genes other than the shared susceptibility to a common atopic background in the family aggregation form of these diseases. Rather, the AD locus identification so far are in close agreement with the psoriasis susceptibility regions such as 1q21. It suggests that these conditions share susceptibility loci in genomic regions encoding genes most relevant for the skin as the target organ. These associations may imply an important role for skin inflammation, immunity and structure sharing, and general effects of proteins expressed by epithelial cells in both diseases [16].

GWAS is feasible through the newly developed high-throughput single nucleotide polymorphism (SNP) genotyping platforms, and the knowledge gained from the HapMap project has revolutionized the discovery of genetic variants associated with complex diseases [17]. In general, GWAS clearly represents a powerful new tool. But the potential of GWAS must be kept in perspective. GWAS presents a lot of logistical, technical, and biostatistical challenges with some important limitations. However, GWAS has the potential to significantly improve the understanding of the genetics and pathogenic mechanisms of complex diseases, such as eczema, if the research is carried out under strict conditions, sufficiently robust, and thoroughly reproduced in an independent population [18]. GWAS for AD consolidated more than 307,000 SNP markers, collected mainly in Germany and 10,000 people from the Family and Case Reference Panel [19]. Within AD GWAS, the association of eczema with the four prevalent *FLG* null mutations could be reconfirmed, and a potential susceptibility SNP located within the gene encoding the filaggrin-related protein hornerin within the epidermal differentiation complex (EDC) was found.

Candidate Gene Association Studies

Candidate gene association studies analyze the distribution of genetic markers, usually SNPs, in unrelated individuals (case–control and case–cohort studies) or their transmission in families (family-based design) [9]. These discussions can be positional, functional, or both. For example, the gene is located in a region for which linkage has been observed in prior screening studies or there is a specific biological hypothesis. More than 100 candidate genes have been investigated for association with AD so far. Assuming publication bias, there are probably more genes for which testing of associations has failed [20]. Only very few associations could be replicated in at least one independent study. Common reasons for the nonreproducibility of the results are inadequate selection of candidate loci and markers, small sample size, inadequate evaluation of the trait of interest and the use of inadequate controls, defects in design and inappropriate statistical modeling, replication failure, and genetic and environmental heterogeneity [8]. Based on the reported data, only *FLG* appears to be represent a potent and consistent AD risk gene across all collections in all populations and in many large independent studies.

Skin Barrier–Related Genetic Mutations

The skin barrier, which consists of the stratum corneum, is the first protective barrier against the external environment. It is well known that the skin barrier acts as a physical barrier that prevents water loss and prevents the invasion of allergens and bacteria, and AD is caused by abnormal function of the skin barrier. In particular, loss-of-function mutation of the filaggrin gene (*FLG*) is known to be an important risk factor for AD [21, 22].

FLG Mutations

Chromosome 1q21 encodes genes related to the EDC, among which loss-of-function mutation of *FLG* is associated with AD [23]. The EDC is a dense cluster of genes, all of which are involved in the terminal differentiation of keratinocytes [24]. The EDC *FLG,* which displays a complex highly repetitive sequence, encodes a key protein in the formation of the outermost keratin layer of the skin [25]. Immunohistochemical and immunoblotting studies showed diminished or absent filaggrin expression in ichthyosis vulgaris (IV) patients [26, 27]. The linkage findings between IV and markers in the EDC region, a genetically determined filaggrin deficiency, were considered and found to be involved in IV. In 2006, two null mutations in *FLG* were identified in IV patients from Irish, Scottish, and European-American populations, which have an estimated combined population allele frequency of approximately 6% [22, 23]. Interestingly, most mutations appear to be population specific, with most so far being identified in those of European ancestry, with other *FLG* gene mutations apparently restricted to Asian populations [28]. All these variants cause frameshifts, premature stop codons, or nonsense mutations, and prevent the production of free filaggrin in the epidermis. Carriers of one *FLG* mutation show a significant decrease in filaggrin expression immunohistochemically, but processed filaggrin is completely absent in homozygotes and compound heterozygotes [23, 28]. After that, both the R501X and the 2282del4 alleles are suggested as strong predisposing factors for AD [22]. Many studies show that *FLG* null alleles particularly affect an early-onset, severe, and persistent course of AD [29]. Surprisingly, *FLG* null alleles are rather common at carrier frequencies of 8% in the general population and up to 48% in AD cases [30, 31]. Therefore, *FLG* mutations are considered the strongest and best replicated genetic risk for AD so far.

Several studies have shown that FLG-deficient eczema increases the risk for allergic sensitization, elevated Ig-E levels, and concomitant asthma and/or allergic rhinitis [32]. This led to the hypothesis that reduction or loss of filaggrin expression mainly causes a dryness and disturbance of the skin barrier, increasing the passage of antigens, allergens, and chemicals through the epidermis, which cause inflammation, depending allergic sensitization due to the immune responses of the host [33, 34]. Thus, it has been suggested that asthma in individuals with AD can be secondary to sensitization, primarily through a defective epidermal barrier. This hypothesis is supported by a recent population-based study in adults demonstrating the association of *FLG* mutations with dry skin regardless of the presence of AD, but an association with increased IgE levels was observed only in atopic individuals [34]. The findings on *FLG* are a milestone in the study of molecular genes for atopic disorders, and the knowledge gained regarding barrier dysfunction is expected to lead to the development of more rational and more effective therapies.

FLG mutations have been identified in patients with AD from Europe, the USA, and Asia including China, Japan, and Korea. To date, more than 40 *FLG* loss-of-function mutations have been reported in Europe and Asia. A study in Koreans has also found that *FLG* nonsense mutations (p.Y1767X, p.K4022X) are associated with AD in Korean [35]. Another Korean study of 322 Korean AD patients reported *FLG* P478S (rs11584340) [36].

SPINK5 and *KLK7* Mutations

Filaggrin, a main barrier protein, is initially synthesized as biologically inactive profilaggrin, which is processed into biologically active filaggrin monomers by several dephosphorylation and proteolytic steps during the transition from granular cells to horny cells [37]. Therefore, dysregulation of filaggrin processing may impair skin barrier function. One of the proteases proposed to be involved in profilaggrin processing is the stratum corneum chymotryptic enzyme (SCCE) [38]. Interestingly, an insertion in the 3′ untranslated region of the kallikrein 7 gene (*KLK7*), which encodes SCCE, has been reported to be associated with eczema in a small cohort of 103 British children [39]. In Korea, the *KLK7* mutation has been reported to be associated with the development of AD [40]. SCCE is putatively regulated by a serine protease inhibitor, lymphoepithelial Kazal-type inhibitor (LEKTI), encoded by *SPINK5* [41, 42]. *SPINK5* is a gene located in chromosome 5q32 and is related to Netherton syndrome, a rare autosomal-recessive disease characterized by congenital erythroderma and ichthyosis, bamboo hair, and atopic manifestations. Serine protease (kallikrein) plays an important role in skin barrier function and is an enzyme that plays an important role in forming the lipid barrier structure and cornified cell envelope. By inhibiting this kallikrein activity, LEKTI regulates proteolytic processes to differentiate keratinocytes and produce normal epidermal structures. The *SPINK5* gene mutation is known to be associated with the development of AD, especially in Asians. *SPINK5* polymorphisms have been reported to be associated with the severity of Chinese AD, and in Japan, a 1258G>A *SPINK5* polymorphism has been associated with AD [43]. In Korea, four *SPINK5* SNPs (rs17718511, rs17860502, rs60978485, rs17718737) were reported to be related to AD in a study involving 631 patients with AD and 459 controls [44]. In contrast, studies in Germany, France, and the Netherlands did not show any association. In a large-scale study of several cohorts, which involved more than 2700 AD subjects and more than 10,000 controls, the *SPINK5* Glu420Lys mutation conferred a risk of AD only when maternally inherited, but it did not appear to be a major eczema risk factor [45]. The *KLK7* insertion was not associated with AD in this large study and in a smaller French study [41], and no evidence was found for significant interaction effects between *KLK7* or *SPINK5* variants and *FLG* mutations [45].

Other Genes Related to the Skin Barrier

The filaggrin-2 (*FLG2*) variation is associated with more persistent AD in African-American patients [46]. Small proline-rich proteins (SPRRs) are cross-bridging proteins in the cornified cell envelope (CE), which provides the main barrier function of stratified squamous epithelia.

The *SPRR3* variant associated with AD carries an extra 24-bp repeat in the central domain, which may alter the physical properties of the CE [47]. Expression of the tight junction (TJ) proteins claudin-1 and claudin-23 is strikingly reduced only in patients with AD. Claudin-1 expression inversely correlated with T_H2 biomarkers. *CLDN1* haplotype-tagging SNPs revealed associations with AD in two North American populations [48].

Inflammatory and Immune Response–Related Gene Polymorphisms

AD is a complex chronic inflammatory response caused by T_H2 bias and immune dysregulation of the T_H17/T_H22 response. Genetic mutations associated with these abnormal immunological responses have been linked to AD.

Pattern-Recognition Receptors and Antimicrobial Peptides

Pattern-recognition receptors (PRRs) recognize pathogen-associated molecular patterns (PAMPs) to protect the body, and antimicrobial peptides (AMPs) play an important role in the elimination of pathogens. Among these PRRs, genetic variations of Toll-like receptors (TLRs) or nucleotide-binding oligomerization domain–like receptors (NLRs) are known to be associated with AD. The *TLR2* R753Q polymorphism defines a subgroup of patients with AD with a severe phenotype [49]. Conversely, in a study of white German subjects, there was no evidence that common *TLR2* or *TLR4* variants or haplotypes were associated with AD in the study population [50].

IL-1 Family Cytokines

Interleukin (IL)-1 family cytokines are cytokines that play an important role in innate immunity in the pathogenesis of AD, including IL-1α, IL-1β, IL-18, and IL-33. These are cytokines that act at the first stage in the inflammatory response of AD [51]. The *IL-18* gene is located on chromosome 11q22 and promotes IL-4 and IL-13 to induce T_H2 response through IgE production [52]. *IL-18* polymorphisms have been suggested in several inflammatory diseases. A Korean research team found that one SNP and the haplotype T–T–C were strongly associated with the allergic type of AD, but not with the nonallergic intrinsic type [53].

Thymic Stromal Lymphopoietin

Thymic stromal lymphopoietin (TSLP) signals through a heterodimeric receptor complex composed of the TSLP receptor and the IL-7Rα chain. It mainly impacts myeloid cells and induces the release of T cell–attracting chemokines from monocytes and enhances the maturation of myeloid (CD11c+) dendritic cells [54]. Therefore, genetic mutations of *TSLP* and IL-7 receptor-α (*IL-7RA*) are known to be associated with AD.

T_H2 Cytokines

T_H2 cytokines are important in the acquired immune response of AD. These include IL-4, IL-5, IL-13, and IL-31. T_H22 cytokine (IL-22) is also an important cytokine in the acute phase of AD [55]. Polymorphisms of *IL-4*, *IL-5*, *IL-13*, IL-4 receptor-α (*IL-4RA*), IL-5 receptor-α (*IL-5RA*), and IL-13 receptor-α (*IL-13RA*) are known to be involved in AD [56, 57]. A variant of signal transducer and activator of transcription 6 (STAT6) as a downstream transcription factor of IL-4 and IL-13 has also been reported to be associated with AD [58].

IL-4 and IL-4 Receptor-α

IL-4 causes isotype switching from IgM/G to IgE in T_H2-stimulated B cells [59]. Several studies have shown that *IL-4* polymorphism occurs at three sites: −590CT (promoter), −34C/T (untranslated region), and dinucleotide repeat (*IL-4R1*, intron 2) [60, 61]. In a Japanese study, the *IL-4* and *IL-4RA* chain genotypes were not significantly associated with either the total prevalence of AD or the prevalence of AD with normal IgE productivity. The distribution of genotypes of *IL-4* − 589C/T differed by the serum IgE levels in patients with AD. The results suggested that polymorphisms in the *IL-4* gene and the *IL-4RA* chain gene play no role in the development of AD patients with normal IgE [62]. An Australian study reported no association between AD and promoter region polymorphism of the *IL4* −590C/T and −34C/T haplotypes [63]. *IL-4RA* is located on chromosome 16p12. IL-4RA performs isotype switching to IgE as receptors for IL-4 and IL-13. *IL-4RA* polymorphism Gln551Arg is associated with adult AD in Japan [64]. However, any SNPs in the *IL-4* and *IL-4R* genes that were associated with AD were not found in a Korean AD cohort (comprising 631 AD patients and 458 controls) [65] and Chinese AD samples [66].

IL-13

IL-13 works similarly to IL-4. *IL-13* is located close to the *IL-4* gene and has structural and functional similarities. There are about seven polymorphic forms of the *IL-13* gene. Among them, Gln110Arg has been associated with AD in Germans, and has been reported to be associated with serum IgE levels in Caucasians [67]. In a Polish study, the promoter −1112C/T polymorphism of the *IL-13* gene was associated with AD [68]. Japanese studies have also found an association with the G4257A polymorphism of the *IL-13* gene [69]. In Korean AD patients, the rs3091307 and rs20541 polymorphisms of the *IL-13* gene were found to be related [65].

T_H1 Cytokines and Other Cytokines

In AD, the T_H1 immune response is reduced. Genetic mutations of *IL-12* and *IL-12R* have been reported to be associated with AD [70, 71]. In addition, genetic variations of various IL-2, IL-6, IL-9, and IL-10 cytokines and their receptors have been reported to be associated with AD.

IL-10

IL-10 is an anti-inflammatory cytokine whose gene is located on chromosome 1q31–32. In AD, production of IL-10 is reduced. One Korean study found that polymorphisms in the *IL-10* promoter were related to AD [72]. Recent Finnish studies have also linked atopy in preschoolers to *IL-10* polymorphisms (rs1800871, rs1800872, rs1800890, and rs1800896) [73].

IL-9

IL-9 is a T_H2-type cytokine first described in a murine model as a potent growth factor for T cells and mast cells. It promotes CD8+ cell proliferation. Moreover, IL-9 is known to induce bronchial epithelial cell mucus and chemokine secretion, promote mast cell proliferation, and increase IgE production in B cells. The rs31563 SNP (−4091G/A) located in the *IL-9* gene is associated with an increased susceptibility to AD. Similarly, the rs3093467 SNP in *IL-9R* seems to be associated with an increased risk of developing nonallergic AD [74].

IL-12B

IL-12 is a cytokine that induces a T_H1 immune response, which can lower the T_H2 response of AD. It is encoded by *IL-12A* (p35) and *IL-12B* (p40), located on chromosome 3 and chromosome 5q31–33, respectively. It has been reported to be associated with asthma, and in connection with AD. Japanese studies reported polymorphisms of the 3′ untranslated region of the *IL-12B* (p40) gene [75]. In Koreans, rs438421 polymorphism of the *IL-12RB1* (TT) gene and rs438421 polymorphism of the *IL-12RB1* (AA) gene are associated with AD [71].

High-Affinity IgE Receptor Mutations

The gene for the high-affinity IgE receptor (FCERI) maps to chromosome 11q13 and has been thought to play an important role in atopic pathogenesis [76]. Several polymorphisms have been reported, including the Leu181Ileu and Gly237Glu variants and the 1109C/T promoter polymorphism, while other studies have confirmed these polymorphisms. However, the same race shows inconsistencies in the association studies for the *FCERI* gene. Cox et al. found an association between *FCERI* gene polymorphism

Table 1 Representative genes associated with AD, classified according to their functions

	Genes	Encoding proteins	Functions
Skin barrier	Filaggrin (*FLG*)	Filaggrin	A central role for cornified envelope formation and lamellar body synthesis
	SPINK5	LEKTI (lymphoepithelial Kazal-type inhibitor)	Serine protease inhibitor
	KLK7	SCCE (stratum corneum chymotryptic enzyme)	Endogenous protease-degrading corneodesmosome
Innate immune responses	*TLR2, TLR4, TLR9*	TLRs (Toll-like receptors)	A pattern-recognition receptor (PRR) enabling the immune system to differentiate various pathogen-associated microbial patterns (PAMPs)
	NOD1, *NOD2* = *CARD15*	NOD1 (intracellular nucleotide-binding oligomerization domain 1) or CARD (caspase recruitment domain), NOD2 or CARD15	PRRs detecting PAMPs
Adaptive immune responses	*IL-4RA*	α chain of IL-4 receptor	T_H2 cytokines inducing allergic inflammation
	IL-13RA	α chain of IL-13 receptor	
	STAT6	STAT6 (signal transducer and activator of transcription 6)	Activates genes involved in IgE synthesis
	FCER1A	Alpha chain of high-affinity IgE receptor	Affects the expression of the α chain
	TSLP	TSLP (Thymic stromal lymphopoietin)	Plays a role in priming naïve T cells in the direction of T_H2 cells through human dendritic cells

and AD from a study with 60 family members [77]. In Korean AD patients, a 66T>C (rs2251746) polymorphism has been reported [78].

The representative genes associated with AD are summarized in Table 1 according to their functions.

References

1. Bieber T. Atopic dermatitis. N Engl J Med. 2008;358(14):1483–94.
2. Nakajima S, Kitoh A, Egawa G, Natsuaki Y, Nakamizo S, Moniaga CS, et al. IL-17A as an inducer for T_H2 immune responses in murine atopic dermatitis models. J Invest Dermatol. 2014;134(8):2122–30.
3. Morar N, Willis-Owen SAG, Moffatt MF, Cookson WOCM. The genetics of atopic dermatitis. J Allergy Clin Immunol. 2006;118(1):24–36.
4. Schultz Larsen F. Atopic dermatitis: a genetic-epidemiologic study in a population-based twin sample. J Am Acad Dermatol. 1993;28(5) Pt 1:719–23.
5. Schultz Larsen FV, Holm NV. Atopic dermatitis in a population based twin series. Concordance rates and heritability estimation. Acta Derm Venereol Suppl. 1985;114:159.
6. Thomsen SF, Ulrik CS, Kyvik KO, Hjelmborg JVB, Skadhauge LR, Steffensen I, et al. Importance of genetic factors in the etiology of atopic dermatitis: a twin study. Allergy Asthma Proc. 2007;28(5):535–9.
7. Moore JH. A global view of epistasis. Nat Genet. 2005;37(1):13–4.
8. Cardon LR, Bell JI. Association study designs for complex diseases. Nat Rev Genet. 2001;2(2):91–9.
9. Altshuler D, Daly MJ, Lander ES. Genetic mapping in human disease. Science. 2008;322(5903):881–8.
10. Hunter KW, Crawford NP. The future of mouse QTL mapping to diagnose disease in mice in the age of whole-genome association studies. Annu Rev Genet. 2008;42:131–41.
11. Scharschmidt TC, Segre JA. Modeling atopic dermatitis with increasingly complex mouse models. J Invest Dermatol. 2008;128(5):1061–4.
12. Risch NJ. Searching for genetic determinants in the new millennium. Nature. 2000;405(6788):847.
13. Bradley M, Söderhäll C, Luthman H, Wahlgren C-F, Kockum I, Nordenskjöld MJ. Susceptibility loci for atopic dermatitis on chromosomes 3, 13, 15, 17 and 18 in a Swedish population. Hum Mol Genet. 2002;11(13):1539–48.
14. Haagerup A, Bjerke T, Schiøtz PO, Dahl R, Binderup HG, Tan Q, et al. Atopic dermatitis—a total genome-scan for susceptibility genes. Acta Derm Venereol. 2004;84(5):346–52.
15. Morar N, Cookson WO, Harper JI, Moffatt MF. Filaggrin mutations in children with severe atopic dermatitis. J Invest Dermatol. 2007;127(7):1667–72.

16. Willis-Owen SA, Morar N, Willis-Owen CA. Atopic dermatitis: insights from linkage overlap and disease co-morbidity. Expert Rev Mol Med. 2007;9(9):1–13.
17. McCarthy MI, Abecasis GR, Cardon LR, Goldstein DB, Little J, Ioannidis JPA, et al. Genome-wide association studies for complex traits: consensus, uncertainty and challenges. Nat Rev Genet. 2008;9(5):356–69.
18. Hardy J, Singleton A. Genomewide association studies and human disease. N Engl J Med. 2009;360(17):1759–68.
19. Esparza-Gordillo J, Weidinger S, Fölster-Holst R, Bauerfeind A, Ruschendorf F, Patone G, et al. A common variant on chromosome 11q13 is associated with atopic dermatitis. Nat Genet. 2009;41(5):596–601.
20. Barnes KC. An update on the genetics of atopic dermatitis: scratching the surface in 2009. J Allergy Clin Immunol. 2010;125(1):16–29. e11.
21. Elias PM, Schmuth M. Abnormal skin barrier in the etiopathogenesis of atopic dermatitis. Curr Opin Allergy Clin Immunol. 2009;9(4):265–72.
22. Palmer CN, Irvine AD, Terron-Kwiatkowski A, Zhao Y, Liao H, Lee SP, et al. Common loss-of-function variants of the epidermal barrier protein filaggrin are a major predisposing factor for atopic dermatitis. Nat Genet. 2006;38(4):441–6.
23. Smith FJ, Irvine AD, Terron-Kwiatkowski A, Sandilands A, Campbell LE, Zhao Y, et al. Loss-of-function mutations in the gene encoding filaggrin cause ichthyosis vulgaris. Nat Genet. 2006;38(3):337–42.
24. Toulza E, Mattiuzzo NR, Galliano M-F, Jonca N, Dossat C, Jacob D, et al. Large-scale identification of human genes implicated in epidermal barrier function. Genome Biol. 2007;8(6):R107.
25. Candi E, Schmidt R, Melino G. The cornified envelope: a model of cell death in the skin. Nat Rev Mol Cell Biol. 2005;6(4):328–40.
26. Fleckman P, Holbrook KA, Dale BA, Sybert VP. Keratinocytes cultured from subjects with ichthyosis vulgaris are phenotypically abnormal. J Invest Dermatol. 1987;88(5):640–5.
27. Fleckman P, Brumbaugh S. Absence of the granular layer and keratohyalin define a morphologically distinct subset of individuals with ichthyosis vulgaris. Exp Dermatol. 2002;11(4):327–36.
28. Sandilands A, Terron-Kwiatkowski A, Hull PR, O'Regan GM, Clayton TH, Watson RM, et al. Comprehensive analysis of the gene encoding filaggrin uncovers prevalent and rare mutations in ichthyosis vulgaris and atopic eczema. Nat Genet. 2007;39(5):650–4.
29. Irvine AD. Fleshing out filaggrin phenotypes. J Invest Dermatol. 2007;127(3):504–7.
30. Baurecht H, Irvine AD, Novak N, Illig T, Bühler B, Ring J, et al. Toward a major risk factor for atopic eczema: meta-analysis of filaggrin polymorphism data. J Allergy Clin Immunol. 2007;120(6):1406–12.
31. Sandilands A, Smith FJD, Irvine AD, McLean WHI. Filaggrin's fuller figure: a glimpse into the genetic architecture of atopic dermatitis. J Invest Dermatol. 2007;127(6):1282–4.
32. McLean WHI, Hull PR. Breach delivery: increased solute uptake points to a defective skin barrier in atopic dermatitis. J Invest Dermatol. 2007;127(1):8–10.
33. Hudson TJ. Skin barrier function and allergic risk. Nat Genet. 2006;38(4):399–400.
34. Weidinger S, Rodríguez E, Stahl C, Wagenpfeil S, Klopp N, Illig T, et al. Filaggrin mutations strongly predispose to early-onset and extrinsic atopic dermatitis. J Invest Dermatol. 2007;127(3):724–6.
35. Park KY, Li K, Seok J, Seo SJ. An analysis of the filaggrin gene polymorphism in Korean atopic dermatitis patients. J Korean Med Sci. 2016;31(7):1136–42.
36. Kim S-Y, Yang SW, Kim H-L, Kim S-H, Kim SJ, Park S-M, et al. Association between P478S polymorphism of the filaggrin gene & atopic dermatitis. Indian J Med Res. 2013;138(6):922–7.
37. Resing KA, Walsh KA, Haugen-Scofield J, Dale BA. Identification of proteolytic cleavage sites in the conversion of profilaggrin to filaggrin in mammalian epidermis. J Biol Chem. 1989;264(3):1837–45.
38. Resing KA, Thulin C, Whiting K, al-Alawi N, Mostad S. Characterization of profilaggrin endoproteinase 1. A regulated cytoplasmic endoproteinase of epidermis. J Biol Chem. 1995;270(47):28193–8.
39. Vasilopoulos Y, Sharaf N, di Giovine F, Simon M, Cork MJ, Duff GW, et al. The 3′-UTR AACCins5874 in the stratum corneum chymotryptic enzyme gene (SCCE/KLK7), associated with atopic dermatitis; causes an increased mRNA expression without altering its stability. J Dermatol Sci. 2011;61(2):131–3.
40. Yoon NY, Wang HY, Jun M, Jung M, Kim DH, Lee NR, et al. Simultaneous detection of barrier- and immune-related gene variations in patients with atopic dermatitis by reverse blot hybridization assay. Clin Exp Dermatol. 2018;43(4):430–6.
41. Descargues P, Deraison C, Bonnart C, Kreft M, Kishibe M, Ishida-Yamamoto A, et al. Spink5-deficient mice mimic Netherton syndrome through degradation of desmoglein 1 by epidermal protease hyperactivity. Nat Genet. 2005;37(1):56–65.
42. Komatsu N, Takata M, Otsuki N, Ohka R, Amano O, Takehara K, et al. Elevated stratum corneum hydrolytic activity in Netherton syndrome suggests an inhibitory regulation of desquamation by SPINK5-derived peptides. J Invest Dermatol. 2002;118(3):436–43.
43. Kato A, Fukai K, Oiso N, Hosomi N, Murakami T, Ishii M. Association of SPINK5 gene polymorphisms with atopic dermatitis in the Japanese population. Br J Dermatol. 2003;148(4):665–9.
44. Namkung J-H, Lee J-E, Kim E, Byun J-Y, Kim S, Shin E-S, et al. Hint for association of single nucleotide polymorphisms and haplotype in SPINK5 gene with atopic dermatitis in Koreans. Exp Dermatol. 2010;19(12):1048–53.
45. Weidinger S, Baurecht H, Wagenpfeil S, Henderson J, Novak N, Sandilands A, et al. Analysis of the individual and aggregate genetic contributions of previously identified serine peptidase inhibitor Kazal type 5 (SPINK5), kallikrein-related peptidase 7 (KLK7), and filaggrin (FLG) polymorphisms to eczema risk. J Allergy Clin Immunol. 2008;122(3):560–8.e4.

46. Margolis DJ, Gupta J, Apter AJ, Ganguly T, Hoffstad O, Papadopoulos M, et al. Filaggrin-2 variation is associated with more persistent atopic dermatitis in African American subjects. J Allergy Clin Immunol. 2014;133(3):784–9.
47. Marenholz I, Rivera VAG, Esparza-Gordillo J, Bauerfeind A, Lee-Kirsch M-A, Ciechanowicz A, et al. Association screening in the Epidermal Differentiation Complex (EDC) identifies an SPRR3 repeat number variant as a risk factor for eczema. J Invest Dermatol. 2011;131(8):1644–9.
48. De Benedetto A, Rafaels NM, McGirt LY, Ivanov AI, Georas SN, Cheadle C, et al. Tight junction defects in patients with atopic dermatitis. J Allergy Clin Immunol. 2011;127(3):773–86.e867.
49. Ahmad-Nejad P, Mrabet-Dahbi S, Breuer K, Klotz M, Werfel T, Herz U, et al. The Toll-like receptor 2 R753Q polymorphism defines a subgroup of patients with atopic dermatitis having severe phenotype. J Allergy Clin Immunol. 2004;113(3):565–7.
50. Weidinger S, Novak N, Klopp N, Baurecht H, Wagenpfeil S, Rummler L, et al. Lack of association between Toll-like receptor 2 and Toll-like receptor 4 polymorphisms and atopic eczema. J Allergy Clin Immunol. 2006;118(1):277–9.
51. Abramovits W, Rivas Bejarano JJ, Valdecantos WC. Role of interleukin 1 in atopic dermatitis. Dermatol Clin. 2013;31(3):437–44.
52. Novak N, Kruse S, Potreck J, Maintz L, Jenneck C, Weidinger S, et al. Single nucleotide polymorphisms of the IL18 gene are associated with atopic eczema. J Allergy Clin Immunol. 2005;115(4):828–33.
53. Kim E, Lee JE, Namkung JH, Park JH, Kim S, Shin ES, et al. Association of the single-nucleotide polymorphism and haplotype of the interleukin 18 gene with atopic dermatitis in Koreans. Clin Exp Allergy. 2007;37(6):865–71.
54. Reche PA, Soumelis V, Gorman DM, Clifford T, Liu M, Travis M, et al. Human thymic stromal lymphopoietin preferentially stimulates myeloid cells. J Immunol. 2001;167(1):336–43.
55. Gittler JK, Shemer A, Suárez-Fariñas M, Fuentes-Duculan J, Gulewicz KJ, Wang CQF, et al. Progressive activation of T_H2/T_H22 cytokines and selective epidermal proteins characterizes acute and chronic atopic dermatitis. J Allergy Clin Immunol. 2012;130(6):1344–54.
56. Novak N, Kraft S, Geiger E, Klüken H, Bieber T, Kruse S, et al. Dichotomic nature of atopic dermatitis reflected by combined analysis of monocyte immunophenotyping and single nucleotide polymorphisms of the interleukin-4/interleukin-13 receptor gene: the dichotomy of extrinsic and intrinsic atopic dermatitis. J Invest Dermatol. 2002;119(4):870–5.
57. Söderhäll C, Bradley M, Kockum I, Luthman H, Wahlgren C-F, Nordenskjöld M. Analysis of association and linkage for the interleukin-4 and interleukin-4 receptor balpha; regions in Swedish atopic dermatitis families. Clin Exp Allergy. 2002;32(8):1199–202.
58. Howell MD, Gao P, Kim BE, Lesley LJ, Streib JE, Taylor PA, et al. The signal transducer and activator of transcription 6 gene (STAT6) increases the propensity of patients with atopic dermatitis toward disseminated viral skin infections. J Allergy Clin Immunol. 2011;128(5):1006–14.
59. Lebman DA, Coffman RL. Interleukin 4 causes isotype switching to IgE in T cell-stimulated clonal B cell cultures. J Exp Med. 1988;168(3):853–62.
60. Dizier M-H, Sandford A, Walley A, Philippi A, Cookson W, Demenais F. Indication of linkage of serum IgE levels to the interleukin-4 gene and exclusion of the contribution of the (–590 C to T) interleukin-4 promoter polymorphism to IgE variation. Genet Epidemiol. 1999;16(1):84–94.
61. Jha AN, Singh VK, Kumari N, Singh A, Antony J, van Tong H, et al. IL-4 haplotype -590T, -34T and intron-3 VNTR R2 is associated with reduced malaria risk among ancestral Indian tribal populations. PLoS One. 2012;7(10):e48136.
62. Tanaka K, Sugiura H, Uehara M, Hashimoto Y, Donnelly C, Montgomery DS. Lack of association between atopic eczema and the genetic variants of interleukin-4 and the interleukin-4 receptor alpha chain gene: heterogeneity of genetic backgrounds on immunoglobulin E production in atopic eczema patients. Clin Exp Allergy. 2001;31(10):1522–7.
63. Elliott K, Fitzpatrick E, Hill D, Brown J, Adams S, Chee P, et al. The –590C/T and –34C/T interleukin-4 promoter polymorphisms are not associated with atopic eczema in childhood. J Allergy Clin Immunol. 2001;108(2):285–7.
64. Oiso N, Fukai K, Ishii M. Interleukin 4 receptor alpha chain polymorphism Gln551Arg is associated with adult atopic dermatitis in Japan. Br J Dermatol. 2000;142(5):1003–6.
65. Namkung J-H, Lee J-E, Kim E, Kim H-J, Seo E-Y, Jang H-Y, et al. Association of polymorphisms in genes encoding IL-4, IL-13 and their receptors with atopic dermatitis in a Korean population. Exp Dermatol. 2011;20(11):915–9.
66. Chang YT, Lee WR, Yu CW, Liu HN, Lin MW, Huang CH, et al. No association of cytokine gene polymorphisms in Chinese patients with atopic dermatitis. Clin Exp Dermatol. 2006;31(3):419–23.
67. Liu X, Nickel R, Beyer K, Wahn U, Ehrlich E, Freidhoff LR, et al. An IL13 coding region variant is associated with a high total serum IgE level and atopic dermatitis in the German multicenter atopy study (MAS-90). J Allergy Clin Immunol. 2000;106(1 Pt 1):167–70.
68. Gleń J, Trzeciak M, Sobjanek M, Bandurski T, Wilkowska A, Nedoszytko B, et al. Interleukin-13 promoter gene polymorphism –1112 C/T is associated with atopic dermatitis in Polish patients. Acta Dermatovenerol Croat. 2012;20(4):231–8.
69. Tsunemi Y, Saeki H, Nakamura K, Sekiya T, Hirai K, Kakinuma T, et al. Interleukin-13 gene polymorphism G4257A is associated with atopic dermatitis in Japanese patients. J Dermatol Sci. 2002;30(2):100–7.
70. Matsui E, Kaneko H, Fukao T, Teramoto T, Inoue R, Watanabe M, et al. Mutations of the IL-12 receptor β2

chain gene in atopic subjects. Biochem Biophys Res Commun. 1999;266(2):551–5.
71. Namkung J-H, Lee J-E, Kim E, Kim S, Kim S, Shin E-S, et al. Association of single nucleotide polymorphisms in the IL-12 (IL-12A and B) and IL-12 receptor (IL-12Rβ1 and β2) genes and gene–gene interactions with atopic dermatitis in Koreans. J Dermatol Sci. 2010;57(3):199–206.
72. Shin HD, Park BL, Kim LH, Kim JS, Kim JW. Interleukin-10 haplotype associated with total serum IgE in atopic dermatitis patients. Allergy. 2005;60(9):1146–51.
73. Korppi M, Nuolivirta K, Lauhkonen E, Holster A, Teräsjärvi J, Vuononvirta J, et al. IL-10 gene polymorphism is associated with preschool atopy and early-life recurrent wheezing after bronchiolitis in infancy. Pediatr Pulmonol. 2017;52(1):14–20.
74. Namkung J-H, Lee J-E, Kim E, Park GT, Yang HS, Jang HY, et al. An association between IL-9 and IL-9 receptor gene polymorphisms and atopic dermatitis in a Korean population. J Dermatol Sci. 2011;62(1):16–21.
75. Tsunemi Y, Saeki H, Nakamura K, Sekiya T, Hirai K, Fujita H, et al. Interleukin-12 p40 gene (IL12B) 3′-untranslated region polymorphism is associated with susceptibility to atopic dermatitis and psoriasis vulgaris. J Dermatol Sci. 2002;30(2):161–6.
76. Shirakawa T, Hashimoto T, Furuyama J, Takeshita T, Morimoto K. Linkage between severe atopy and chromosome 11q13 in Japanese families. Clin Genet. 1994;46(3):228–32.
77. Cox HE, Moffatt MF, Faux JA, Walley AJ, Coleman R, Trembath RC, et al. Association of atopic dermatitis to the beta subunit of the high affinity immunoglobulin E receptor. Br J Dermatol. 1998;138(1):182–7.
78. Park KY, Park MK, Kim EJ, Lee M-K, Seo SJ. FCεRI gene promoter polymorphisms and total Ige levels in susceptibility to atopic dermatitis in Korea. J Korean Med Sci. 2011;26(7):870–4.

Skin Barrier-Related Pathogenesis of Atopic Dermatitis

Eung Ho Choi

Introduction

The skin barrier consists of corneocytes in the stratum corneum (SC) functioning as bricks, intercorneocyte lipids as mortar, corneodesmosomes as rivets, and tight junctions (TJs), which connect the lateral sides of the upper granular cells [1]. Recently, studies have shown that skin barrier dysfunction is a very important cause of atopic dermatitis (AD) [2–4]. Congenital skin barrier damage became known as a primary cause of AD after a 2006 report noted that a loss-of-function mutation of the filaggrin gene (*FLG*) is very important in white AD patients in northwestern European countries [5]. The cause of AD has been largely classified into an "outside-in model," in which skin barrier dysfunction acts primarily, and an "inside-out model," in which an abnormal immune response occurs first, thereby impairing skin barrier function. In recent years, however, the two mechanisms have been shown to work together to create an "outside-inside-outside model" [2]. In other words, the combination of a vulnerable skin barrier and an abnormal immune response acts as a cause of AD.

E. H. Choi (✉)
Department of Dermatology, Yonsei University Wonju College of Medicine, Wonju, Korea (Republic of)
e-mail: choieh@yonsei.ac.kr

Representative etiologies of AD proposed in connection with abnormal skin barrier function are as follows: (1) reduction of ceramides in SC intercellular lipids from the SC lipid barrier [6]; (2) an *FLG* mutation causing a deficiency of filaggrin protein in the protein barrier [7]; (3) activation of serine proteases (SPs; kallikrein [KLK]) causing desquamation of corneocytes and a reduction in SP inhibitors [8]; and (4) a tight junction abnormality [9]. If we consider that the most frequently prescribed treatment for AD patients in clinics is a moisturizer (emollient) to replenish the damaged SC and to resolve skin dryness caused by the decrease of SC hydration, it is possible to explain the importance of skin barrier dysfunction in the pathogenesis of AD.

Lipid Barrier Impairment: Abnormal SC Intercellular Lipids

SC intercellular lipid lamellae perform the role of an epidermal permeability barrier as the most important function of the skin barrier. The lipid lamellae are composed of ceramides, cholesterol, and fatty acids in an equimolar ratio. Among them, ceramides are the most important lipid accounting for more than 50% [10] (Table 1). In the SC, ceramides play an important role in confining moisture in the SC [11].

K. H. Lee et al. (eds.), *Practical Insights into Atopic Dermatitis*,
https://doi.org/10.1007/978-981-15-8159-5_7

In patients with AD, ceramides, the main component that forms the SC intercellular lipids, is significantly reduced in eczema lesions as well as in nonlesional skin showing only dry skin, in comparison with healthy controls without atopy. In particular, ceramide 1, which has the longest chain structure, decreases the most [12]. AD patients show an inverse correlation between ceramide levels and transepidermal water loss (TEWL) as the most basic measurement for skin barrier function. Also, the epidermis of a ceramide-deficient mouse shows a simultaneous decrease of SC hydration and barrier function [13]. Thus, an important cause of the dry skin complaint in almost all AD patients is the reduction of ceramides in the SC and the reduction of natural moisturizing factors (NMFs), as filaggrin degradation products [14] (Fig. 1). However, unlike filaggrin proteins, the reduction of ceramides has not been considered as a congenital cause in patients with AD. In other words, ceramide levels in infants with AD are reduced in lesional skin but not in nonlesional skin in comparison with a control group. Therefore, ceramide reduction in AD has been thought to be a secondary phenomenon due to an inflammatory response. In addition, no mutations in the genes associated with ceramide reduction have been reported.

Table 1 Major components of SC lipids

Lipid species	Weight (%)	Molar ratio
Ceramides	50	1
Cholesterol	25	1
Free fatty acids	25	1

Recently, however, long-chain ceramides have been shown to be reduced, but short-chain ceramides have been shown to be increased in nonlesional skin of AD patients [15, 16]. Long-chain ceramides play a more decisive role in the permeability barrier function. Elongases ELOVL1 and ELOVL2, enzymes that produce very long-chain fatty acids, are important for the elongation of free fatty acids with more than 16 carbon atoms in the epidermis [17]. It has been reported that the protein expression of these elongases is reduced in the epidermis of AD patients [18]. These elongation processes are inhibited by the T_H2 cytokines IL-13 and IL-4, making it difficult to produce very long-chain ceramides in the epidermis of AD patients [19].

Most SC intercellular lipids are produced in the granular layer, are stored in lamellar bodies (LBs), and then migrate to be secreted into the interface between the SC and the stratum granulosum (SG). Recently, it has been found that transmembrane protein 79/mattrin (Tmem79/Matt) is involved in secretion of the contents of LBs. Tmem79 is a 5-transmembrane protein present in LBs. Tmem79-deficient mice have increased serum IgE and natural dermatitis, similar to human AD [20]. Also, a missense mutation of *TMEM79* has been reported to have a small but significant association with AD occurrence [21].

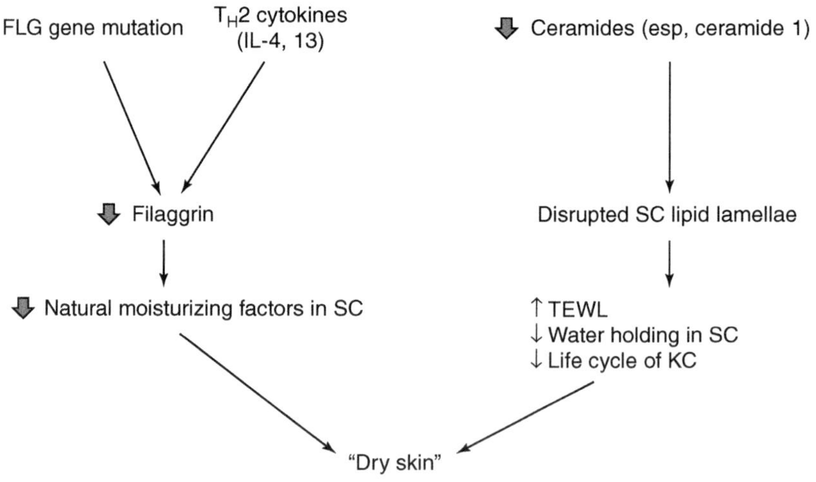

Fig. 1 Pathogenesis of dry skin in patients with atopic dermatitis. (Cited from Choi EH, Yoon NY. Pathogenesis of atopic dermatitis. J Korean Med Assoc. 2014;57:218–225.)

Protein Barrier Impairment

Deficiency of Filaggrin and Its Metabolites

Filaggrin is present in the form of profilaggrin, a protein that forms keratohyalin granules in the granular layer of the epidermis. Profilaggrin breaks down into filaggrin in the terminal differentiation process of keratinocytes and then aggregates keratin filaments to form a solid and flat structure of corneocytes while forming cornified cell envelopes, allowing corneocytes to act as bricks in the skin barrier structure. Then, the filaggrins move into the SC and the polymers turn into monomers and break down into amino acids, which change into free amino acids, pyrrolidone carboxylic acid (PCA), urocanic acid (UCA), and various organic acids. Proteolytic enzymes such as caspase 14, calpain 1, and bleomycin hydroxylase act in this process [22, 23] (Fig. 2).

Among natural moisturizing factors (NMFs), free amino acids constitute 40% and PCA 12%. These filaggrin metabolites play a variety of roles not only in SC hydration, but also in the normalization of the SC pH, the permeability barrier, SC integrity, and antibacterial and anti-inflammatory effects. In recent reports, patients with ichthyosis vulgaris and FLG-deficient mice (*Flg−/−*) that had a congenital filaggrin deficiency showed cellular structural abnormalities, inadequate lamellar content loading, an abnormal SC intercellular lipid membrane structure, and tight junction abnormalities. This could explain why a lack of filaggrin, the constituent protein of corneocytes, also leads to the loss of permeability barrier function [24, 25].

Since it was reported that only filaggrin among epidermal differentiation proteins was reduced in nonlesional skin of patients with AD [26], several studies have focused on lack of filaggrin as a cause of AD. To date, more than 30 loss-of-function mutations of *FLG* have been reported in Europe and Asia [27]. Among patients with AD, *FLG* mutations have been reported in more than 40% of northwestern European Caucasians, about 30% of Chinese, about 25% of Japanese, and about 10% of Koreans. Of these *FLG* variations, only R501X and E2422X have been reported commonly in northwestern Europeans and Asians, so the *FLG* variation is distinct from race [28–31]. AD patients with *FLG* mutations develop AD at a young age, have more severe symptoms, more often have symptoms that persist in adulthood, and have more atopic marches that progress to respiratory atopic disease [32]. *FLG* mutations reduce filaggrin protein production, weakening cornified envelope formation, decreasing adhesion between corneocytes, and increasing TEWL, thereby reducing overall skin barrier function. Eventually, this increases the

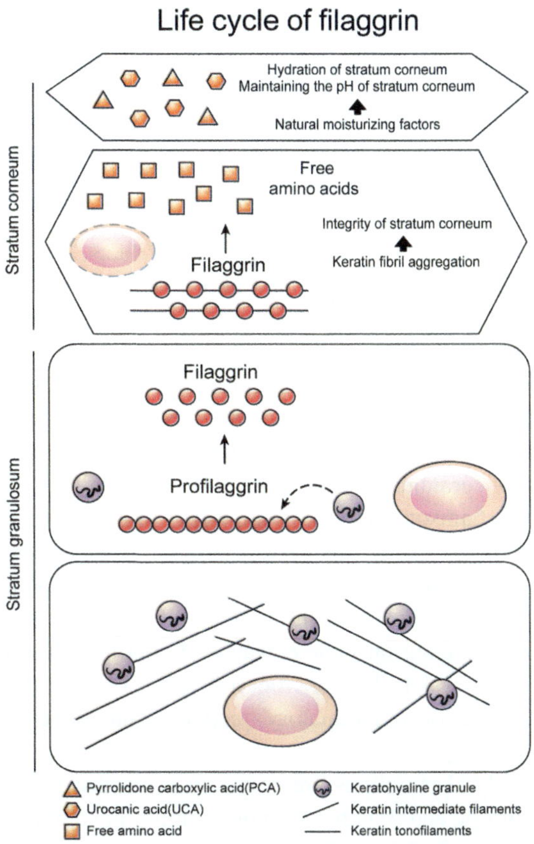

Fig. 2 Life cycle of filaggrin. Filaggrin exists as profilaggrin within keratohyalin granules in the granular layer of the epidermis. It is degraded to filaggrin during the terminal differentiation process. Then, moving to the upper part of the stratum corneum (SC), filaggrin degrades into amino acids and plays a crucial role in maintaining SC hydration and pH by forming natural moisturizing factors including pyrrolidone carboxylic acid or urocanic acid. (From Choi EH, et al. J Skin Barrier Res 2013;15:13–23, with permission from the Korean Society for Skin Barrier Research)

penetration of external allergens into the body, and so sensitization occurs easily, which leads to an allergic reaction. In addition, the contents of LBs become inadequate due to atrophy of the cytoskeleton, the SC pH increases due to the decrease of trans-UCA, and dry skin is induced due to the decrease of amino acid and PCA, which are filaggrin degradation products, resulting in AD [33]. Elevated skin pH induces corneodesmosome degradation by increasing serine protease (kallikrein) activity, leading to excessive desquamation of corneocytes, but on the other hand, it attenuates the activity of enzymes required for ceramide synthesis, thereby reducing ceramide levels in the SC. Eventually, this mechanism increases the T_H2 inflammatory response and increases antigen penetration through the skin [19, 25, 34] (Fig. 3). Studies in AD animal models and humans have shown that normalizing only the elevated SC pH in AD can restore skin barrier function and reduce the degree of inflammatory response and eczema [34–37].

FLG mutations are common in northwestern Europe and Asia but are not common in southern Europe and are not found in some African countries. In recent studies, another skin barrier protein, filaggrin2 (FLG2), has been reduced in the epidermis of AD patients, and nonsense mutations in *FLG2* have been reported to be associated with persistent AD in African patients [38]. Since the structure, expression, and biological properties of filaggrin 2 are very similar to those of filaggrin, filaggrin also appears to play an important role in skin barrier function [39]. Mice with homozygous frameshift mutations of *FLG* show marked cell infiltration and increased serum IgE after allergen exposure [40].

Serine Protease Inhibitor Deficiency

Corneocytes are continuously slowly desquamated on the surface of the SC, which is physiologically important for skin homeostasis. The desquamation of corneocytes is mainly regulated by the proteolysis of kallikrein-related peptidases such as KLK5, KLK7, and KLK14 [41]. Since the activity of these proteases is pH dependent, it increases with increasing SC pH. The skin surface pH is higher in AD patients than in normal healthy controls. Increasing the SC pH promotes SP activity, which induces the desquamation of corneocytes, and increases the activity of protease-activated receptor-2 (PAR2), thereby precipitating allergic inflammation with a T_H2 immune response. Allergens such as house dust mites and cockroaches, which are the main causes of AD and asthma, have been shown to activate PAR2, delaying recovery of damaged skin barriers and exacerbating AD [42]. However, the protein that inhibits SP action is LEKTI (lympho-epithelial Kazal type-related inhibitor) and is the product of the SP inhibitor Kazal type 5 gene (*SPINK5*). These KLKs and LEKTIs are both stored in LBs and are secreted together into the SC intercellular space.

Two genetic polymorphisms involved in increasing KLK activity are associated with the pathogenesis of AD. Those are the gain-of-function mutation of the *KLK7* gene and the loss-of-function mutation of the *SPINK5* gene. A 4-bp insertion polymorphism of *KLK7* [43] and a mutation of *SPINK5* located on chromosome 5q32 [44] were reported in patients with AD. The increased allergic inflammatory response in these patients may be explained by the inability to adequately inhibit the action of activated SPs. It has also been reported that a SNP of the gene encoding PAR2 (*F2RL1*) is associated with Korean AD. This mutation appears to increase the stability of *F2RL1* mRNA transcription. These findings indicate that an inherited variation in protease activity in the SC is linked to the pathogenesis of AD in certain populations, such as Asians.

Tight Junction Abnormality

Tight junctions are present in epithelial cells and function as a barrier that fixes the membrane side of neighboring cells to each other and prevents the flow of water and body fluid through the cell side space. Tight junctions consist of transmembrane proteins such as claudin and occludin and

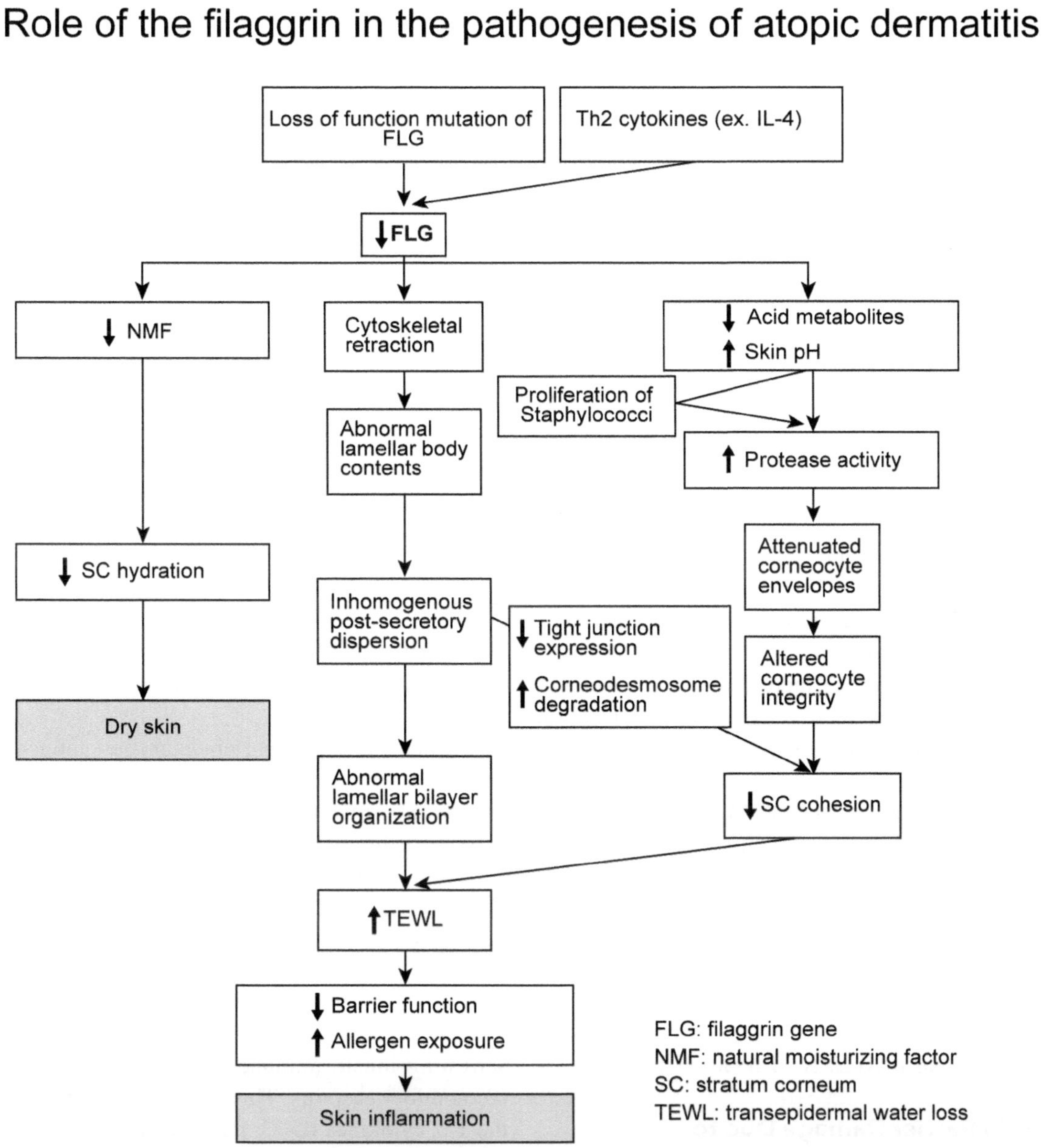

Fig. 3 Role of filaggrin in the pathogenesis of atopic dermatitis. Filaggrin gene mutations reduce filaggrin protein production, which in turn reduces the production of natural moisturizing factors (NMFs), leading to reduced SC hydration, resulting in dry skin. Due to the atrophy of the cytoskeleton, the contents of lamellar bodies become inadequate, resulting in abnormal formation of SC lipid lamellae and then increasing TEWL. On the other hand, the SC pH is increased by decreasing trans-UCA, which increases the activity of SPs (kallikreins). This increases the breakdown of corneodesmosomes and induces excessive desquamation, thereby increasing TEWL. Eventually, this increases the penetration of external allergens into the body, and so sensitization occurs easily, which leads to an allergic reaction

cytosolic scaffold proteins such as zonula occludens [45, 46]. In normal skin, tight junctions are observed in the granule layer and increase rapidly after skin damage. Tight junctions are also essential for the differentiation (keratinization) of epidermal cells. In diseases with abnormal keratinization, such as psoriasis and ichthyosis vulgaris, tight junctions are also expressed in the lower part of the epidermis [47]. After the SC is damaged, the calcium ion concentration decreases along with the transepidermal loss of the body fluid between the SC and SG, and then the tight junctions of the upper granule layer are opened [48]. Immediately, the dendrites of Langerhans cells, which are located just below the tight junctions, stretch above them. At this time, the high molecular weight protein antigens that pass through the damaged SC are captured by the dendrites of Langerhans cells and then are recognized and migrate to regional lymph nodes. The serine protease component of these protein antigens activates PAR2 present in the keratinocyte membrane. On the other hand, bacteria that penetrate the SC activate Toll-like receptors (TLRs). After that, in keratinocytes, several chemokines and cytokines such as TNF-α, IL-1, and TSLP are secreted to promote the development of AD and aggravate the disease [49]. Claudin 1 deficiency in mice showed a marked decrease of skin barrier function increasing TEWL without structural damage [50]. In addition, tight junction protein expression is markedly decreased in the skin of AD patients compared to normal healthy people. Claudin 1 gene (*CDN1*) mutations have been reported in AD patients, and the cause of frequent herpes virus infection in AD patients has been explained by the reduction of claudin-1 in tight junction proteins [9, 51].

Correlation Between the Immune Response and Skin Barrier Function

Skin Barrier Damage Due to the Immune Response

Several studies have shown that immune cells affect the skin barrier through cytokine production [52, 53]. Blocking signal transduction of the T_H2 cytokines IL-4 and IL-13 alleviates AD [54]. IL-4 and IL-13 have been shown to inhibit the production of cornified envelope components such as filaggrin, keratin, loricrin, and involucrin, cell adhesion molecules such as desmogleins, and zona occludens 1 and ceramide lipids [54]. Other T_H2 cytokines (IL-31 and IL-33) also decrease the expression of *FLG* [55].

Cutaneous inflammatory reactions reduce epidermal lipid biosynthesis and affect skin barrier function. Cytokines such as IL-4 have been reported to affect lipid metabolism in the epidermis [56]. IL-4, IFNγ, and TNF-α affect the activity of lipid-related enzymes such as acid sphingomyelinase, β-glucocylcerebrosidase, and acid ceramidase. TNF-α, a proinflammatory cytokine, and IFNγ, a T_H1 cytokine, reduced acid sphingomyelinase and β-glucocylcerebrosidase at the mRNA level and reduced ceramide levels at the epidermis. Tawade et al. reported that IFNγ treatment in human keratinocyte cultures and epidermis reduced the mRNA of elongases and ceramide synthase, thereby reducing ceramides with long-chain fatty acids [18].

Activation of the Immune Response Due to Skin Barrier Dysfunction

It has become clear that epicutaneous antigens are potent sensitizers that cause allergic diseases. Mouse experiments have shown that food allergies and asthma can be induced through skin sensitization, which is more easily induced when skin barriers are damaged [34, 36, 40, 57]. Antigen exposure through the skin causes sensitization, while oral antigen exposure induces immune tolerance [58, 59]. SC damage allows foreign antigens to easily penetrate into the skin, activating innate immune receptors and pattern recognition receptors. This induces production of the T_H2 cytokines IL-33, IL-24, and TSLP.

Conclusion

When skin barrier damage occurs, whether innate or acquired, foreign antigens easily penetrate into the skin through the damaged barrier. The penetrating antigens react with the immune cells in the skin, causing an inflammatory response in the skin, and even a systemic immune response. This is called an outside-in hypothesis and explains

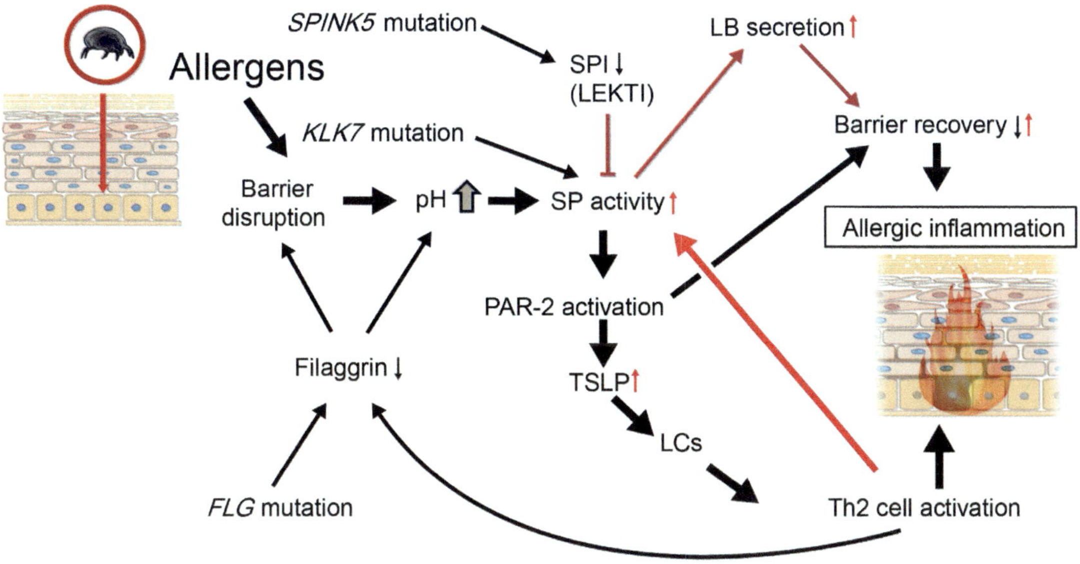

Fig. 4 Barrier-related pathogenesis of atopic dermatitis. (From Choi EH, et al. Lee's Illustrated Skin Barrier with permission from the authors)

why people with AD develop an "atopic march" that progresses to food allergies, asthma, and allergic rhinitis in succession. And the inflammatory skin reactions break the skin barrier again, making allergic diseases occur more easily (Fig. 4). Therefore, maintaining and preserving skin barrier function is very important for the treatment of AD as well as to prevent an atopic march.

References

1. Kirschner N, Brandner JM. Barriers and more: functions of tight junction proteins in the skin. Ann NY Acad Sci. 2012;1257(1):158–66.
2. Elias PM, Steinhoff M. "Outside-to-inside"(and now back to "outside") pathogenic mechanisms in atopic dermatitis. J Invest Dermatol. 2008;128(5):1067–70.
3. Peng W, Novak N. Pathogenesis of atopic dermatitis. Clin Exp Allergy. 2015;45(3):566–74.
4. Choi EH, Yoon NY. Pathogenesis of atopic dermatitis. J Korean Med Assoc. 2014;57(3):218–25.
5. Palmer CN, Irvine AD, Terron-Kwiatkowski A, Zhao Y, Liao H, Lee SP, et al. Common loss-of-function variants of the epidermal barrier protein filaggrin are a major predisposing factor for atopic dermatitis. Nat Genet. 2006;38(4):441–6.
6. Melnik B, Hollmann J, Plewig G. Decreased stratum corneum ceramides in atopic individuals—a pathobiochemical factor in xerosis? Br J Dermatol. 1988;119(4):547–9.
7. Irvine AD, McLean WHI. Breaking the (un)sound barrier: filaggrin is a major gene for atopic dermatitis. J Invest Dermatol. 2006;126(6):1200–2.
8. Kato A, Fukai K, Oiso N, Hosomi N, Murakami T, Ishii M. Association of SPINK5 gene polymorphisms with atopic dermatitis in the Japanese population. Br J Dermatol. 2003;148(4):665–9.
9. De Benedetto A, Rafaels NM, McGirt LY, Ivanov AI, Georas SN, Cheadle C, et al. Tight junction defects in patients with atopic dermatitis. J Allergy Clin Immunol. 2011;127(3):773–86.e867.
10. Weerheim A, Ponec M. Determination of stratum corneum lipid profile by tape stripping in combination with high-performance thin-layer chromatography. Arch Dermatol Res. 2001;293(4):191–9.
11. Lampe MA, Burlingame AL, Whitney J, Williams ML, Brown BE, Roitman E, et al. Human stratum corneum lipids: characterization and regional variations. J Lipid Res. 1983;24(2):120–30.
12. Imokawa G, Abe A, Jin K, Higaki Y, Kawashima M, Hidano A. Decreased level of ceramides in stratum corneum of atopic dermatitis: an etiologic factor in atopic dry skin? J Invest Dermatol. 1991;96(4):523–6.
13. Nakajima K, Terao M, Takaishi M, Kataoka S, Goto-Inoue N, Setou M, et al. Barrier abnormality due to ceramide deficiency leads to psoriasiform inflammation in a mouse model. J Invest Dermatol. 2013;133(11):2555–65.
14. Jung M, Choi J, Lee S-A, Kim H, Hwang J, Choi EH. Pyrrolidone carboxylic acid levels or caspase-14 expression in the corneocytes of lesional skin correlates with clinical severity, skin barrier function and lesional inflammation in atopic dermatitis. J Dermatol Sci. 2014;76(3):231–9.

15. van Smeden J, Janssens M, Kaye ECJ, Caspers PJ, Lavrijsen AP, Vreeken RJ, et al. The importance of free fatty acid chain length for the skin barrier function in atopic eczema patients. Exp Dermatol. 2014;23(1):45–52.
16. Kim D, Lee NR, Park S-Y, Jun M, Lee K, Kim S, et al. As in atopic dermatitis, nonlesional skin in allergic contact dermatitis displays abnormalities in barrier function and ceramide content. J Invest Dermatol. 2017;137(3):748–50.
17. Vasireddy V, Uchida Y, Salem N Jr, Kim SY, Mandal MNA, Reddy GB, et al. Loss of functional ELOVL4 depletes very long-chain fatty acids (> or =C28) and the unique omega-O-acylceramides in skin leading to neonatal death. Hum Mol Genet. 2007;16(5):471–82.
18. Tawada C, Kanoh H, Nakamura M, Mizutani Y, Fujisawa T, Banno Y, et al. Interferon-γ decreases ceramides with long-chain fatty acids: possible involvement in atopic dermatitis and psoriasis. J Invest Dermatol. 2014;134(3):712–8.
19. Briot A, Deraison C, Lacroix M, Bonnart C, Robin A, Besson C, et al. Kallikrein 5 induces atopic dermatitis-like lesions through PAR2-mediated thymic stromal lymphopoietin expression in Netherton syndrome. J Exp Med. 2009;206(5):1135–47.
20. Sasaki T, Shiohama A, Kubo A, Kawasaki H, Ishida-Yamamoto A, Yamada T, et al. A homozygous nonsense mutation in the gene for Tmem79, a component for the lamellar granule secretory system, produces spontaneous eczema in an experimental model of atopic dermatitis. J Allergy Clin Immunol. 2013;132(5):1111–20. e4
21. Saunders SP, Goh CSM, Brown SJ, Palmer CNA, Porter RM, Cole C, et al. Tmem79/Matt is the matted mouse gene and is a predisposing gene for atopic dermatitis in human subjects. J Allergy Clin Immunol. 2013;132(5):1121–9.
22. Hoste E, Kemperman P, Devos M, Denecker G, Kezic S, Yau N, et al. Caspase-14 is required for filaggrin degradation to natural moisturizing factors in the skin. J Invest Dermatol. 2011;131(11):2233–41.
23. Kamata Y, Taniguchi A, Yamamoto M, Nomura J, Ishihara K, Takahara H, et al. Neutral cysteine protease bleomycin hydrolase is essential for the breakdown of deiminated filaggrin into amino acids. J Biol Chem. 2009;284(19):12829–36.
24. Gruber R, Elias PM, Crumrine D, Lin T-K, Brandner JM, Hachem J-P, et al. Filaggrin genotype in ichthyosis vulgaris predicts abnormalities in epidermal structure and function. Am J Pathol. 2011;178(5):2252–63.
25. Kawasaki H, Nagao K, Kubo A, Hata T, Shimizu A, Mizuno H, et al. Altered stratum corneum barrier and enhanced percutaneous immune responses in filaggrin-null mice. J Allergy Clin Immunol. 2012;129(6):1538–46.e6.
26. Seguchi T, Cui CY, Kusuda S, Takahashi M, Aisu K, Tezuka T. Decreased expression of filaggrin in atopic skin. Arch Dermatol Res. 1996;288(8):442–6.
27. Weidinger S, Kabesch M. Clinical impact of current genetics findings. atopic dermatitis in childhood and adolescence, vol. 15. Basel: Karger Publishers; 2011. p. 21–38.
28. Morar N, Cookson WOCM, Harper JI, Moffatt MF. Filaggrin mutations in children with severe atopic dermatitis. J Invest Dermatol. 2007;127(7):1667–72.
29. Nomura T, Akiyama M, Sandilands A, Nemoto-Hasebe I, Sakai K, Nagasaki A, et al. Specific filaggrin mutations cause ichthyosis vulgaris and are significantly associated with atopic dermatitis in Japan. J Invest Dermatol. 2008;128(6):1436–41.
30. Li M, Liu Q, Liu J, Cheng R, Zhang H, Xue H, et al. Mutations analysis in filaggrin gene in northern China patients with atopic dermatitis. J Eur Acad Dermatol Venereol. 2013;27(2):169–74.
31. Greisenegger E, Novak N, Maintz L, Bieber T, Zimprich F, Haubenberger D, et al. Analysis of four prevalent filaggrin mutations (R501X, 2282del4, R2447X and S3247X) in Austrian and German patients with atopic dermatitis. J Eur Acad Dermatol Venereol. 2010;24(5):607–10.
32. Barker JNWN, Palmer CNA, Zhao Y, Liao H, Hull PR, Lee SP, et al. Null mutations in the filaggrin gene (FLG) determine major susceptibility to early-onset atopic dermatitis that persists into adulthood. J Invest Dermatol. 2007;127(3):564–7.
33. Kezic S, O'Regan GM, Yau N, Sandilands A, Chen H, Campbell LE, et al. Levels of filaggrin degradation products are influenced by both filaggrin genotype and atopic dermatitis severity. Allergy. 2011;66(7):934–40.
34. Lee H-J, Lee NR, Kim B-K, Jung M, Kim DH, Moniaga CS, et al. Acidification of stratum corneum prevents the progression from atopic dermatitis to respiratory allergy. Exp Dermatol. 2017;26(1):66–72.
35. Lee H-J, Yoon NY, Lee NR, Jung M, Kim DH, Choi EH. Topical acidic cream prevents the development of atopic dermatitis- and asthma-like lesions in murine model. Exp Dermatol. 2014;23(10):736–41.
36. Lee H-J, Lee NR, Jung M, Kim DH, Choi EH. Atopic march from atopic dermatitis to asthma-like lesions in NC/Nga mice is accelerated or aggravated by neutralization of stratum corneum but partially inhibited by acidification. J Invest Dermatol. 2015;135(12):3025–33.
37. Lee NR, Lee H-J, Yoon NY, Kim D, Jung M, Choi EH. Acidic water bathing could be a safe and effective therapeutic modality for severe and refractory atopic dermatitis. Ann Dermatol. 2016;28(1):126–9.
38. Margolis DJ, Gupta J, Apter AJ, Ganguly T, Hoffstad O, Papadopoulos M, et al. Filaggrin-2 variation is associated with more persistent atopic dermatitis in African American subjects. J Allergy Clin Immunol. 2014;133(3):784–9.
39. Makino T, Mizawa M, Yamakoshi T, Takaishi M, Shimizu T. Expression of filaggrin-2 protein in the epidermis of human skin diseases: a comparative analysis with filaggrin. Biochem Biophys Res Commun. 2014;449(1):100–6.
40. Fallon PG, Sasaki T, Sandilands A, Campbell LE, Saunders SP, Mangan NE, et al. A homozygous

frameshift mutation in the mouse Flg gene facilitates enhanced percutaneous allergen priming. Nat Genet. 2009;41(5):602–8.
41. Deraison C, Bonnart C, Lopez F, Besson C, Robinson R, Jayakumar A, et al. LEKTI fragments specifically inhibit KLK5, KLK7, and KLK14 and control desquamation through a pH-dependent interaction. Mol Biol Cell. 2007;18(9):3607–19.
42. Jeong SK, Kim HJ, Youm J-K, Ahn SK, Choi EH, Sohn MH, et al. Mite and cockroach allergens activate protease-activated receptor 2 and delay epidermal permeability barrier recovery. J Invest Dermatol. 2008;128(8):1930–9.
43. Zhao LP, Di Z, Zhang L, Wang L, Ma L, Lv Y, et al. Association of SPINK5 gene polymorphisms with atopic dermatitis in Northeast China. J Eur Acad Dermatol Venereol. 2012;26(5):572–7.
44. Rihs H-P, Kowal A, Raulf-Heimsoth M, Degens P-O, Landt O, Brüning T. Rapid detection of the SPINK5 polymorphism Glu420Lys by real-time PCR technology. Clin Chim Acta. 2005;355(1-2):185–9.
45. Morita K, Miyachi Y, Furuse M. Tight junctions in epidermis: from barrier to keratinization. Eur J Dermatol. 2011;21(1):12–7.
46. Tsukita S, Furuse M. Claudin-based barrier in simple and stratified cellular sheets. Curr Opin Cell Biol. 2002;14(5):531–6.
47. O'Neill CA, Garrod D. Tight junction proteins and the epidermis. Exp Dermatol. 2011;20(2):88–91.
48. Baek JH, Lee SE, Choi KJ, Choi EH, Lee SH. Acute modulations in stratum corneum permeability barrier function affect claudin expression and epidermal tight junction function via changes of epidermal calcium gradient. Yonsei Med J. 2013;54(2):523–8.
49. Kubo A, Nagao K, Amagai M. Epidermal barrier dysfunction and cutaneous sensitization in atopic diseases. J Clin Invest. 2012;122(2):440–7.
50. Furuse M, Hata M, Furuse K, Yoshida Y, Haratake A, Sugitani Y, et al. Claudin-based tight junctions are crucial for the mammalian epidermal barrier: a lesson from claudin-1-deficient mice. J Cell Biol. 2002;156(6):1099–111.
51. De Benedetto A, Slifka MK, Rafaels NM, Kuo IH, Georas SN, Boguniewicz M, et al. Reductions in claudin-1 may enhance susceptibility to herpes simplex virus 1 infections in atopic dermatitis. J Allergy Clin Immunol. 2011;128(1):242–6.e5.
52. Howell MD, Kim BE, Gao P, Grant AV, Boguniewicz M, DeBenedetto A, et al. Cytokine modulation of atopic dermatitis filaggrin skin expression. J Allergy Clin Immunol. 2009;124(3 Suppl 2):R7–R12.
53. Levin J, Fallon Friedlander S, Del Rosso JQ. Atopic dermatitis and the stratum corneum: part 3: the immune system in atopic dermatitis. J Clin Aesthet Dermatol. 2013;6(12):37–44.
54. Thaçi D, Simpson EL, Beck LA, Bieber T, Blauvelt A, Papp K, et al. Efficacy and safety of dupilumab in adults with moderate-to-severe atopic dermatitis inadequately controlled by topical treatments: a randomised, placebo-controlled, dose-ranging phase 2b trial. Lancet. 2016;387(10013):40–52.
55. Cornelissen C, Marquardt Y, Czaja K, Wenzel J, Frank J, Lüscher-Firzlaff J, et al. IL-31 regulates differentiation and filaggrin expression in human organotypic skin models. J Allergy Clin Immunol. 2012;129(2):426–33.e4338.
56. Hatano Y, Terashi H, Arakawa S, Katagiri K. Interleukin-4 suppresses the enhancement of ceramide synthesis and cutaneous permeability barrier functions induced by tumor necrosis factor-alpha and interferon-gamma in human epidermis. J Invest Dermatol. 2005;124(4):786–92.
57. Spergel JM. From atopic dermatitis to asthma: the atopic march. Ann Allergy Asthma Immunol. 2010;105(2):99–117.
58. Du Toit G, Sayre PH, Roberts G, Sever ML, Lawson K, Bahnson HT, et al. Effect of avoidance on peanut allergy after early peanut consumption. N Engl J Med. 2016;374(15):1435–43.
59. Perkin MR, Logan K, Tseng A, Raji B, Ayis S, Peacock J, et al. Randomized trial of introduction of allergenic foods in breast-fed infants. N Engl J Med. 2016;374(18):1733–43.

Immune-Meidated Pathogenesis of Atopic Dermatitis

Chang Ook Park and Tae-Gyun Kim

Innate Immune Response

Atopic dermatitis is a chronic recurrent inflammatory skin disease whose cause is not well known, but it is reported to be induced by a combination of genetic causes, abnormal skin barrier, and immunological factors. Moreover, environmental elements are highly likely to contribute to the current increasing prevalence of atopic dermatitis [1].

Histological findings of atopic dermatitis can be classified into acute and subacute/chronic phases. Histological characteristics of an acute phase are spongiosis of the epidermis and the infiltration of various immune cells. As atopic dermatitis develops into a subacute/chronic phase, there are more lichenified lesions and acanthosis, which is thickening of the epidermis. In the moderate to severe phase of atopic dermatitis, numerous immune cells are significantly infiltrated [2]. Since there are innate immune cells such as eosinophils and mast cells infiltrated in combination with the acquired immune cells like dendritic cells and T cells, many researches are being actively conducted on those various and new innate immune cells (Table 1).

C. O. Park (✉) · T.-G. Kim
Department of Dermatology, Cutaneous Biology Research Institute, Yonsei University College of Medicine, Seoul, Korea (Republic of)
e-mail: copark@yuhs.ac

Innate Immune Cell

Eosinophil

Since the Eosinophil level is elevated in serum and skin lesions of atopic dermatitis, eosinophil appears to play a critical role in causing atopic dermatitis. It is also known that there is a correlation between the number of infiltrated eosinophils and the severity of atopic dermatitis. Furthermore, eosinophils may contribute to the chronicity of atopic dermatitis, due to its increase in skin lesions of chronic atopic dermatitis. Patients with atopic dermatitis have an elevated level of Th2 cytokines, such as IL-4, IL-5, and IL-13, which affect production, survival, infiltration of eosinophils [3]. In the epidermal lesion of atopic dermatitis, thymic stromal lymphopoietin (TSLP), which induces Th2 immune response, is increased. Thus, it is possible that TSLP directs eosinophils infiltrating into the skin lesions of atopic dermatitis patients [4]. Once eosinophils are stimulated, it leads to a release of various inflammation mediators, such as eosinophil cationic protein, eosinophil-derived neurotoxin, and major basic protein. In addition, eosinophils involve inflammation of atopic dermatitis by releasing a variety of cytokines and chemokines, such as IL-1β, IL-6, IL-31, CXCL1, CXCL8, CCL2, CCL18, and CCL26 [3].

K. H. Lee et al. (eds.), *Practical Insights into Atopic Dermatitis*,
https://doi.org/10.1007/978-981-15-8159-5_8

Table 1 Innate immune cells in atopic dermatitis

Cell type	Induced by major cytokines from the epidermis	The most produced cytokines and chemokines	Transcription factor
Mast cells	TSLP	IL-5, IL-13, IL-6, GM-CSF, CXCL8, CCL1	GATA-2, PU.1
Basophils	TSLP	IL-4, IL-6, CXCL12, CCL12, CCL3	C/EBPα
Eosinophils	TSLP	IL-6, CXCL8, CXCL1, CCL2	GATA-1, PU.1
NKT cells	TSLP	IL-4, IL-13	PLZF, GATA-3
ILCs	TSLP, IL-25, IL-33	IL-5, IL-13	RORα, GATA-3

C/EBPα CCAAT enhancer-binding protein α, *CCL* CC chemokine ligand, *CXCL* CXC chemokine ligand, *GATA-2* GATA binding protein 2, *GATA-3* GATA binding protein 3, *GM-CSF* Granulocyte-macrophage colony-stimulating factor, *IL* interleukin, *ILC* Innate lymphoid cell, *NKT* natural killer T, *PLZF* Promyelocytic leukemia zinc finger protein, *PU.1* Purine-rich box-1, *RORα* Retinoic acid–related orphan receptor α, *RORγt* Retinoic acid-related orphan receptor γt, *TSLP* Thymic stromal lymphopoietin

Mast Cell

The role of mast cells has not yet been known well; however, it has been reported to have a higher level of mast cells in skin lesions of atopic dermatitis patients. If the atopic dermatitis patient gets exposed to an allergen, FcεRI of mast cells combines with allergen-specific IgE. Then mast cells become degranulated and exhibit the symptoms by releasing histamine, heparin, serotonin, prostaglandins, leukotriens, major basic protein, and platelet-activating factor. Such histamine and tryptase from mast cells induce itchiness and secondary damage on the skin barrier. Mast cells further infiltrate into the lesions and aggravate atopic dermatitis symptoms. By interaction of chemokine and adhesion molecules in vascular endothelial cells, mast cells guide T cells to the lesion. Mast cells activated by the elevated TSLP milieu are stimulated to release Th2 cytokines. Mast cells also secrete IL-5, IL-13, IL-6, GM-CSF, CXCL8, CCL1, and so on [3].

Basophil

Basophils, initially known as counterparts residing in the blood of mast cells in skin tissues, also get degranulated when their FcεRI, like the ones in mast cells, adhere to allergen-specific IgE. The increased TSLP in atopic dermatitis then activates basophils and secrete Th2 cytokines. Basophils can release IL-4, IL-6, CXCL12, CCL12, CCL3, etc. [3].

Innate T Cell

Recently, there has been a number of studies actively going on about innate T cells, which display different patterns from those of conventional T cells. Unlike the conventional ones, innate T cells do not have memory about immunity. So that is why one of the newly named innate T cells is called natural killer T (NKT) cells. NKT cells own markers for both natural killer cells and T cells. In the case of human NKT cells, they have invariant T cell receptors (TCR) consisted of Vα24-Jα18 TCRα chain and Vβ11 chain. These receptors of NKT cells recognize glycolipid, which is related with CD1d, in a way of pattern recognition receptor (PRR) that binds to the very initial condition of a well-conserved part, transcending the species. Various stimulants make NKT cells release Th1 (IFN-γ), Th2 (IL-4, IL-13), and Th17 (IL-17) [3]. There are also a lot of NKT cells infiltrating into the lesions of atopic dermatitis patients, and increased TSLP in

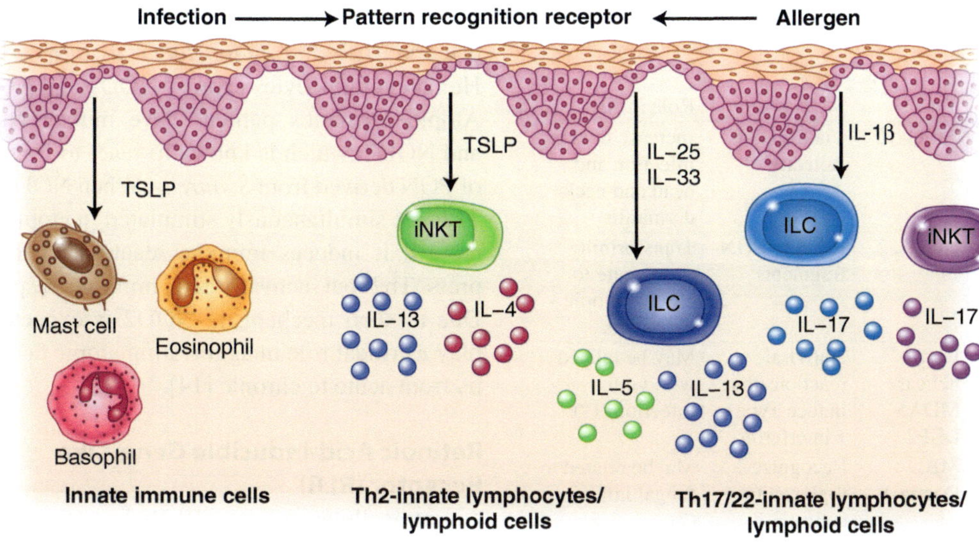

Fig. 1 The photomechanism of innate immune cells in atopic dermatitis

atopic dermatitis patients activates NKT cells to secrete Th2 cytokines [5, 6].

Innate Lymphoid Cell (ILC)

Even though they do not have markers for B cells and T cells that are present in a number of peripheral tissues, innate lymphoid cells (ILC) are named as such because there are cells found similar to lymphocytes in a morphological way. There are many studies on ILC as well [7]. As it has been proved in experiments of atopic dermatitis mice, ILCs can induce allergic inflammation even in a condition without conventional B cells and T cells. In a sense that ILC can cause skin inflammation regardless of acquired immune mechanisms, it has been emphasizing the importance of innate immune mechanisms once again in the field of atopic dermatitis immunology [7]. Stimulated by various factors, ILCs produce Th1 (IFN-γ), Th2 (IL-4, IL-13), and Th17 (IL-17), like NKT cells. Not only an increased level of ILC in the atopic dermatitis skin lesions but also TSLP, IL-25, and IL-23 released from the epidermis of atopic dermatitis patients activate ILC cells and lead to the release of Th2 cytokines [8] (Fig. 1).

Pattern Recognition Receptor (PRR)

Pattern recognition receptors (PRR) recognize the most well-conserved pathogen-associated molecular patterns that numerous pathogens commonly have. Atopic dermatitis patients are vulnerable to bacterial and viral infections because various PRRs participate in the stimulation of infectious agents in atopic dermatitis (Table 2).

Toll-like Receptor (TLR)

TLR, the most well-known type of PRR, varies from TLR1 through TLR10 in human bodies. TLR1, 2, 4–6, and 10 exist on the cell surface, while TLR2, 7–9 inside cells. There is TLR in innate immune cells or keratinocyte, and the activated TLR stimulates transcription factors like activator protein (AP)-1 and nuclear factor (NF)-κB and causes a release of cytokines, chemokines, antimicrobial peptides (AMP) that react

Table 2 Pattern recognition receptors in atopic dermatitis

PRR type	Type	Mechanism	Role in AD
TLR	TLR1-10	Via MyD88 Activate AP-1& NF-κB	Increase in skin infection and head and neck dermatitis
NLR	NOD1, 2	React to PGN fragments	Transforming from acute to chronic atopic dermatitis
RLR	RIG-I-helicase MDA5 LGP2	Antiviral reactions that induce Type 1 interferon	May be related with viral infections (?)
CLR	MBL Dectin-1	Recognize β-glucan to activate NF-κB	Maybe related to fungal infections (?)

AP activator protein, *CLR* C-type lectin receptor, *LGP2* laboratory of genetics and physiology 2, *MBL* mannan-binding lectin, *MDA5* melanoma differentiation-associated protein 5, *MyD88* myeloid differentiation factor 88, *NF* nuclear factor, *NLR* NOD-like receptor, *NOD* nucleotide-binding oligomerization domain-containing protein, *PRR* pattern recognition receptor, *RIG* retinoic acid-inducible gene, *RLR* Retinoic acid-inducible gene-like receptor, *TLR* Toll-like receptor

to various types of infections [9]. In the case of atopic dermatitis, there is an elevated level of Th2 cytokines, causing a reduction in TLR expression and thus increased skin infections in atopic dermatitis patients [10]. Moreover, many atopic dermatitis patients are low in Vitamin D, which induces antimicrobial peptides through TLR [11]. Since atopic dermatitis patients who have affected in head and neck area tend to be low in vitamin D [12], they become sensitive to the infection by fungi such as *Malassezia*. This mechanism is likely to be the reason why atopic dermatitis patients get vulnerable to skin infections.

NOD-Like Receptor (NLR)

NOD (nucleotide-binding oligomerization domain-containing protein)-like receptors are intracellular ones. There are NOD1 and NOD2, which both react to pieces of bacterial breakdown products, peptidoglycans (PGN). NOD1 reacts to Gram-negative bacteria selectively, while NOD2 recognize muramyl dipeptide on PGN of various bacteria, including *Staphylococcus aureus* [13]. Human keratinocytes express NOD1 and NOD2. Atopic dermatitis patients have mutant NOD1 and NOD2, which is known to react to fragment of PGN derived from *S. aureus*. When NOD2 and TLR are simultaneously stimulated in atopic dermatitis, it induces immune reactions that suppress Th2 but activate Th1 immune response. Due to such mechanism, NOD2 is expected to play a critical role in aggravating atopic dermatitis from acute to chronic [14].

Retinoic Acid-Inducible Gene-Like Receptor (RLR)

An intracellular receptor, RLRs have C-terminal helicase domains that recognize viral genome RNA and transfer signals via the N-terminal CARD domain. There are retinoic acid-inducible gene (RIG)-I-helicase, MDA5, LGP2, etc. in RLR. An active form of RLR is highly important in antiviral immune reactions that induce Type 1 interferon. Although it has not been known much about the role of RLR in atopic dermatitis, it is speculated to be involved in viral infections of atopic dermatitis patients [10, 14].

C-Type Lectin Receptor (CLR)

CLR specifically recognizes sugar in bacteria, fungi, and viruses. Mannan-binding lectin (MBL) is one of the most representative CLRs. A cell membrane-penetrating receptor, dectin-1 recognizes β-glucan on cell walls of fungi to activate NF-κB and thus release a number of inflammatory cytokines. It has not been defined much about the roles of CLR in atopic dermatitis, however, it is expected to be related to numerous infections [10, 14].

Antimicrobial Peptide (AMP)

AMP, a significant element for innate immunity, was derived from lysozyme found by Fleming in the 1920s. Since then, over 200 types of AMP have been found and registered. A majority of AMPs are cationic peptides, which display a wide range of antimicrobial reactions and present

Table 3 Antimicrobial peptides in atopic dermatitis

AMP type	Function	Role in AD
Defensin (α,β)	hBD-1: constitutive hBD-2: induced hBD-3: induced	Suppress an induction of hBD-2 and hBD-3: Decrease in antimicrobial reaction
Cathelicidin (LL-37)	LL-37: induced	Suppress an induction of LL-37: Decrease in antimicrobial reaction
RNase7	RNase7: constitutive	Suppress an induction of RNase7: Decrease in antimicrobial reaction
Dermcidin	Dermcidin: constitutive	Suppress secretion of dermcidin from sweat: Decrease in antimicrobial reaction
S100A7 S100A8 S100A9	S100A7: constitutive S100A8: induced S100A9: induced	Act as DAMP: induce inflammation reaction

AMP antimicrobial peptide, *hBD* human β-defensin, *DAMP* damage-associated molecular pattern

in every epithelial cell. AMP is known to bind to anionic components of the bacterial cell membrane and to kill bacteria by destroying their cell membrane. Keratinocytes are the major cells that express AMP on normal skin tissues. Once skin gets damaged, keratinocytes induce AMP. AMPs in atopic dermatitis skin show a much less level of AMP expression than that of psoriasis skin (Table 3) [15].

Defensin

There are α-defensin and β-defensin in humans, and β-defensin is an essential antimicrobial peptide for skin antimicrobial activities. β-defensin-1 (hBD-1) in human bodies constitutively present in normal conditions. Although hBD-2 and hBD-3 are induced in conditions with inflammation or infections, they present in a very low level in normal status. There is no difference in hBD-1 between atopic dermatitis and psoriasis; however, the induced AMPs such as hBD-2 and hBD-3 show a lower expression level in atopic dermatitis than psoriasis. The mechanism is reported that Th2 cytokines in atopic dermatitis suppress the expression of hBD-2 and hBD-3 in atopic dermatitis patients [16].

Cathelicidin (LL-37)

While cathelicidin (LL-37) presents in a significantly low level in normal keratinocytes, they are AMP induced in case of inflammation or damage. LL-37 works together with hBD-1 to amplify antimicrobial activities. An expression of LL-37 is known to be more reduced in atopic dermatitis than in psoriasis [15].

RNase7

RNase7 is also an AMP that presents constitutively in normal skin. Rnase7 shows strong antimicrobial activity to *S. aureus*. An expression of RNase7 is known to be reduced in atopic dermatitis than in psoriasis [15].

Dermcidin

Dermcidin is an AMP that presents constitutively in the sweat gland, unlike the abovementioned AMP that is expressed in keratinocytes. Dermcidin in human sweats shows antimicrobial reactions to *S. aureus* and *Candida albicans*. Sweats of atopic dermatitis patients show a reduced expression level of dermcidin than those of normal people [17].

S100A7 (Psoriasin), S100A8, S100A9

S100A7 (psoriasin), an AMP that exist constitutively in normal skin, becomes induced in case of skin inflammation or damage. S100A7 is known to have antimicrobial effects against *Escherichia coli*. Unlike other AMPs, atopic dermatitis skin shows an increased expression of S100A7, S100A8, and S100A9, which are not only antimicrobial peptides but also damage-associated molecular patterns (DAMP) molecules that transfer signals associated with innate immune reaction caused by inflammation or external damage. In the presence of S100A8/A9 that are increased in atopic dermatitis, keratinocytes produce IL-33 that induces Th2 immune response in atopic dermatitis [18]. In psoriasis, the increased AMP, LL-37, also stimulates plasmacytoid dendritic cell (pDC) and causes inflammation, which is likely to be DAMP-associated inflammation [19].

Adaptive Immune Response

Atopic dermatitis is a chronic inflammatory skin disease showing recurrent eczematous skin lesions characterized by early age of onset, persistent itch, and concomitant systemic allergic features such as allergic asthma and an increased level of immunoglobulin E. In our body, different T cell immune responses such as Th1 and Th2 should be balanced to maintain immune homeostasis. However, changes in T cell immune homeostasis have a profound effect on the development of atopic dermatitis. Various clinical observations and studies have shown that T cells play the most important role in the development of atopic dermatitis [20]. In particular, skin-homing memory T cells play an important role in the recurrent phase of atopic dermatitis [21]. It can be confirmed with the fact that eczema does not occur without T cells, and atopic dermatitis is improved by suppressing activated T cells with topical calcineurin inhibitors in animal models. This section examines Th1/Th2 imbalance, T reg cells, Th17 cells, and Th22 cells in atopic dermatitis. We also look at acquired immunological factors involved in the development of atopic dermatitis, such as dendritic cells and cytokines produced by T cells that affect T cell activation.

T Cell

Th1/Th2 Cell Imbalance

Atopic dermatitis lesions are infiltrated by a number of CD4+ T cells, which is one of the characteristic findings of atopic dermatitis [2]. In particular, atopic dermatitis is caused by Th2 cells among CD4+ T cells, and accordingly, diseases such as ulcerative colitis and inflammatory bowel disease can be accompanied. Acute lesions of atopic dermatitis are caused by Th2/Th22 responses [22]. On the other hand, chronic lesions are caused by Th1 responses, and Th0 cells (those that share the activity of Th1 and Th2 cells) and Th1 cells play a major role. Depending on the responses, cytokines are also diverse. Th2 cytokines such as IL-4, IL-5, IL-13 are increased in acute lesions, and interferon-gamma (IFN-γ), IL-12, IL-5, granulocyte macrophage colony-stimulating factor (GM-CSF) are increased in chronic lesions [23, 24]. However, although Th1 responses are important in chronic lesions, the main cells infiltrating atopic dermatitis lesions are Th2 cells [25].

The percentage of Th1 cells in chronic atopic dermatitis was only 0.09 compared to Th2 cells. Th2 cells accounted for 64.6% of the total T cells and 4.8% of Th1 cells [26]. In other words, although the Th1 response predominates as the lesion becomes chronic, it can be confirmed that Th2 cells are an important factor for the development and persistence of atopic dermatitis.

In addition, IL-5 produced by Th2 cells is involved in eosinophil development and survival, and GM-CSF inhibits cell death of monocytes and plays a role in sustaining atopic dermatitis [21]. The change from acute to chronic lesions is thought to be due to the action of IL-12 produced in eosinophils or inflammatory dendritic epidermal cells (IDEC) [27].

Cytokines

IL-4 and IL-13

IL-4 is the most important cytokine among Th2 cytokines and plays an important role in the differentiation of Th2 cells and the production of IgE. In rat experiments with genetic modifications to overexpress IL-4, all skin findings of atopic dermatitis including pruritus, infiltration of inflammatory cells, and susceptibility to bacterial infection, increased levels of IgG1 and IgE, were demonstrated [28]. IL-4 receptors are expressed in T cells, B cells, mast cells, and macrophages [29]. When IL-4 is engaged to these receptors, low-affinity IgE receptors are expressed on the surface of B cells, monocytes, and macrophages. When IL-4 stimulates IL-4 receptors in B cells, Janus kinase-1 and -3 are activated, leading to the activation of STAT6, increasing the production of IgE [21]. IL-4 acts on Th0 cells to promote differentiation and growth into Th2 cells, and newly differentiated and grown Th2 cells produce IL-4, amplifying and sustaining Th2 responses. In addition, IL-4 inhibits the production of IFN-γ and prevents the differentiation into Th1 cells [21, 22].

IL-4 and IL-13 promote microbial invasion by inhibiting the production of antimicrobial peptides in the epidermis, as well as inhibiting the production of lipids in the stratum corneum, causing epidermal barrier damage [29]. It also inhibits the expression of major epidermal differentiation complexes such as filaggrin, loricrin, and involucrin, and inhibits keratinocyte differentiation through the STAT3 pathway. The use of Janus kinase inhibitors in animal models of atopic dermatitis inhibited STAT3 activation and restored skin barrier function [30]. In addition, a clinical trial using topical tofacitinib, a local Janus kinase inhibitor, has demonstrated its effectiveness [31]. Those results suggest that JAK inhibition would block the mechanism of action of IL-4 and IL-13.

In addition, IL-4 and IL-13 induce the expression of TSLP, which contributes to the association of barrier abnormality and Th2 response in keratinocytes [32]. TSLP derived from keratinocytes strongly activates dendritic cells which stimulate Th2 cells by expressing OX40L on the surface [27, 32]. IL-4 and IL-13 also induce the expression of adhesion molecules in vascular endothelial cells to recruit various inflammatory cells into the skin. In recent clinical trials, duplimumab, which inhibits IL-4 and IL-13 as a monoclonal antibody against anti-IL-4 receptor alpha, has shown therapeutic effects and safety [33, 34].

IL-5

IL-5 is a cytokine involved in the infiltration and increase of eosinophils. The mRNA of IL-4 was increased in acute lesions and decreased when the lesion became chronic, but IL-5 mRNA was increased in both acute and chronic lesions [35]. IL-5 produces eosinophil colony-stimulating factor and eosinophil growth-stimulating factor to increase blood eosinophils and increase eosinophil survival. Eosinophils activated by IL-5 release various pro-allergic mediators such as eosinophilic cationic protein, major basic protein, and reactive oxygen species to mediate allergic inflammatory reactions and skin damage.

IL-18

In a sterile mouse model, IL-18 played a role in the development of spontaneous atopic dermatitis-like lesions [36]. In addition, maternal blood and umbilical cord IL-18 levels have been shown to be important determinants of atopic dermatitis. Increases in serum IL-18 and IL-18 receptors have been shown to be associated with atopic dermatitis severity [37]. IL-18 is a Th1 cytokine produced by various cells such as keratinocytes, mast cells, IDEC, monocyte-derived dendritic cells [38]. Of these, keratinocytes and mast cells produce IL-18 in response to the allergens such as house dust mites or to the bacteria such as *staphylococcus aureus* [39]. In this process, cytotoxic T cells secrete perforin and granzyme B to activate pro-IL-18.

In acute atopic dermatitis lesions, IL-18 promotes Th2 production by activating basophils, mast cells, and CD4+ T cells without IL-12. On the other hand, chronic lesions stimulate Th1 cells with IL-12 to produce IFN-γ. In addition, IL-18 contributes to CD4+ T cells and NKT cell-dependent IgE production. In patients with atopic dermatitis, corticotropin-releasing hormone reduces IL-18 expression in monocyte-derived dendritic cells independent of receptors, suggesting that stress may increase IL-18 and exacerbate atopic dermatitis symptoms [40].

IL-31

IL-31, a new Th2 cytokine, is a major inflammatory factor that causes itching in atopic dermatitis. In atopic dermatitis, IL-31 protein and RNA were increased, and serum IL-31 levels were proportional to disease severity [21]. Also, IL-31 interferes with the final differentiation of the epidermis and promotes inflammatory precursor cytokine secretion [41]. In addition, IL-31 can affect the composition of lipids and impair epidermal barrier function, which is known to decrease the expression of filaggrin and loricrin, thereby preventing the final differentiation of the epidermis.

IL-31 works by binding to a heterodimeric receptor composed of the IL-31 receptor (IL-31RA) and the oncostatin M receptor beta complex. IL-31RA is found in keratinocytes, macrophages, eosinophils, and nerve fibers in patients with atopic dermatitis, and the dorsal root ganglion of healthy people. The IL-31/IL-31RA complex activates signaling pathways such as the JAK-STAT pathway, mitogen-activated protein kinase, and phosphatidyl-inositol-3-kinase pathway. A recent study showed the efficacy and safety of the human anti-IL-31RA monoclonal antibody in reducing itching of atopic dermatitis [42]. This suggests that the itching-inducing effect of IL-31 occurs through IL-31RA. Some studies have shown that the itching-inducing effect of IL-31 is indirectly mediated by keratinocytes and secondary itching-causing agents, not skin neuroreceptors [43].

IL-33

IL-33 is an IL-1 family cytokine produced by innate immune cells. It is produced when stimulated by allergens or microorganisms and acts by binding to the ST2 receptor [20]. In the in vitro experiments, IL-33 acted on Th2 cells and generated IL-5 and IL-13 [44]. On the other hand, it increased the number of blood eosinophils and serum immunoglobulins in the in vivo experiments. In addition, ST2 receptors are also present in mast cells and mast cells stimulated by IL-33 were found to produce chemokines and cytokines such as IL-5, IL-6, IL-10, IL-13, CXCL8, and CCL1 [45]. In addition, it has been reported that IL-33 mRNA is increased about 10 times in the skin of atopic patients compared to that of healthy people. As such, IL-33 produced by keratinocytes and innate immune cells plays an important role in the expression of Th2 cytokines and is thought to play an important role in the initiation of Th2 response. In this process, it was found that type 2 innate lymphoid cells play an important role [21]. The Th2 cytokines and their roles related to atopic dermatitis are summarized in Fig. 2.

Treg Cell

Treg cells are immunosuppressive cells that inhibit both Th1 and Th2 responses and are characterized by high expression of the IL-2 receptor alpha receptor (CD25) and the transcription factor FOXP3 [21]. According to Dudda et al., in the Foxp3 deficient Scurfy mouse model, the ability of Treg cells to actively migrate to the skin and suppress skin inflammation was impaired [46]. According to these results, it seems that Treg cells play an important role in maintaining homeostasis of skin immunity.

Some studies have shown that Treg cells are reduced in skin lesions of atopic dermatitis [47–50]. In addition, *Staphylococcus aureus* can further exacerbate skin inflammation by inhibiting the function of Treg cells. However, research on Treg cells in atopic dermatitis has many contradictory results, so further researches will be needed to elucidate the pathophysiological role of Tregs in atopic dermatitis immune responses.

Th17 Cell

Th17 cells contribute to the onset of acute lesions of atopic dermatitis [21]. IL-17 is thought to play a role in the differentiation of Th2 cells. Th17 cells produce IL-17 and IL-22 to induce the production of S100 protein, antibacterial peptide, and various inflammatory cytokines. As Th2 cytokines inhibit IL-17 production, IL-17 gradually decreases in chronic atopic dermatitis lesions. IL-17 is lower in patients with atopic dermatitis than in patients with psoriasis, which is thought to be due to the inhibitory effect of Th2 cytokines [51]. The relative deficiency of IL-17 in atopic dermatitis lesions is associated with a decrease in antimicrobial peptides and an increase in susceptibility to skin infection.

Increased Th17 counts and increased IL-17 expression in atopic dermatitis lesions and serum are associated with disease severity, and this association is particularly pronounced in intrinsic atopic dermatitis [52]. In the transcriptome analysis of intrinsic and extrinsic atopic dermatitis patients, intrinsic atopic dermatitis patients showed stronger Th17 and Th22 activation than extrinsic atopic dermatitis patients. Unlike those with atopic dermatitis in Europe or the United States, patients with atopic dermatitis in Asia also showed more severe epidermal hyperplasia and

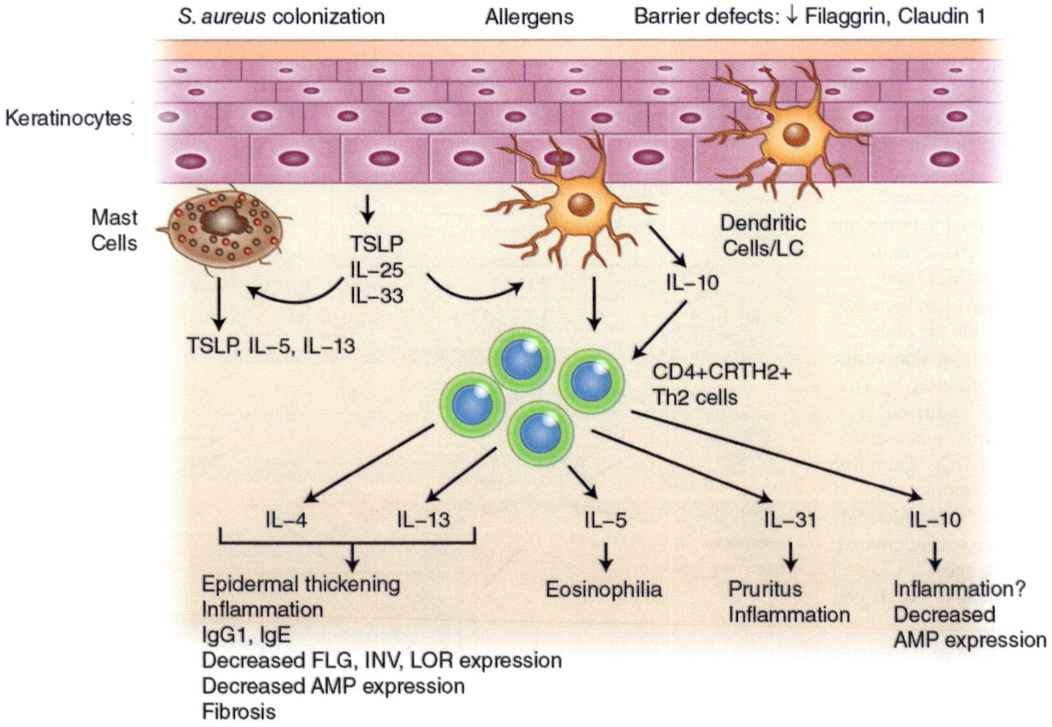

Fig. 2 The role of Th2 cytokines expressed in atopic dermatitis. Langerhans cells and dendritic cells promote the differentiation of Th2 cells, whereby activated or differentiated Th2 cells secrete IL-4, IL-5, IL-13, IL-31. Each cytokine decreases antimicrobial peptides (AMP) and several proteins important for skin barrier function (filaggrin (FLG), loricrin (LOR), involucrin (INV)), causes inflammation and fibrosis. The function of IL-10 is still controversial

hyperkeratosis in patients with extrinsic atopic dermatitis and were found to show strong Th17 and Th22 activation similar to psoriasis [53]. However, another study conducted in Europe and the United States showed that the number of Th17 cells and the expression of IL-17 were decreased in patients with severe atopic dermatitis [24]. Therefore, further study is needed to understand the role of Th17 cells in atopic dermatitis.

Th22 Cell

Existing theories that atopic dermatitis occurs by activation of Th2 cannot explain the epidermal hyperplasia seen in chronic atopic dermatitis. However, as new subtypes of T cells have recently been discovered, the main cause of epidermal hyperplasia in atopic dermatitis is thought to be mediated by Th2/Th22 (Fig. 3). Recent studies have shown that Th22 cells produce IL-22, which is involved in skin barrier damage and epidermal hyperplasia [26, 54].

In atopic dermatitis patients, both Th2 and Th22 cells are involved in the defect of the skin barrier. IL-22, similar to Th2 cytokines, inhibits the major final differentiation protein and damages the epidermal barrier [21]. In addition, IL-22 increases IL-6 secretion by increasing S100A7, S100A8, and S100A9 gene expression, which suppresses epidermal differentiation and shows an inflammatory effect in atopic dermatitis lesions [21]. In addition, IL-22 and IL-17 increase the expression of S100 protein and antibacterial peptide in the epidermis. The secretion of IL-22 is immediately induced by

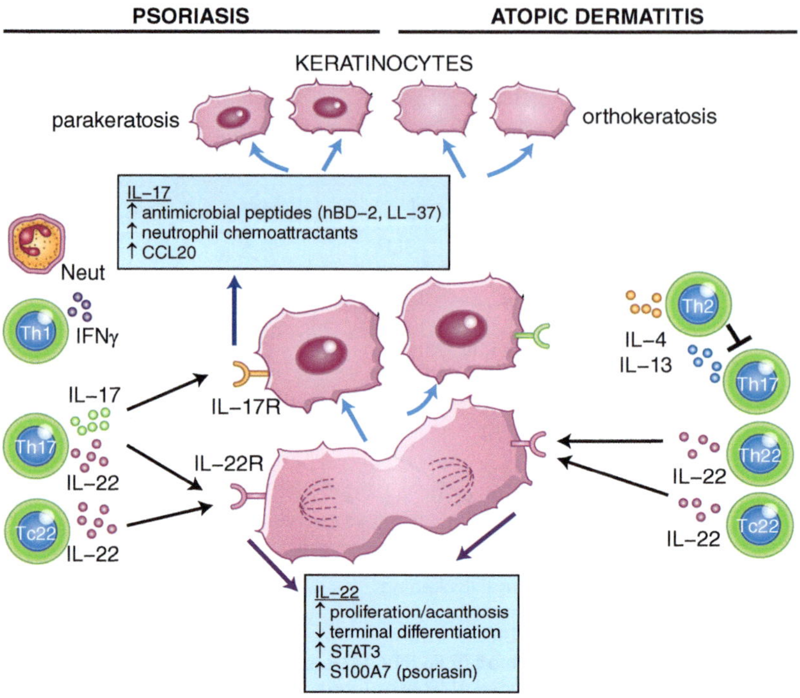

Fig. 3 Expression of Th22 cells in psoriasis and atopic dermatitis. In psoriasis, Th1 cells express IFN-r, Th17 cells produce IL-17 and IL-22, and the induced Th22 cells produce IL-22. As IL-17 increases, antimicrobial peptides and CCL20 increase, and epidermal thickening occurs due to an increase in IL-22. On the other hand, in atopic dermatitis, IL-17 is inhibited by Th2 cytokines, and IL-22 is significantly increased by Th22 and Tc22. Therefore, in chronic atopic dermatitis, the epidermal thickening is exacerbated by IL-22, and histologically, it is shaped like psoriasis

Staphylococcus aureus exotoxin and house dust mite and amplifies chronic skin inflammation in patients with atopic dermatitis [55]. In addition, IL-22 stimulates CCL17 production in human keratinocytes and promotes T cell skin migration [55]. Depending on the patient's age and disease activity, the activity of Th22 cells is also different, and in the case of infant atopic dermatitis, Th1/Th2 cell imbalance is mainly found, but in adult atopic dermatitis, the Th2/Th22 cell subtype is expressed [23]. The immunological mechanism of T cells in atopic dermatitis is summarized in Fig. 4.

Dendritic Cell

Dendritic cells play an important role in inducing the development of atopic dermatitis by uptaking antigens and presenting them to T cells [27]. Unlike dendritic cells of other skin diseases, Langerhans cells and IDEC of atopic dermatitis express FcεRI (high-affinity IgE receptor) [56]. Langerhans cells with Birbeck granules are present in both lesions and non-lesions of atopic dermatitis patients. When IgE and FcεRI are combined by allergens, Langerhans cells produce IL-16 and monocyte chemotactic protein to induce CD4+ T cells into the skin. In addition, Langerhans cells sensitize T cells by presenting antigens to T cells, activate not only memory Th2 cells, but also migrate to lymph nodes so that naïve T cells differentiate into Th2 cells. This Th2 immune response and amplification of the immune response plays an important role in the initial formation of atopic dermatitis lesions. In addition, Langerhans cells could prime Th22 cells which are important T cell subset in atopic dermatitis [57]. Thus, Langerhans cells would be crucial dendritic cell population in atopic dermatitis pathomechanisms.

On the other hand, in the case of chronic lesions, IDEC on the inflammatory site plays an important role. The monocytes that have migrated to the skin differentiate into IDEC to produce pro-inflammatory cytokines IL-1, IL-6, and TNF-α. IDEC is known to infiltrate within the first 48 h in an atopic patch model. In atopic dermatitis, IDEC functions as an antigen presenter and secretes IL-12 and IL-18 to convert Th2 cells into Th1/0 cells. Th1/0 cells produce IFN-γ, IL-5, and IL-31, which are important in the chronic

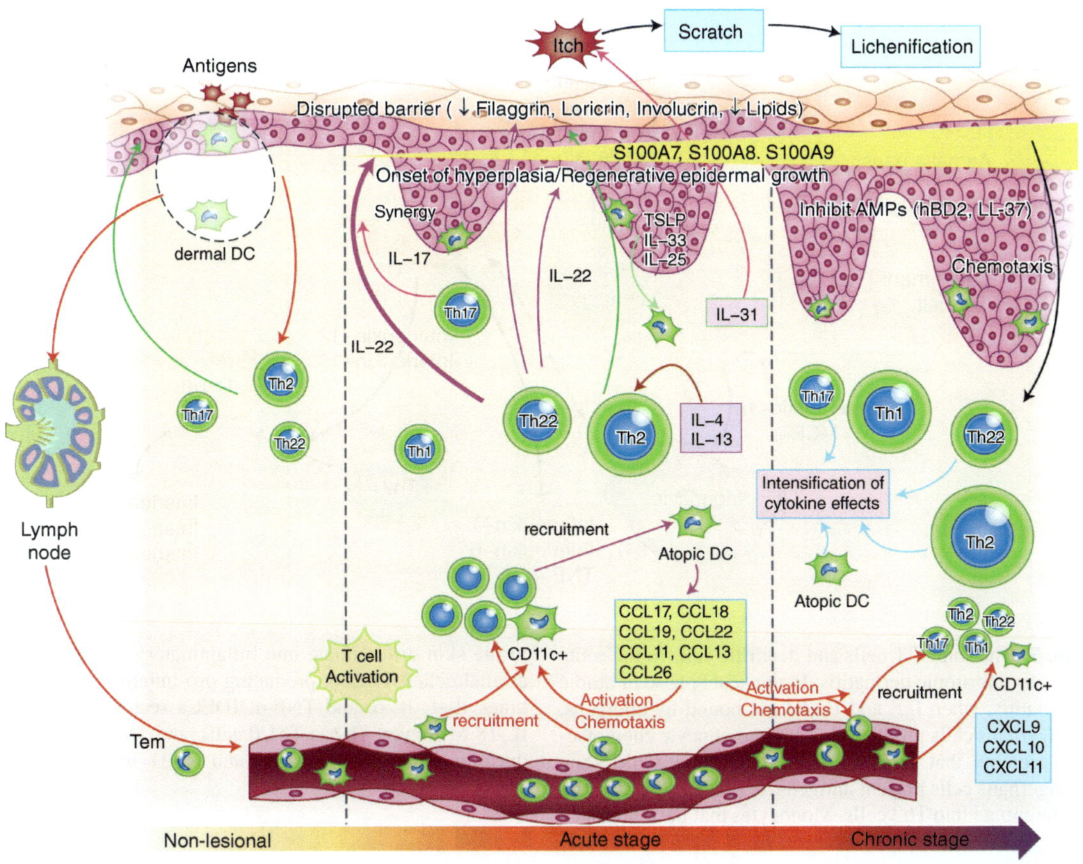

Fig. 4 Immunological mechanism of atopic dermatitis by time, considering Th17 and Th22. IL-4 and IL-13 are increased in the non-lesional area of atopic dermatitis, and thus the skin barrier is easily damaged. Damage to the skin barrier makes allergens easily permeable, and when allergens meet Langerhans cells and dendritic cells, Th2 and Th22 cells are activated and the acute phase of atopic dermatitis begins. From the acute phase, the weak activation of Th1 and Th17 cells begins to occur and the activity gradually increases as the chronic phase progresses. With the continuous activation of Th2 and Th22 cells, a typical clinical pattern of chronic atopic dermatitis appears, and IL-22 together with IL-17 increases the expression of S100A7, S100A8, and S100A9 proteins, causing hyperproliferation of the epidermis

phase. Accordingly, in the early stage of atopic dermatitis, an inflammatory reaction caused by the Th2 immune response is induced, and Th1 immune response occurs by IDEC appearing on the inflammatory site as it progresses to a chronic site [27] (Fig. 5).

Compared to the other DCs, low frequency of plasmacytoid dendritic cells (pDC) are observed in atopic dermatitis skin lesions [58]. After allergen stimulation, the modified immune function of pDC in atopic dermatitis patients is thought to contribute to the local deficiency of type 1 IFN, resulting in increased susceptibility to viral infection in atopic dermatitis patients. In addition, pDC stimulates differentiation of Th22 cells in chronic atopic dermatitis lesions.

In epidermal dendritic cells of patients with atopic dermatitis, the expression of IFN-γ receptors and the response to IFN-γ are increased. Activated epidermal Langerhans cells and dermal dendritic cells produce CCL17 and CCL22, respectively, to induce and amplify Th2 responses [59]. In addition, Langerhans cells and dermal dendritic cells induce differentiation into Th22 cells, and IL-6 and TNF-a secreted from dendritic cells have been suggested as contrib-

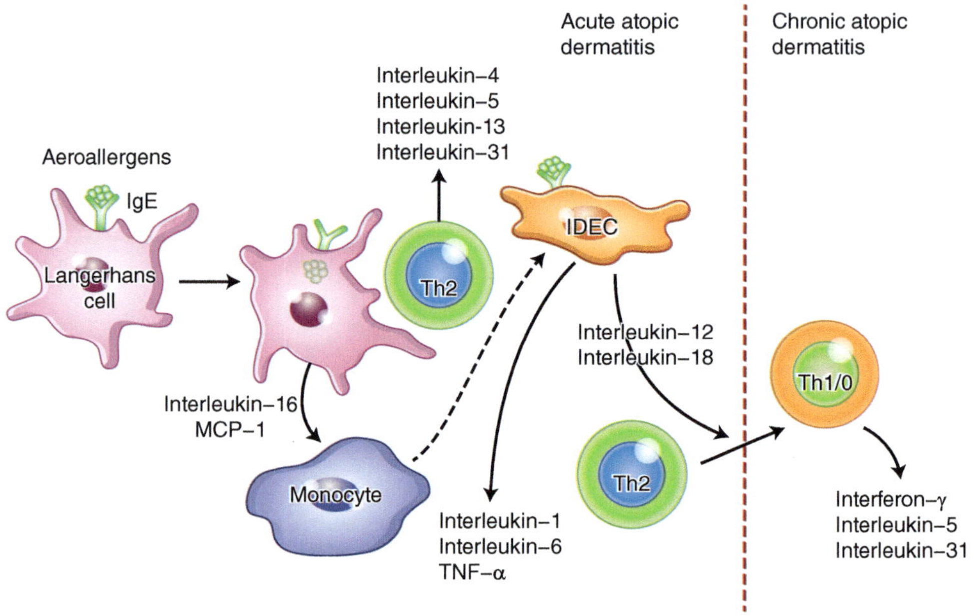

Fig. 5 The role of T cells and dendritic cells in the acute and chronic atopic dermatitis. In the acute phase of atopic dermatitis, when IgE and FcεRI are bound by allergens, Langerhans cells produce IL-16 and monocyte chemotactic proteins that induce CD4+ T cells into the skin. Langerhans cells present antigens to T cells, sensitize and differentiate into Th2 cells. Monocytes that have migrated to the skin differentiate into inflammatory dendritic epidermal cells (IDECs), producing pro-inflammatory cytokines IL-1, IL-6, and TNF-α. IDECs secrete IL-12 and IL-18 to convert Th2 to Th1/0 cells, and Th1/0 cells produce important IFN-γ, IL-5, and IL-31 in the chronic phase

uting factors [57]. Langerhans cells, IDEC, and pDC express histamine receptor H4. In atopic dermatitis lesions, histamine secretion is relatively increased in mast cells, which induces activation of dendritic cells expressing the H4 histamine receptor, contributing to the atopic inflammation [60].

B Cell

In atopic dermatitis, B cells also play an important role and are found in the dermis of atopic dermatitis lesions. B cells present antigen to CD4+ T cells to activate T cells [21]. Th2 cytokine IL-4 promotes IgE production by promoting immunoglobulin substitution in B cells and induces adhesion molecules and recruitment of various immune cells to the skin. B cells also produce CCL17, CCL22, and IL-16 to attract T cells into atopic dermatitis lesions. It has been reported that atopic dermatitis has been improved in some patients by administering rituximab, a monoclonal antibody against CD20, which is mainly expressed on the surface of B cells [61].

In patients with atopic dermatitis, IgE is significantly increased with allergic sensitization. IgE stimulates FcεRI expressing cells such as mast cells and basophils, contributing to IgE-mediated inflammatory responses [21]. In addition, IgE contributes to the autoallergic inflammatory response in patients with certain atopic dermatitis subtypes. However, the role of IgE in the pathophysiology of atopic dermatitis is thought to be less important than that of T cells. In a recent meta-analysis that analyzed two randomized clinical trials and 13 clinical case groups, omalizumab, a monoclonal antibody that selectively binds to IgE in the blood in atopic dermatitis, showed a limited effect that only 43% of atopic dermatitis patients clinically responded [62].

Chemokines

CCL27 (C-C motif chemokine ligand 27), a cutaneous T cell-attracting chemokine, is highly expressed in atopic dermatitis and induces skin-homing CLA (cutaneous lymphocyte antigen)+ CCR10+ T cells into the skin [63]. CCR10 is a receptor for CCL27, and these two substances were highly expressed in biopsy of atopic dermatitis patients. CCL27 is mostly produced by keratinocytes and is produced under the influence of proinflammatory cytokines. In the mouse experiment, it was observed that when the CCL27 was neutralized, inflammation of the skin was reduced. In addition, suppression of CCL27 reduces inflammation and T cell skin infiltration [64].

The thymus and activation-regulated chemokine (TARC), also known as CCL17, is a key chemokine expressed in vascular endothelial and dendritic cells that promotes the Th2 response through CCR4 and is involved in T cell infiltration into the skin [65]. The number of CCR4+ lymphocytes in serum has been reported to be related to the severity of atopic dermatitis, serum IgE levels, and eosinophil levels. In addition, a recent meta-analysis suggested that serum CCL17 is the most reliable marker for atopic dermatitis [66].

CCL22, a macrophage–derived chemokine, is a chemotactic factor for CCR4 expressing T cells that function similarly to CCL17. Th2 chemokines CCL17 and CCL22 are mainly produced in Langerhans cells. The levels of CCL17 and CCL22 reflect the extent of skin barrier damage and induce skin-homing T cells into atopic dermatitis lesions. H4R antagonist inhibits CCL17 and CCL22 chemokine production by Langerhans cells in patients with atopic dermatitis [59].

Monokines are induced by fractalkine, IFN-γ-inducible protein 10, IFN-γ, and are highly increased in keratinocytes. Monokines are responsible for transporting Th1 cells to the epidermis in chronic atopic dermatitis. In addition, CC chemokines, macrophage chemoattractant protein-4, eotaxin, RANTES (regulated on activation, normal T cell expressed and secreted) also contributes to macrophage, eosinophil, and T cell infiltration in acute and chronic atopic dermatitis skin lesions [33].

References

1. Akdis CA, Akdis M, Trautmann A, Blaser K. Immune regulation in atopic dermatitis. Curr Opin Immunol. 2000;12(6):641–6.
2. Bieber T. Atopic dermatitis. N Engl J Med. 2008;358(14):1483–94.
3. Park CO, Noh S, Jin S, Lee NR, Lee YS, Lee H, et al. Insight into newly discovered innate immune modulation in atopic dermatitis. Exp Dermatol. 2013;22(1):6–9.
4. Noh JY, Shin JU, Park CO, Lee N, Jin S, Kim SH, et al. Thymic stromal lymphopoietin regulates eosinophil migration via phosphorylation of l-plastin in atopic dermatitis. Exp Dermatol. 2016;25(11):880–6.
5. Wu WH, Park CO, Oh SH, Kim HJ, Kwon YS, Bae BG, et al. Thymic stromal lymphopoietin-activated invariant natural killer T cells trigger an innate allergic immune response in atopic dermatitis. J Allergy Clin Immunol. 2010;126(2):290–9.
6. Sun Z, Kim JH, Kim SH, Kim HR, Zhang K, Pan Y, et al. Skin-resident natural killer T cells participate in cutaneous allergic inflammation in atopic dermatitis. J Allergy Clin Immunol. Epub 2021. S0091-6749(21)00097-X. https://doi.org/10.1016/j.jaci.2020.11.049. Online ahead of print. PMID: 33516870
7. McKenzie AN. Type-2 innate lymphoid cells in asthma and allergy. Ann Am Thorac Soc. 2014;11(Suppl 5):S263–70.
8. Kim BS, Siracusa MC, Saenz SA, Noti M, Monticelli LA, Sonnenberg GF, et al. TSLP elicits IL-33-independent innate lymphoid cell responses to promote skin inflammation. Sci Transl Med. 2013;5(170):170ra16.
9. Kumar H, Kawai T, Akira S. Pathogen recognition by the innate immune system. Int Rev Immunol. 2011;30(1):16–34.
10. Kuo IH, Yoshida T, De Benedetto A, Beck LA. The cutaneous innate immune response in patients with atopic dermatitis. J Allergy Clin Immunol. 2013;131(2):266–78.
11. Liu PT, Stenger S, Li H, Wenzel L, Tan BH, Krutzik SR, et al. Toll-like receptor triggering of a vitamin D-mediated human antimicrobial response. Science. 2006;311(5768):1770–3.
12. Noh S, Park CO, Bae JM, Lee J, Shin JU, Hong CS, et al. Lower vitamin D status is closely correlated with eczema of the head and neck. J Allergy Clin Immunol. 2014;133(6):1767–70.

13. Caruso R, Warner N, Inohara N, Núñez G. NOD1 and NOD2: signaling, host defense, and inflammatory disease. Immunity. 2014;41(6):898–908.
14. Skabytska Y, Kaesler S, Volz T, Biedermann T. The role of innate immune signaling in the pathogenesis of atopic dermatitis and consequences for treatments. Semin Immunopathol. 2016;38(1):29–43.
15. Clausen ML, Slotved HC, Krogfelt KA, Andersen PS, Agner T. In vivo expression of antimicrobial peptides in atopic dermatitis. Exp Dermatol. 2016;25(1):3–9.
16. Ong PY, Ohtake T, Brandt C, Strickland I, Boguniewicz M, Ganz T, et al. Endogenous antimicrobial peptides and skin infections in atopic dermatitis. N Engl J Med. 2002;347(15):1151–60.
17. Kimata H. Increase in dermcidin-derived peptides in sweat of patients with atopic eczema caused by a humorous video. J Psychosom Res. 2007;62(1):57–9.
18. Jin S, Park CO, Shin JU, Noh JY, Lee YS, Lee NR, et al. DAMP molecules S100A9 and S100A8 activated by IL-17A and house-dust mites are increased in atopic dermatitis. Exp Dermatol. 2014;23(12):938–41.
19. Lande R, Gregorio J, Facchinetti V, Chatterjee B, Wang YH, Homey B, et al. Plasmacytoid dendritic cells sense self-DNA coupled with antimicrobial peptide. Nature. 2007;449(7162):564–9.
20. Brandt EB, Sivaprasad U. Th2 cytokines and atopic dermatitis. J Clin Cell Immunol. 2011;2:3.
21. Werfel T, Allam JP, Biedermann T, Eyerich K, Gilles S, Guttman-Yassky E, et al. Cellular and molecular immunologic mechanisms in patients with atopic dermatitis. J Allergy Clin Immunol. 2016;138(2):336–49.
22. Czarnowicki T, Krueger JG, Guttman-Yassky E. Skin barrier and immune dysregulation in atopic dermatitis: an evolving story with important clinical implications. J Allergy Clin Immunol Pract. 2014;2(4):371–9.
23. Czarnowicki T, Esaki H, Gonzalez J, Malajian D, Shemer A, Noda S, et al. Early pediatric atopic dermatitis shows only a cutaneous lymphocyte antigen (CLA)(+) TH2/TH1 cell imbalance, whereas adults acquire CLA(+) TH22/TC22 cell subsets. J Allergy Clin Immunol. 2015;136(4):941–51 e3.
24. Czarnowicki T, Gonzalez J, Shemer A, Malajian D, Xu H, Zheng X, et al. Severe atopic dermatitis is characterized by selective expansion of circulating TH2/TC2 and TH22/TC22, but not TH17/TC17, cells within the skin-homing T-cell population. J Allergy Clin Immunol. 2015;136(1):104–15 e7.
25. Noda S, Krueger JG, Guttman-Yassky E. The translational revolution and use of biologics in patients with inflammatory skin diseases. J Allergy Clin Immunol. 2015;135(2):324–36.
26. Nograles KE, Zaba LC, Shemer A, Fuentes-Duculan J, Cardinale I, Kikuchi T, et al. IL-22-producing "T22" T cells account for upregulated IL-22 in atopic dermatitis despite reduced IL-17-producing TH17 T cells. J Allergy Clin Immunol. 2009;123(6):1244–52 e2.
27. Novak N, Koch S, Allam JP, Bieber T. Dendritic cells: bridging innate and adaptive immunity in atopic dermatitis. J Allergy Clin Immunol. 2010;125(1):50–9.
28. Chan LS, Robinson N, Xu L. Expression of interleukin-4 in the epidermis of transgenic mice results in a pruritic inflammatory skin disease: an experimental animal model to study atopic dermatitis. J Invest Dermatol. 2001;117(4):977–83.
29. Leung DY, Guttman-Yassky E. Deciphering the complexities of atopic dermatitis: shifting paradigms in treatment approaches. J Allergy Clin Immunol. 2014;134(4):769–79.
30. Amano W, Nakajima S, Kunugi H, Numata Y, Kitoh A, Egawa G, et al. The Janus kinase inhibitor JTE-052 improves skin barrier function through suppressing signal transducer and activator of transcription 3 signaling. J Allergy Clin Immunol. 2015;136(3):667–77 e7.
31. Bissonnette R, Papp KA, Poulin Y, Gooderham M, Raman M, Mallbris L, et al. Topical tofacitinib for atopic dermatitis: a phase IIa randomized trial. Br J Dermatol. 2016;175(5):902–11.
32. Ziegler SF. Thymic stromal lymphopoietin and allergic disease. J Allergy Clin Immunol. 2012;130(4):845–52.
33. Simpson EL, Bieber T, Guttman-Yassky E, Beck LA, Blauvelt A, Cork MJ, et al. Two phase 3 trials of dupilumab versus placebo in atopic dermatitis. N Engl J Med. 2016;375(24):2335–48.
34. Beck LA, Thaci D, Hamilton JD, Graham NM, Bieber T, Rocklin R, et al. Dupilumab treatment in adults with moderate-to-severe atopic dermatitis. N Engl J Med. 2014;371(2):130–9.
35. Homey B, Steinhoff M, Ruzicka T, Leung DY. Cytokines and chemokines orchestrate atopic skin inflammation. J Allergy Clin Immunol. 2006;118(1):178–89.
36. Konishi H, Tsutsui H, Murakami T, Yumikura-Futatsugi S, Yamanaka K, Tanaka M, et al. IL-18 contributes to the spontaneous development of atopic dermatitis-like inflammatory skin lesion independently of IgE/stat6 under specific pathogen-free conditions. Proc Natl Acad Sci U S A. 2002;99(17):11340–5.
37. Jin JJ, Zou YX, Zeng SW. Risk factors for and expression of immune and inflammatory factors in atopic dermatitis in Chinese population: a birth cohort study. Mol Cell Probes. 2016;30(3):168–73.
38. Lee JH, Cho DH, Park HJ. IL-18 and cutaneous inflammatory diseases. Int J Mol Sci. 2015;16(12):29357–69.
39. Inoue Y, Aihara M, Kirino M, Harada I, Komori-Yamaguchi J, Yamaguchi Y, et al. Interleukin-18 is elevated in the horny layer in patients with atopic dermatitis and is associated with Staphylococcus aureus colonization. Br J Dermatol. 2011;164(3):560–7.
40. Park CO, Lee HJ, Lee JH, Wu WH, Chang NS, Hua L, et al. Increased expression of CC chemokine ligand 18 in extrinsic atopic dermatitis patients. Exp Dermatol. 2008;17(1):24–9.
41. Cornelissen C, Marquardt Y, Czaja K, Wenzel J, Frank J, Luscher-Firzlaff J, et al. IL-31 regulates differentiation and filaggrin expression in human

organotypic skin models. J Allergy Clin Immunol. 2012;129(2):426–33, 33.e1–8.
42. Nemoto O, Furue M, Nakagawa H, Shiramoto M, Hanada R, Matsuki S, et al. The first trial of CIM331, a humanized antihuman interleukin-31 receptor A antibody, in healthy volunteers and patients with atopic dermatitis to evaluate safety, tolerability and pharmacokinetics of a single dose in a randomized, double-blind, placebo-controlled study. Br J Dermatol. 2016;174(2):296–304.
43. Hawro T, Saluja R, Weller K, Altrichter S, Metz M, Maurer M. Interleukin-31 does not induce immediate itch in atopic dermatitis patients and healthy controls after skin challenge. Allergy. 2014;69(1):113–7.
44. Schmitz J, Owyang A, Oldham E, Song Y, Murphy E, McClanahan TK, et al. IL-33, an interleukin-1-like cytokine that signals via the IL-1 receptor-related protein ST2 and induces T helper type 2-associated cytokines. Immunity. 2005;23(5):479–90.
45. Allakhverdi Z, Smith DE, Comeau MR, Delespesse G. Cutting edge: the ST2 ligand IL-33 potently activates and drives maturation of human mast cells. J Immunol. 2007;179(4):2051–4.
46. Dudda JC, Perdue N, Bachtanian E, Campbell DJ. Foxp3+ regulatory T cells maintain immune homeostasis in the skin. J Exp Med. 2008;205(7):1559–65.
47. Loser K, Beissert S. Regulatory T cells: banned cells for decades. J Invest Dermatol. 2012;132(3 Pt 2):864–71.
48. Oh SH, Park CO, Wu WH, Kim JY, Jin S, Byamba D, et al. Corticotropin-releasing hormone downregulates IL-10 production by adaptive forkhead box protein 3-negative regulatory T cells in patients with atopic dermatitis. J Allergy Clin Immunol. 2012;129(1):151–9.
49. Jin S, Shin JU, Noh JY, Kim H, Kim JY, Kim SH, et al. DOCK8: regulator of Treg in response to corticotropin-releasing hormone. Allergy. 2016;71(6):811–9.
50. Lee N, Shin JU, Jin S, Yun KN, Kim JY, Park CO, et al. Upregulation of CD47 in regulatory T cells in atopic dermatitis. Yonsei Med J. 2016;57(6):1435–45.
51. Moy AP, Murali M, Kroshinsky D, Duncan LM, Nazarian RM. Immunologic overlap of helper T-cell subtypes 17 and 22 in erythrodermic psoriasis and atopic dermatitis. JAMA Dermatol. 2015;151(7):753–60.
52. Suarez-Farinas M, Dhingra N, Gittler J, Shemer A, Cardinale I, de Guzman Strong C, et al. Intrinsic atopic dermatitis shows similar TH2 and higher TH17 immune activation compared with extrinsic atopic dermatitis. J Allergy Clin Immunol. 2013;132(2):361–70.
53. Noda S, Suarez-Farinas M, Ungar B, Kim SJ, de Guzman Strong C, Xu H, et al. The Asian atopic dermatitis phenotype combines features of atopic dermatitis and psoriasis with increased TH17 polarization. J Allergy Clin Immunol. 2015;136(5):1254–64.
54. Noh S, Jin S, Park CO, Lee YS, Lee N, Lee J, et al. Elevated galectin-10 expression of IL-22-producing T cells in patients with atopic dermatitis. J Invest Dermatol. 2016;136(1):328–31.
55. Jang M, Kim H, Kim Y, Choi J, Jeon J, Hwang Y, et al. The crucial role of IL-22 and its receptor in thymus and activation regulated chemokine production and T-cell migration by house dust mite extract. Exp Dermatol. 2016;25(8):598–603.
56. Novak N, Valenta R, Bohle B, Laffer S, Haberstok J, Kraft S, et al. FcepsilonRI engagement of Langerhans cell-like dendritic cells and inflammatory dendritic epidermal cell-like dendritic cells induces chemotactic signals and different T-cell phenotypes in vitro. J Allergy Clin Immunol. 2004;113(5):949–57.
57. Fujita H, Nograles KE, Kikuchi T, Gonzalez J, Carucci JA, Krueger JG. Human Langerhans cells induce distinct IL-22-producing CD4+ T cells lacking IL-17 production. Proc Natl Acad Sci U S A. 2009;106(51):21795–800.
58. Wollenberg A, Wagner M, Gunther S, Towarowski A, Tuma E, Moderer M, et al. Plasmacytoid dendritic cells: a new cutaneous dendritic cell subset with distinct role in inflammatory skin diseases. J Invest Dermatol. 2002;119(5):1096–102.
59. Miyano K, Matsushita S, Tsuchida T, Nakamura K. Inhibitory effect of a histamine 4 receptor antagonist on CCL17 and CCL22 production by monocyte-derived Langerhans cells in patients with atopic dermatitis. J Dermatol. 2016;43(9):1024–9.
60. Dijkstra D, Stark H, Chazot PL, Shenton FC, Leurs R, Werfel T, et al. Human inflammatory dendritic epidermal cells express a functional histamine H4 receptor. J Invest Dermatol. 2008;128(7):1696–703.
61. Simon D, Hosli S, Kostylina G, Yawalkar N, Simon HU. Anti-CD20 (rituximab) treatment improves atopic eczema. J Allergy Clin Immunol. 2008;121(1):122–8.
62. Wang HH, Li YC, Huang YC. Efficacy of omalizumab in patients with atopic dermatitis: a systematic review and meta-analysis. J Allergy Clin Immunol. 2016;138(6):1719–22 e1.
63. Vestergaard C, Deleuran M, Gesser B, Gronhoj Larsen C. Expression of the T-helper 2-specific chemokine receptor CCR4 on CCR10-positive lymphocytes in atopic dermatitis skin but not in psoriasis skin. Br J Dermatol. 2003;149(3):457–63.
64. Homey B, Alenius H, Muller A, Soto H, Bowman EP, Yuan W, et al. CCL27-CCR10 interactions regulate T cell-mediated skin inflammation. Nat Med. 2002;8(2):157–65.
65. Morita E, Takahashi H, Niihara H, Dekio I, Sumikawa Y, Murakami Y, et al. Stratum corneum TARC level is a new indicator of lesional skin inflammation in atopic dermatitis. Allergy. 2010;65(9):1166–72.
66. Thijs J, Krastev T, Weidinger S, Buckens CF, de Bruin-Weller M, Bruijnzeel-Koomen C, et al. Biomarkers for atopic dermatitis: a systematic review and meta-analysis. Curr Opin Allergy Clin Immunol. 2015;15(5):453–60.

Evironmental Factors Related To Atopic Dermatitis

Jaeyong Shin

Environmental factors related to atopic dermatitis

- Atopic dermatitis is caused by the interaction of genetic factors, skin barrier functions, abnormalities in the immune system, environmental factors, etc.
- Hygiene Hypothesis: The balance of Th1/Th2 immunity leads to Th2 causing allergic diseases.
- Industrialization, warming, and westernized lifestyle are factors that cause and worsen atopic dermatitis.
- The synthesis and degradation of filaggrin protein is one of the important diseases of atopic dermatitis.
- Psychological and social stress are involved in the occurrence and deterioration of atopic dermatitis.

Introduction

Although the causes of atopic dermatitis are not known for certain, it is said to be the result of complex interactions such as genetic factors, skin barrier functions, immune system abnormalities, and environmental factors. An epidemiological survey on the prevalence of atopic dermatitis in Korea shows a tendency to increase as industrialization and westernization progress compared to the past, and these results are also consistently observed in data from various westernized countries. So far, many studies have been conducted on the mechanism of atopic dermatitis, but the exact cause has yet to be determined.

Characteristics of AD Pathogenesis

Atopic dermatitis is caused by exposure to various environmental factors in people with genetic predispositions and is known to induce immune responses, especially Th2 lymphocytes, resulting in a particular IgE for allergens and causing an overreaction. The recent rapid increase in the prevalence of atopic dermatitis is related to the increase in the environmental change of atopic dermatitis, rather than to the possibility of rapid genetic change itself.

The hygiene hypothesis of AD was proposed on the basis of the high prevalence rate of atopic dermatitis in developed countries with westernized lifestyles in which society is advanced and economic standards, compared to undeveloped countries [1]. According to the hygiene hypothesis, the immune response is skewed toward the

J. Shin (✉)
Department of Preventive Medicine,
Yonsei University College of Medicine, Seoul,
Korea (Republic of)
e-mail: drshin@yuhs.ac

K. H. Lee et al. (eds.), *Practical Insights into Atopic Dermatitis*,
https://doi.org/10.1007/978-981-15-8159-5_9

Th2 reaction at a time when the immune system is not fully completed, and as it grows, the Th1 reaction is gradually induced and balanced through proper stimulation by microorganisms [2]. However, it explains that maintaining too hygienic conditions reduces the chance of exposure to microbial infections, leaving the immune system where the Th2 reaction prevails, resulting in allergic diseases such as asthma and atopic dermatitis. It is appropriate to explain the possibility that conditions in hygiene before and after birth have a profound effect on determining the immune response to a substance, and it has opened a new chapter in understanding the immune response after birth.

Many epidemiological studies so far support the hygiene hypothesis. It is known that the higher the risk of infection, such as the higher the number of siblings in the family [3], the younger the child goes to nursery schools with more children [4], is related to the less occurrence rate of allergic diseases such as asthma or atopic dermatitis. However, the hygiene hypothesis alone cannot explain the occurrence of atopic dermatitis as the prevalence rate of atopic dermatitis is rather high in underdeveloped countries, and atopic dermatitis is often high in population groups with poor socioeconomic conditions in advanced countries.

There are also reports that as a highly industrialized society develops, environmental factors that could be directly irritated to the skin gradually increase. In other words, the increase in indoor and outdoor environmental pollutants, the decrease in breastfeeding, the increase in powdered milk, the increase in pollen (plants), and the infection of the respiratory virus are cited as possible reasons for AD, but many studies still need to reveal the causal relationship.

In the case of allergic diseases, symptoms do not appear if the human body is not exposed to certain environmental causes, even if it has a genetic predisposition. In other words, individuals are exposed to environmental factors with sensitivity, causing allergic symptoms. These indoor and outdoor allergy substances include house dust mites, cats, dogs, pollen (plants, polyen), and fungi, and act as factors that can cause or worsen asthma, rhinitis, or atopic dermatitis. Recently, it has been revealed that indoor and outdoor air pollutants are also a risk factor for allergies. Indoor air pollutants are mainly caused by new material volatile chemicals related to gases or buildings that occur when wood, coal, oil, and gas are burned, which are used for cooking or heating, and by substances emitted from smoking. Pollutants for outdoor air pollutants are pollutants emitted from heating, power plants, and factories, as well as car fumes.

Hygiene Hypothesis

Individuals born with genetic factors do not necessarily have allergic symptoms. The hygiene hypothesis explains that in order to establish a form in which human body immune responses can cause allergies, the specific factors that protect the human body from allergic diseases are extinguished as the sanitary environment improves, leading to the occurrence of allergic diseases. Based on an epidemiological study by David Strachan in 1989, younger siblings are less prone to allergic diseases than older siblings. It suggests that the younger siblings may be more frequently exposed to infections through older siblings and this may be related to the less occurrence of atopic diseases. Multiple Th2 cytokines (IL-4, IL-5, IL-9, IL-13), due to allergen stimuli in allergic disease patients, increase the production of IgE in B-lymphocytes, thereby increasing the likelihood of developing allergic diseases, and relatively, the Th1 cytokine (TNF-alpha, IFN-r, IL-2), secreted from Th1 lymphocytes [5].

In the neonatal period, the immune system is not yet fully complete as Th2 cytokines are increased. During the period, the appropriate stimulus by microorganisms reduces Th2 cytokines, causing Th1/Th2 to balance. This hypothesis provides the basis for the immunological mechanism that the balance of Th1/Th2 immunity remains centered on Th2, which is appropriate for explaining the possibility of having a profound effect on the determination of immune response in accordance with the sanitary conditions before and after birth. This has opened a new chapter in understanding the post-birth immune response. However, several other epidemiological findings suggest that the incidence of allergic diseases is not necessarily consistent, raising the possibility that the decrease in the occurrence of allergic diseases may be affected by the distribution of endotoxins or intestinal bacteria from germs, not by pathogens. In addition, hygiene hypotheses are strongly related to asthma, allergic rhinitis, and allergen sensitization, while some analyze that they are relatively less related to atopic dermatitis, so further research is needed on how much sanitary hypothesis contributes to the occurrence of atopic dermatitis.

Immaturity of Skin Barrier

"Outside–Inside" Hypothesis

Regardless of the increased incidence of AD, the most cases occur around the age of one. However, the prevalence decreases as they gradually grow and reach adulthood. Therefore, it is possible to assume that atopic dermatitis is highly influenced by changes in the environment. However, overall immaturity or immaturity in the body is also an important factor in the development. In other words, the factors associated with the occurrence of atopic dermatitis can be considered as an immaturity of body function, such as skin barrier function, mucous membrane immunity, systemic immunity, and digestive enzymes. Among them, damage to the skin barrier function is also regarded as an important cause of atopic dermatitis in recent years.

The skin is an organ, which is constantly in contact with the external environment and is responsible for the primary defense function. The epidermal permeability barrier, which controls the permeability of water and other electrolytes, is the most important function of the skin and is handled by the stratum corneum, the outermost layer of the epidermis. The concept and study of skin barriers began when Elias [6] presented the "Brick & Mortar Model." The disease of atopic dermatitis can be explained from two main perspectives: damage to the epidermal barrier and immunological change. Contrary to the conventional "inside–outside" hypothesis, in which immunological changes come first and secondary to eczema changes in the epidermis, the damaged skin barrier acts as an important initial response to the occurrence of atopic dermatitis by allowing antigen to penetrate easily through the skin, increasing interaction with antigenous cells and immune cells in the dermis. This is contrary to the conventional "inside–outside" hypothesis that skin barrier damage in atopic dermatitis is the result of inflammatory reactions to irritants and allergens. Neither hypothesis can be explained, but it is likely that the two hypotheses will work differently depending on the stage at which atopic dermatitis occurs and whether it is severe, internal or external [6].

Mutation of Filaggrin Gene

If skin barrier damage is involved in the development of atopic dermatitis primarily, genes that control the function of the skin barrier will play an important role sequentially. There are many studies that genes are responsible for the skin barrier. These studies show that the mutation of filaggrin genes is the beginning of atopic dermatitis [7]. The clinical patterns of patients with filaggrin mutations are analyzed. The results show that patients with mutations often develop early, show severe symptoms, and tend to show atopic march [8]. The synthesis and deterioration of the feline protein, which serves as an important barrier in the stratum corneum of the epidermis (the stratum plays the most important role as a physical epidermal barrier), has resulted in a major disability in the normal epidermal barrier role. This important finding has been found to cause atopic dermatitis by making external allergens more easily pass through the stratum and cause infection in the body.

Atopic March

Atopic diseases begin in infants at the early stage, in the form of eczema called atopic dermatitis and progress to asthma or allergic rhinitis, a respiratory atopic disease. We call this as atopic march [9]. It is assumed that atopic dermatitis in the younger period has a greater possibility to have allergic respiratory diseases, because of skin barrier damage. If there is damage to the skin barrier accompanied by atopic dermatitis, various kinds of irritants or allergens are easily penetrated through the damaged epidermis, leading to the Th2 immune response. If the Th2 cells move to the respiratory tract, they will cause systemic hypersensitivity. Finally, if the allergen is inhaled into the respiratory atopic disease, asthma or allergic rhinitis is likely to occur [9].

Correlation Between Atopic Dermatitis and Environmental Factors

Recently, it is suggested that causes of atopic dermatitis are closely related to environmental factors such as industrialization and changes in lifestyle. The reason why asthma, allergic rhinitis, and atopic dermatitis have soared since the 1980s, is because of environmental problems caused by industrialization. Pollution due to the operation of industrial facilities, exhaust fumes from automobiles, consumption of fossil fuels for heating or cooking purposes, changes in the indoor environment due to global warming and Westernized lifestyles, and changes in food consumption patterns are cited as causes and aggravation of atopic dermatitis.

Air Pollution

Air pollution and air quality management, which cause various health problems in the human body, have become a global concern. There are various environmental factors, but recently, the increase in environmental pollutant emissions due to economic development and urbanization and the expansion of the use of harmful chemicals are likely to serve as one of the causes of atopic dermatitis [10].

Causes of indoor and outdoor air pollution include factories, car exhaust fumes, cigarette smoke, cooking combustion, building materials, paints, various indoor consumer goods, and pollutants are formulatively: sulfur dioxide (SO2), nitrogen oxide (NO), ozone (Ozone), volatile organic compounds (VOC), formaldehyde (Formaldehyde) [11].

The results of epidemiological studies on the prevalence of air pollution and atopic dermatitis are mainly data on asthma among atopic diseases rather than atopic dermatitis. According to a study report in France in 2005 [12], it reported that an increase in atopic diseases in children exposed to pollution in the long term. Another study in Taiwan in 2002 [13] compared the amount of pollution in the two cities. It showed that there were many allergic diseases in cities with high pollution. Epidemiological surveys in Ethiopia [14] also reported that there were more atopic dermatitis in urban areas than in rural areas, while a study of air pollution in Russia in 2001 [15] showed that air pollution is not related to the increased prevalence of AD. Even though it is still controversial whether air pollution is related to AD, it sounds reasonable since developed countries have a higher incidence rate of AD.

Sick Building Syndrome, Sick House Syndrome

Sick building syndrome (SBS) is defined that indoor air pollution induces various kinds of respiratory and skin clinical symptoms. Among symptoms, if it is related to living, it is separately defined as Sick house syndrome (SHS) [16].

Recently, media outlets have shown increasing interest in the link between atopic dermatitis and new house syndrome. New house syndrome is commonly referred to as various organic compounds and pollutants from new buildings or newly remodeled environments that have caused tenants to develop various pathological symptoms on their bodies. The main causes can be found in defects in ventilation and heating systems, building materials, various volatile organic compounds, and urinary materials.

A causative agent for house syndrome is a volatile chemical. Among them, formaldehyde is a representative causative substance. Formaldehyde is a colorless gas with an irritating smell that melts well in water. Spray paint, mainly for preservatives or adhesives (architecture, furniture industry) and interior decoration, is the main problem, and formaldehyde is released indoors for many years in the case of new houses using building materials containing formaldehyde.

It is relatively common to complain of multiple symptoms immediately after moving into a new house, such as worsening existing allergic diseases such as atopic dermatitis and asthma, or repeated skin diseases for no particular reason. Among the symptoms of sick house syndrome, the stimulus response is mainly caused by irritation of the eyes, nose, larynx, and airway mucous membrane, such as eye pain and itching, sore throat, and coughing, and other nonspecific symptoms include complaining of headaches or easily fatigue and lethargy. Symptoms of sick house syndrome tend to be large in individual differences, which are more severe in infants or elderly people with weak immune system, and in patients with allergic diseases, the symptoms worsen. In particular, there are reports of increased incidence of atopic dermatitis in homes with newborn babies. In particular, it has recently become a social problem in Korea, but there is a lack of objective research data on whether living in a new house is directly related to the increase in atopic dermatitis [17].

There is no specific test for diagnosing sick house syndrome. It is diagnosed through a questionnaire, including the history of moving into a new house, related symptoms, lifestyle, and reactions to chemicals. Treatment is required for each symptom that occurs after moving to a new house, and efforts should be made to remove indoor pollutants if possible at the same time. Reducing the use of materials that can cause indoor air pollution is the most effective way, preferably using natural materials, eco-friendly plywood without formaldehyde treatment, and using natural finishing materials can reduce symptoms. Indoor ventilation is also important, and windows or doors should be opened to become natural ventilation, and frequent ventilation should be carried out in the event of activities that pollute indoor air, such as cooking. It is also recommended that bake out be implemented when moving into a new house.

Bake-out is a method of removing harmful substances by increasing the indoor temperature of a building. It is also helpful to choose a house that has been built for more than 3 years, rather than a new one, if you are suffering from an allergic disease.

However, indoor air pollutants are exposed to anyone but do not cause problems in everyone. It is assumed that they cause abnormal symptoms, especially in children, the elderly, patients with underlying diseases, and that they have a significant impact on people with [18] genetic predisposition or socioeconomic low class.

Heavy Metal and Water Pollution

It is still controversial that the relationship between the concentration of heavy metals in human blood, urine, and hair and atopic dermatitis. The most representative heavy metal reported in relation to atopic dermatitis is mercury. The link between mercury concentration in urine and atopic dermatitis was observed in the study of the association with acute lesions and total IgE [18]. This was especially more problematic when dental prostheses were treated in the Amalgam. This is presumed to cause or worsen allergic reactions through immune responses that induce the secretion of Th2 cytokine through exposure to mercury. In addition, some studies have shown that the higher the concentration of residual chlorine in the water, the worse the atopic dermatitis. However, the role of heavy metals and water quality, associated with the occurrence or deterioration of atopic dermatitis, needs further study.

Climate Change

In general, mild and warm climates are known to have a good effect on symptoms of atopic dermatitis. However, the ongoing and long-term climate change caused by global warming is believed to cause an increase in atopic diseases (especially asthma and allergic rhinitis) due to an increase in allergens such as air pollutants and pollen. A number of epidemiological surveys recently explain the causes of the increase in atopic dermatitis prevalence in several ways. In addition to genetic effects and hygienic hypotheses, what is commonly mentioned is that changes in living conditions have led to an increase in atopic dermatitis due to westernized lifestyles (especially changes in food and residential environment) and the increase in pollution accompanying an industrialized society. In particular, climate change is one of the most important factors that can lead to changes in the living environment associated with human diseases [19, 20].

It is reported that rapid changes in climate and temperature, cold seasons or areas where the sun is hard to see, have an adverse effect on atopic dermatitis [21, 22]. In a large-scale epidemiological study of infants, the prevalence of atopic dermatitis increases with higher latitudes, lower air temperatures, lower indoor humidity. In contrast, warmer climate and more sunlight are reported to reduce the prevalence of atopic dermatitis [23, 24]. Therefore, although many people are generally thought to have atopic dermatitis in cold regions, the correlation between climate change and atopic dermatitis may vary depending on whether it is a long-term or temporary change. The impact of long-term climate change on human diseases can be thought of in many ways, but most importantly, it is a problem that can be caused by global warming, which has recently become a universal problem. The effects of greenhouse gases, especially carbon dioxide (CO_2), have been increasing air temperature slightly, and the increase in air temperature caused by climate change is known to increase the concentration of pollutants in the atmosphere [25, 26].

Typical air pollutants include nitrogen dioxide (NO2), sulfur dioxide (SO2), ozone (O3), carbon monoxide (CO), and fine dust (particulate matter). These pollutants have been reported in various epidemiological studies to be closely related to the increase in allergic diseases and worsening symptoms [27, 28]. Another factor to consider is that rising global temperatures increase the production of pollen that can cause allergic diseases, and by changing the timing and duration of the pollen season, inhalation allergens increase. It is assumed that pollutants can change the epidermis to affect the immune response, increase the antigenicity of the antigen, and act with inhaled allergens such as pollen to increase the allergic disease. Therefore, climate-induced changes in the environment are thought to induce the Th2 immune response, which can lead to the deterioration of atopic dermatitis. The major problem with climate change is that not only does the climate progresses at a very slow pace, but carbon dioxide exists in the atmosphere for a very long time, so even if greenhouse gas emissions are suddenly curbed, the situation of global warming that has already been going on will continue for a considerable period of time [20].

It explains that the reason why there are more allergic diseases in urban areas is because pollen antigens can break into airways more easily due to the inflammatory effects of ozone, fine dust, and sulfur dioxide. It is also thought that air pollutants can increase the separation of antigens from pollen grains and absorb pollen grains to keep them in the body for a long time.

Meanwhile, improving the indoor environment in a short period of time can induce improvement of atopic dermatitis. It is known that AD patients in high latitude is associated with severe symptoms. It has been reported that temporary movement to warm areas will improve symptoms and that UV rays in warm areas will be closely related to the symptom improvement of atopic dermatitis. Therefore, short-term or temporary climate change that increases air temperature is applied to the treatment of atopic dermatitis.

Many patients get worse in the winter and improve in the summer, which is believed to be due to reduced humidity caused by cold outdoor air and indoor heating. It can also include the secretion of a lot of sebum and sweat, ultraviolet rays, exposure to water while swimming, reduced infection, and reduced stress during summer vacation. However, the same effect may worsen the condition in other patients with atopic dermatitis. Exposure to ultraviolet rays without proper skin protection can be harmful and increased outdoor activity reduces exposure to indoor antigens, but sweating caused by heat or exercise exacerbates clinical patterns in most patients. In general, cold and dry climates exacerbate atopic dermatitis due to the dry action of the skin indirectly. Hot and humid weather can also act as a worsening factor, as the chances of fever and secondary infection increase. And rapid changes in temperature and humidity can also exacerbate atopic dermatitis, as the skin immediately lacks the ability to adapt. The effects of these climates are secondary to most patients and vary from individual to individual.

Clothing

One of the most representative mechanisms in which clothing affects atopic dermatitis is the irritation caused by physical contact with the clothing's fiber and skin [29]. Skin symptoms can be exacerbated by synthetic materials such as nylon and materials. They can irritate the skin such as wool or linnen37. Research as shown that there are far more materials that can worsen atopic dermatitis than effective materials for dermatitis.

It can be observed that eczema lesions with distinct boundaries in atopic dermatitis are adjacent to the fiber label, seams, and joints of the garment, or are confined to contact areas of a particular garment. This stimulus may be caused by mechanical and chemical stimuli (remaining enzymes of cleaning agents or agents containing enzymes, stimuli by fibrous softener, fibrous manufacturing finishes using formaldehyde, chemicals for trimming fibers). Crawling on the carpet can also irritate the skin.

Comfortable and ventilated pure cotton materials are recommended. Noodles also have the advantage of having excellent absorption of sweat. Therefore, clothes that come into direct contact with the skin have a softer surface than wool or synthetic fibers made of coarse fibers. Also, cutting the nails short is recommended as a way to reduce skin irritation. Most atopic dermatitis lesions are scratched and scratched to relieve itching temporarily, but in the long run, there is a vicious cycle of skin itching more. Long fingernails can cause this vicious cycle to occur faster, and skin damage after scratching can become more severe, causing secondary infections to become a problem.

Psychosomatic Aspect

It is known that psychological and social factors as well as biological factors of atopic dermatitis affect the progress of the disease. Among atopic dermatitis patients, mental stress is associated with immunological reactions [30]. Changes in the immune system include abnormal Th1/Th2 ratio and the decrease in the number of NK cells. The changes make patients more vulnerable to atopic dermatitis [31].

A study showed that atopic dermatitis patients had higher levels of anxiety than healthy people. Also, the rate of experiencing stress events in the last 6 months was higher in patients with psoriasis (48%) and atopic dermatitis (38%) than in healthy subjects (11.54%) [32].

In patients with atopic dermatitis, the reactivity of hypothalamus-brachial (HPA) axis induced by mental stress is reduced, which suggests that stress may exacerbate atopic dermatitis [33].

Since mental stress can act as an aggravating factor for atopic dermatitis, efficient management of the stress of patients with atopic dermatitis is very important in improving the quality of life of patients. Therefore, controlling patient stress must be included in the prevention or treatment of atopic dermatitis.

In addition, the more severe the symptoms of atopic dermatitis is associated with the more affected the child's personality formation and instability, the fewer friends and the difficulties of friendship, and the effects of physical health. Therefore, if atopic dermatitis is severe, it is necessary for all societies, including parents, to recognize and mediate in improving their children's difficulty in forming a friendship relationship.

References

1. Strachan DP. Hay fever, hygiene, and household size. BMJ. 1989;299(6710):1259.
2. Weiss ST. Eat dirt—the hygiene hypothesis and allergic diseases. N Engl J Med. 2002;347(12):930–1.
3. Ball TM, Castro-Rodriguez JA, Griffith KA, Holberg CJ, Martinez FD, Wright AL. Siblings, day-care attendance, and the risk of asthma and wheezing during childhood. N Engl J Med. 2000;343(8):538–43.

4. Krämer U, Heinrich J, Wjst M, Wichmann HJ. Age of entry to day nursery and allergy in later childhood. Lancet. 1999;353(9151):450–4.
5. Prescott SL, Macaubas C, Smallacombe T, Holt BJ, Sly PD, Holt PG. Development of allergen-specific T-cell memory in atopic and normal children. Lancet. 1999;353(9148):196–200.
6. Elias PM, Steinhoff M. "Outside-to-inside"(and now back to "outside") pathogenic mechanisms in atopic dermatitis. J Invest Dermatol. 2008;128(5):1067–70.
7. Seguchi T, Chang-Yi C, Kusuda S, Takahashi M, Aisu K, Tezuka TJ. Decreased expression of filaggrin in atopic skin. Arch Dermatol Res. 1996;288(8):442–6.
8. Palmer CN, Irvine AD, Terron-Kwiatkowski A, et al. Common loss-of-function variants of the epidermal barrier protein filaggrin are a major predisposing factor for atopic dermatitis. Nat Genet. 2006;38(4):441–6.
9. Spergel JM. From atopic dermatitis to asthma: the atopic march. Ann Allergy Asthma Immunol. 2010;105(2):99–106.
10. Ahn K, Immunology C. The role of air pollutants in atopic dermatitis. J Allergy Clin Immunol. 2014;134(5):993-999.
11. Bernstein JA, Alexis N, Barnes C, et al. Health effects of air pollution. J Allergy Clin Immunol. 2004;114(5):1116–23.
12. Pénard-Morand C, Charpin D, Raherison C, et al. Long-term exposure to background air pollution related to respiratory and allergic health in schoolchildren. Clin Exp Allergy. 2005;35(10):1279–87.
13. Yu J, Lue K, Lu K, et al. The relationship of air pollution to the prevalence of allergic diseases in Taichung and Chu-Shan in 2002. J Microbiol Immunol Infect. 2005;38(2):123.
14. Yemaneberhan H, Flohr C, Lewis S, et al. Prevalence and associated factors of atopic dermatitis symptoms in rural and urban Ethiopia. Clin Exp Allergy. 2004;34(5):779–85.
15. Dotterud L, Odland J, Falk E. Atopic diseases among schoolchildren in Nikel, Russia, an Arctic area with heavy air pollution. Acta Derm Venereol. 2001;81(3):198–201.
16. Norback D. An update on sick building syndrome. Curr Opin Allergy Clin Immunol. 2009;9(1):55–9.
17. Herbarth O, Fritz GJ, Rehwagen M, et al. Association between indoor renovation activities and eczema in early childhood. Int J Hyg Environ Health. 2006;209(3):241–7.
18. Weidinger S, Krämer U, Dunemann L, et al. Body burden of mercury is associated with acute atopic eczema and total IgE in children from southern Germany. J Allergy Clin Immunol. 2004;114(2):457.
19. Epstein PR. Climate change and human health. N Engl J Med. 2005;353(14):1433–6.
20. Shea K, Truckner R, Weber R, Peden D. Climate change and allergic disease. J Allergy Clin Immun. 2008;122(3):443–53.
21. Rajka G. Atopic dermatitis: correlation of environmental factors with frequency. Int J Dermatol. 1986;25(5):301–5.
22. Vocks E, Busch R, Fröhlich C, Borelli S, Mayer H, Ring J. Influence of weather and climate on subjective symptom intensity in atopic eczema. Int J Biometeorol. 2001;45(1):27–33.
23. Suárez-Varela MM, Alvarez LG-M, Kogan MD, et al. Climate and prevalence of atopic eczema in 6-to 7-year-old school children in Spain. ISAAC phase III. Int J Biometeorol. 2008;52(8):833–40.
24. Weiland S, Hüsing A, Strachan D, Rzehak P, Pearce N, ISAAC Phase One Study Group. Climate and the prevalence of symptoms of asthma, allergic rhinitis, and atopic eczema in children. Occup Environ Med. 2004;61(7):609–15.
25. Noyes PD, McElwee MK, Miller HD, et al. The toxicology of climate change: environmental contaminants in a warming world. Environ Int. 2009;35(6):971–86.
26. Reid CE, Gamble JL. Aeroallergens, allergic disease, and climate change: impacts and adaptation. Ecohealth. 2009;6:458–70.
27. Ring J, Krämer U, Schäfer T, et al. Environmental risk factors for respiratory and skin atopy: results from epidemiological studies in former East and West Germany. Int Arch Allergy Immunol. 1999;118(2–4):403–7.
28. Schäfer T, Heinrich J, Wjst M, et al. Indoor risk factors for atopic eczema in school children from East Germany. Environ Res. 1999;81(2):151–8.
29. Park Y-H. A consumer survey on the efface of clothing materials on atopic determatitis. J Korean Soc Cloth Text. 2008;32(7):1116–28.
30. Buske-Kirschbaum A, Gierens A, Höllig H, Hellhammer D. Stress-induced immunomodulation is altered in patients with atopic dermatitis. J Neuroimmunol. 2002;129(1–2):161–7.
31. Höglund CO, Axen J, Kemi C, et al. Changes in immune regulation in response to examination stress in atopic and healthy individuals. Clin Exp Allergy. 2006;36(8):982–92.
32. Vargas EL, Peña MP, Vargas AM. Influence of anxiety in diverse cutaneous diseases. Actas Dermosifiliogr. 2006;97(10):637–43.
33. Buske-Kirschbaum A, von Auer K, Krieger S, Weis S, Rauh W, Hellhammer D. Blunted cortisol responses to psychosocial stress in asthmatic children: a general feature of atopic disease? Psychosom Med. 2003;65(5):806–10.

Food, Inhalant, and Microbial Allergens

Jung-Won Park

Allergens, in addition to others, are important aggravating factors for atopic dermatitis (AD). This chapter will summarize the important culprit allergens in AD and their roles in the pathogenesis of AD. Diagnostic and effective avoidance and immune-modulating treatment strategies will also be discussed.

Food Allergens

Food allergens are especially important in pediatric AD patients. About one-third of all pediatric AD patients are aggravated by exposure to causative food allergens. Egg, milk, peanut, soybean, wheat, and fish account for more than 90% of all culprit allergens that aggravate AD in pediatric patients. Previously, food allergy has been regarded as the preceding causative etiology of AD; however, recent studies have shown that eczematous skin lesions precede food allergy [1], and skin sensitization rather than gastrointestinal sensitization may be more important for the pathogenesis of food allergy in AD patients. Indeed, AD patients usually have an impaired skin barrier and are vulnerable to epicutaneous sensitization to food or other inhalant allergens [2], and AD cohort studies have indicated that sensitization to allergens at 1 year of age is an important predicting factor of asthma and food allergy at an age of 3 years [3]. Interestingly, pilot studies suggest that prophylactic use of a skin emollient may prevent the development of AD and following allergy march [4]. Furthermore, research with an epicutaneous ovalbumin-sensitized mouse model demonstrated that mechanical skin injury (stripping skin with tape) promotes food anaphylaxis by driving intestinal mast cell expansion via IL-33 production from skin keratinocytes [5]. Notwithstanding, epicutaneous sensitization to allergens can also be induced in healthy subjects with an intact skin barrier. Recently, an outbreak of various immediate-type wheat food allergy diseases was recorded among subjects who had used facial soap containing hydrolyzed wheat protein on intact facial skin in Japan [6]. This episode confirms that epicutaneous sensitization can induce food allergy, even in individuals with an intact skin barrier.

Identification of culprit food allergens and avoidance are the essential treatment strategies for pediatric AD patients. The golden standard for diagnosis of food allergy is a double-blind placebo-controlled food challenge test. However, this test is not easy to perform in real practice as it

J.-W. Park (✉)
Severance Hospital, Yonsei University College of Medicine, Seoul, Korea (Republic of)

Division of Allergy and Immunology, Department of Internal Medicine, Institute of Allergy, Yonsei University College of Medicine, Seoul, Korea (Republic of)
e-mail: PARKJW@yuhs.ac

K. H. Lee et al. (eds.), *Practical Insights into Atopic Dermatitis*,
https://doi.org/10.1007/978-981-15-8159-5_10

Table 1 Diagnostic values for ImmunoCAP sIgE and skin prick tests for food allergy with 95% predictive values for a positive oral food challenge test in children

	ImmunoCAP (sIgE [kIU/L])	Skin prick test (wheals [mm])
Cow's milk	≥15 ≥5, if younger than 1 YO	≥8
Egg white	≥7 ≥2, if younger than 2 YO	≥7
Peanut	≥14	≥8
Fish	≥20	
Wheat	≥26	
Tree nuts	≥15	

requires preparation of allergen extracts, facilities, and experienced professionals. Therefore, practical diagnosis based on compatible clinical history and quantification of specific IgE by ImmunoCAP has been suggested for pediatric AD patients of Western countries. The cornerstone aspects of causality assessment are an appropriate temporal relation between exposure of causative foods and onset of allergic symptoms, reproducibility, specificity of causative allergens, and biologic plausibility [7]. Table 1 shows the diagnostic value of sIgE levels with 95% positive predictive values [8]. However, the diagnostic level of specific IgE may be different in Asian countries and in adult AD patients. Usually, the likelihood of an allergic reaction increases as sIgE levels increase; nonetheless, sIgE levels do not predict the severity of clinical reactions. Indeed, many pediatric food allergy patients develop clinical tolerance with decreased sIgE levels, and thus, many clinician monitor sIgE levels over time for the prediction of remission of pediatric food allergy patients: [9] If sIgE to egg, milk, and peanut falls below 2 kU/L without a recent history of severe exacerbation, food challenge test can be performed to confirm remission [8].

Recently, oral immunotherapy for food allergens, such as peanut, egg, and cow's milk, has been actively administered in pediatric AD patients with food allergy at several hospitals. There are, however, still controversies on the efficacy and safety thereof [10, 11].

Inhalant Allergens

For AD after adolescence, inhalant allergens are more important aggravating factors. The most important inhalant allergens are house dust mite, pet dander, and pollen allergens: in temperate climate, *Dermatophagoides farinae* and *D. pteronyssinus* are the dominant species of house dust mites, whereas in tropical areas, *Blomia tropicalis* is dominant. AD patients sensitized to inhalant allergens are at high risk for respiratory allergic diseases, such as allergic rhinitis and asthma. As previously described, AD patients can be sensitized to allergens via the skin, and subjects can be extensively exposed to house dust mites or pet dander allergens through the skin, in addition to the respiratory tract. While it may be implausible to identify which route is more important for sensitization to inhalant allergens for respiratory allergic diseases, allergen sensitization patterns may differ according to the route of sensitization: One study showed that patients with AD are more frequently sensitized to minor allergens of house dust mites than respiratory allergy only patients [12]. Similarly, cat allergen sensitization patterns may also different between AD and respiratory allergy only patients. For respiratory allergy only patients, Fel d 1 has been recognized as the dominant allergen, whereas AD patients may be more frequently sensitized to Fel d 2 (albumin class) and Fel d 4 (lipocalin class) [13]. Furthermore, some allergens of house dust mites or pollen exhibit protease activity. Group 1 major allergens of house dust mites have cysteine protease activity, and contact with these allergens can disrupt the tight junctions of the epithelium and exacerbate skin barrier impairment in AD patients [14, 15].

Direct epicutaneous exposure to house dust mite can aggravate AD. Atopy patch tests with house dust mites induce exacerbated lesions showing infiltration of eosinophils and sIgE-positive Langerhans cells in the dermis, similar to AD lesions [16, 17]. Although the results of patch tests correlate well with clinical features and sIgE levels, the diagnosis of sensitization to inhalant allergens is still based on the skin prick test or serologic sIgE measurement with compatible clinical history. Respiratory exposure to inhalant allergens is also important. One randomized clinical trial (RCT) proved that inhalation of standardized house dust mites can aggravate AD lesions [18]. Exposure to pet dander usually exacerbates AD lesions in patients with pet dander sensitization. Aggravation of facial eczematous lesions in the pollen season is also frequently found in AD patients with pollinosis, and an environmental chamber study described the worsening of AD severity with grass pollen allergy upon grass pollen exposure [19].

The causal relationship between house dust mites and AD has been proven by several RCTs on avoidance strategies or immunotherapy. A double-blind placebo-controlled RCT study, which adapted three different environmental control modules for house dust mite avoidance, such as mattress encasement, benzyl tannate spray, and use of a high filtration vacuum cleaner, proved the effectiveness thereof [20]. Another RCT study evaluated the effect of mattress encasement only with adult AD patients. This study showed that mattress encasement was effective in both house dust mite-sensitized and non-sensitized AD patients, suggesting that this option is also also effective for the reduction of other inhalant allergens or nonspecific stimulants [21]. Although there is some controversy [22], positive RCT results of allergen-specific immunotherapy have also been reported with subcutaneous and sublingual immunotherapy for house dust mite-sensitized AD patients [23, 24].

Microbial Allergens

Dysbiosis is one of the cardinal features of AD. Research has shown that AD skin lesions have decreased bacterial diversity and that *Staphylococcus aureus* is more abundant than non-lesion skin. AD skin lesions show decreases in commensal bacteria, such as coagulase-negative *Staphylococcus*. Moreover, an abundance of *S. aureus* has been found to be correlated with AD severity and to increase markedly upon acute exacerbation. Recently, methicillin-resistant *S. aureus (MRSA)* consists 10~30% of isolated *S. aureus* from AD patient, and MRSA colonization is associated with more profound changes in the composition of commensal bacteria in AD patients. Management of MRSA is now an emerging challenge in AD patients. *S. aureus* produces staphylococcal enterotoxin A and B, enzymes, and other virulent proteins that induce inflammation and cause skin barrier dysfunction. These enterotoxins can act as superantigens and directly interacting with T-cell receptor. Finally, they can activate T cells and induce Th2 inflammation in AD and allergen sensitization [25]. *S. aureus* colonization may also induce food allergy via epicutaneous sensitization of egg, milk, and peanuts in children with AD [26]. Also, sIgE levels to staphylococcal enterotoxins have been shown to be positively correlated with the severity of AD and density of colonization [27]. Furthermore, these enterotoxin sIgE may also represent the biologic marker of Th2 inflammation aggravated by these organisms. Enterotoxins may also act as classical allergens and stimulate mast cells to release histamine [28].

Antibiotics and bleach bath are prescribed at the acute stage of AD exacerbation. However, the benefit is usually limited, showing only temporal improvement in bacterial diversity.

The majority of AD patients usually exhibit colonization of *Malassezia* species and high non-*Malassezia* diversity, with more prevalent colonization of *Candida albicans, Cryptococcus*, and *Aspergillus* species, compared to healthy controls [29]. Fungal colonization is more prevalent in head and neck type male AD patients [30], as *Malassezia* grows fast in sebum-rich areas, such as the head and neck and as sebaceous gland activity increases in males during adolescent or young age. Reactions to fungi can be divided into humoral and cell-mediated immunity. Colonization of *Malassezia* may produce chemokines and activate local antigen-presenting cells to finally activate Th2 inflammation. Adult AD patients frequently have high levels of *Malassezia* and/or *Candida* sIgE, compared to healthy controls. Fungal proteins also act as allergens that can activate mast cells and basophils. Short-course antifungal antibiotics may be beneficial for these patients.

In conclusion, sensitization to food and inhalant allergens is an important aggravating or causative factor for AD, and dysbiosis of microorganisms can also damage skin barrier tightness and facilitate to the proliferation of vicious products that not only act as allergens but also aggravate Th2 inflammation in AD lesions. Appropriate treatment strategies targeting culprit allergens, such as avoidance, allergen-specific immunotherapy, and short-course antibiotic treatments, are suggested.

References

1. Davidson WF, Leung DYM, Beck LA, Berin CM, Boguniewicz M, Busse WW, et al. Report from the National Institute of Allergy and Infectious Diseases workshop on "Atopic dermatitis and the atopic march: mechanisms and interventions". J Allergy Clin Immunol. 2019;143:894–913.
2. Tham EH, Leung DY. Mechanisms by which atopic dermatitis predisposes to food allergy and the atopic march. Allergy Asthma Immunol Res. 2019;11:4–15.
3. Tran MM, Lefebvre DL, Dharma C, Dai D, Lou WYW, Subbarao P, et al. Predicting the atopic march: results from the Canadian healthy infant longitudinal development study. J Allergy Clin Immunol. 2018;141:601–7.e8.
4. Lowe AJ, Leung DYM, Tang MLK, Su JC, Allen KJ. The skin as a target for prevention of the atopic march. Ann Allergy Asthma Immunol. 2018;120:145–51.
5. Galand C, Leyva-Castillo JM, Yoon J, Han A, Lee MS, McKenzie ANJ, et al. IL-33 promotes food anaphylaxis in epicutaneously sensitized mice by targeting mast cells. J Allergy Clin Immunol. 2016;138:1356–66.
6. Yagami A, Aihara M, Ikezawa Z, Hide M, Kishikawa R, Morita E, et al. Outbreak of immediate-type hydrolyzed wheat protein allergy due to a facial soap in Japan. J Allergy Clin Immunol. 2017;140:879–81.e7.
7. Hill AB. The environment and disease: association or causation? Proc R Soc Med. 1965;58:295–300.
8. Nowak-Wegrzyn A, Assa'ad AH, Bahna SL, Bock SA, Sicherer SH, Teuber SS. Work Group report: oral food challenge testing. J Allergy Clin Immunol. 2009;123:S365–83.
9. Shek LP, Soderstrom L, Ahlstedt S, Beyer K, Sampson HA. Determination of food specific IgE levels over time can predict the development of tolerance in cow's milk and hen's egg allergy. J Allergy Clin Immunol. 2004;114:387–91.
10. Ebisawa M, Ito K, Fujisawa T. Japanese guidelines for food allergy 2017. Allergol Int. 2017;66:248–64.
11. Burks AW, Jones SM, Wood RA, Fleischer DM, Sicherer SH, Lindblad RW, et al. Oral immunotherapy for treatment of egg allergy in children. N Engl J Med. 2012;367:233–43.
12. Park KH, Lee J, Lee JY, Lee SC, Sim DW, Shin JU, et al. Sensitization to various minor house dust mite allergens is greater in patients with atopic dermatitis than in those with respiratory allergic disease. Clin Exp Allergy. 2018;48:1050–8.
13. Wisniewski JA, Agrawal R, Minnicozzi S, Xin W, Patrie J, Heymann PW, et al. Sensitization to food and inhalant allergens in relation to age and wheeze among children with atopic dermatitis. Clin Exp Allergy. 2013;43:1160–70.
14. Wan H, Winton HL, Soeller C, Tovey ER, Gruenert DC, Thompson PJ, et al. Der p 1 facilitates transepithelial allergen delivery by disruption of tight junctions. J Clin Invest. 1999;104:123–33.
15. Nakamura T, Hirasawa Y, Takai T, Mitsuishi K, Okuda M, Kato T, et al. Reduction of skin barrier function by proteolytic activity of a recombinant house dust mite major allergen Der f 1. J Invest Dermatol. 2006;126:2719–23.
16. Langeveld-Wildschut EG, Thepen T, Bihari IC, ven Reijsen FC, de Vries IJ, Bruijnzeel PL, et al. Evaluation of the atopy patch test and the cutaneous late-phase reaction as relevant models for the study of allergic inflammation in patients with atopic eczema. J Allergy Clin Immunol. 1996;98:1019–27.
17. Langeveld-Wildschut EG, Bruijnzeel PL, Mudde GC, Versluis C, Van Ieperen-Van Dijk AG, Bihari IC, et al. Clinical and immunologic variables in skin of patients with atopic eczema and either positive or negative atopy patch test reactions. J Allergy Clin Immunol. 2000;105:1008–16.
18. Tupker RA, De Monchy JG, Coenraads PJ, Homan A, van der Meer JB. Induction of atopic dermatitis by inhalation of house dust mite. J Allergy Clin Immunol. 1996;97:1064–70.
19. Werfel T, Heratizadeh A, Niebuhr M, Kapp A, Roesner LM, Karch A, et al. Exacerbation of atopic dermatitis on grass pollen exposure in an environmental challenge chamber. J Allergy Clin Immunol. 2015;136:96–103.e9.
20. Tan BB, Weald D, Strickland I, Friedman PS. Double-blind controlled trial of effect of housedust-mite allergen avoidance on atopic dermatitis. Lancet. 1996;347:15–8.
21. Holm L, Ohman S, Bengtsson A, van Hage-Hamsten M, Sheynius A. Effectiveness of occlusive bedding in the treatment of atopic dermatitis—a placebo-controlled tiral of 12 months' duration. Allergy. 2001;56:152–8.
22. Tam H, Calderon MA, Manikam L, Nankervis H, García Núñez I, Williams HC, et al. Specific allergen immunotherapy for the treatment of atopic eczema (Review). Cochrane Database Syst Rev. 2016;2016:CD008774.
23. Bae JM, Choi YY, Park CO, Chung KY, Lee KH. Efficacy of allergen-specific immunotherapy

for atopic dermatitis: a systematic review and meta-analysis of randomized controlled trials. J Allergy Clin Immunol. 2013;132:110–7.
24. Pajno GB, Caminiti L, Vita D, Barberio G, Salzano G, Lombardo F, et al. Sublingual immunotherapy in mite-sensitized children with atopic dermatitis: a randomized, double-blind, placebo-controlled study. J Allergy Clin Immunol. 2007;120:164–70.
25. Kim J, Kim BE, Ahn K, Leung DYM. Interactions between atopic dermatitis and *staphylococcus aureus* infection: clinical implications. Allergy Asthma Immunol Res. 2019;11:593–603.
26. Jones AL, Curran-Everett D, Leung DYM. Food allergy is associated with *Staphylococcus aureus* colonization in children with atopic dermatitis. J Allergy Clin Immunol. 2016;137:1247–8.e3.
27. Bunikowski R, Mielke M, Skarabis H, Herz U, Bergmann RL, Wahn U, et al. Prevalence and role of serum IgE antibodies to the Staphylococcus aureus-derived superantigens SEA and SEB in children with atopic dermatitis. J Allergy Clin Immunol. 1999;103:119–24.
28. Leung DY, Harbeck R, Bina P, Reiser RF, Yang E, Norris DA, et al. Presence of IgE antibodies to staphylococcal exotoxins on the skin of patients with atopic dermatitis. Evidence for a new group of allergens. J Clin Invest. 1993;92:1374–80.
29. Zhang E, Tanaka T, Tajima M, Tsuboi R, Nishikawa A, Sugita T. Characterization of the skin fungal microbiota in patients with atopic dermatitis and in healthy subjects. Microbiol Immunol. 2011;55:625–32.
30. Brodska P, Panzner P, Pizinger K, Schmid-Grendelmeier P. IgE-mediated sensitization to malassezia in atopic dermatitis: more common in male patients and in head and neck type. Dermatitis. 2014;25:120–6.

Role of Infection and Microbial Factors

Sang Eun Lee

Changes in Cutaneous Microbiome in Atopic Dermatitis

Cutaneous Microbiome in Healthy Skin

The skin has many species of bacteria, fungi, and viruses that have adapted to utilize the sparse nutrients available on the skin [1]. Since the shotgun metagenomic DNA sequencing was utilized, which has enabled to assess the skin microbiota at the kingdom, species, strain, or gene level, the diversity of the cutaneous microbiome has been revealed. The composition of bacterial communities varies by body sites and these differences are influenced by pH, temperature, and moisture levels [2]. Species of *Cutibacterium* and fungi, mainly of the genus *Malassezia* are predominant in oily sites, whereas moist sites have fewer Cutibacterium and relatively more Staphylococcus [1, 3]. These commensal skin microorganisms have been demonstrated to control innate and adaptive skin immune systems [4–10].

During the early-life, microbiota of the individuals is rapidly changed and established. The exposure to microbiota begins in utero and expands rapidly after birth. The mode of delivery and subsequent environmental exposures influence the composition of the microbiota in the infant [11]. A recent study demonstrated that exposure of neonatal mice skin to a commensal microbiota induces accumulation of activated regulatory T cells in the skin that results in the subsequent tolerance to this same antigen-containing microbiota in later life, suggesting that commensal microbiota exposure in the early period of life shapes the skin's immune system [12]. Meanwhile, the skin microbiota of a healthy adult has been shown to remain constant over time, despite the changes in environment [13]. Normal skin flora is not harmful to their host (commensal). Some skin flora even offers the beneficial effects on the host by preventing the colonization of transient pathogenic organisms either by competing for nutrients, secreting antimicrobial peptides, or interacting with immunes cells such as dendritic cells and T cells [6, 14–19]. The protective role of skin commensal bacteria against AD will be discussed in the later section.

Dysbiosis in Atopic Dermatitis Skin

An altered microbial state in the skin has been demonstrated to be associated with various inflammatory skin diseases, such as AD, psoriasis, rosacea, and acne vulgaris [20–24]. The key components in the pathogenesis of AD are

S. E. Lee (✉)
Department of Dermatology, Gangnam Severance Hospital, Yonsei University College of Medicine, Seoul, Korea (Republic of)
e-mail: jennifer823@yuhs.ac

K. H. Lee et al. (eds.), *Practical Insights into Atopic Dermatitis*,
https://doi.org/10.1007/978-981-15-8159-5_11

impaired skin barrier function, Th2-deviated immune reactions, and dysbiosis. Skin barrier abnormalities and dysregulated Th2 immune responses can lead to dysbiosis and conversely, dysbiosis can cause barrier damage and inflammation. Inherited or acquired filaggrin deficiency is common in patients with AD; therefore, the degradation products of filaggrin including trans-urocanic acid are reduced, resulting in the increased skin surface pH that renders the skin infection vulnerable [25]. Levels of natural moisturizing factor in the stratum corneum have been shown to control the adhesion of *Staphylococcus aureus* (*S. aureus*) to corneocytes [26]. AD patients also show disturbances of antimicrobial lipids in the skin [27]. The increased prevalence of *S. aureus* on lesional skin and anterior nares of AD patients with *FLG* mutations compared with AD patients without *FLG* mutations supports that barrier abnormalities lead to cutaneous dysbiosis [28]. Th2 cytokines attenuate the expression of antimicrobial peptides, predisposing AD skin to *S. aureus* infection [29]. In addition, Th2 cytokines such as interleukin(IL)-4 have been shown to promote the binding by *S. aureus*, that is mediated by fibronectin and fibrinogen [30]. A recent study from Callewaert et al. reported that inhibition of IL-4 and IL-13 signaling by Dupilumab decreased *S. aureus* abundance and increased bacterial diversity in patients with AD, suggesting the contribution of dysregulated Th2 immunity to the dysbiosis of AD [31]. Dysbiosis in AD is characterized by the colonization by *S. aureus* and a decreased diversity of microbiome [20–22]. *S. aureus* skin colonization is s characteristic of lesional and non-lesional skin in AD and is generally accepted to be associated with increased disease severity and flares of AD [20–22]. In the first section, we will focus on the role of *S. aureus* in the pathogenesis of AD, the involvement of other skin commensal bacteria that promote health and protect against *S. aureus* in the AD pathogenesis, and the potential of targeting cutaneous microbiomes for therapeutic intervention in AD.

The Role of *Staphylococcus aureus* in the AD Pathogenesis

The role of *S. aureus* as a potential trigger factor for AD has been extensively explored. A recent meta-analysis revealed that the prevalence of *S. aureus* skin colonization in AD patients was 70% on lesional skin, 39% on non-lesional skin, and 62% on the nose [32]. It has been demonstrated that disease flare is accompanied by *S. aureus* dominance in both lesional and non-lesional skin and *S. aureus* colonization precedes the disease flare [33]. A previous study using ADAM17-deficiency mice that developed eczematous dermatitis with naturally occurring dysbiosis also demonstrated that dysbiosis precedes the eczematous dermatitis and the inoculation of *S. aureus* induces eczematous dermatitis [34]. These findings suggest a role of dysbiosis with *S. aureus* dominance is a driving factor in the development of eczematous inflammation.

Virulent Factors from *Staphylococcus aureus*

S. aureus commonly colonizes the epidermis, and many virulent factors of *S. aureus* have been demonstrated to trigger skin inflammation. Virulence factors of *S. aureus* are secreted out or located on the surface of the cell wall. *S. aureus* secretes toxins with superantigen activity, various cytotoxins, and enzymes (Table 1) [35]. Superantigens from *S. aureus* include toxic shock syndrome toxin-1 (TSST-1) and staphylococcal enterotoxins A, B, and C (SEA, SEB, and SEC) and superantigens bind both the major histocompatibility complex class II on antigen-presenting cells and the T cell receptor on T cells, inducing an overactive immune responses and cytokines production [36]. Indeed, SEB has been shown to induce eczema when it is applied to healthy and atopic skin by a T cell–superantigen-mediated mechanism [37]. In addition, SEB and TSST-1 can stimulate Th2 cells to secrete IL-31 that induces itch and barrier disruption by inhibiting keratinocytes differentiation [38].

Table 1 Virulence factors from *Staphylococcus aureus*

Classes/toxin	Effect on skin barrier	Effect on immune dysregulation
Superantigens		
Toxic shock syndrome toxin-1		Excessive T cell cytokine production and toxicity
Staphylococcal enterotoxins		• Activation of Langerhans cells • Mast cell degranulation • Recruitment of eosinophils
Cytotoxins		
α-toxin	• Interacting with lipid sphingomyelin • Lysis of keratinocytes • Alteration of E-cadherin integrity	
β-toxin	Hydrolyzes sphingomyelin	
δ-toxin	Permeabilizes ceramide hydrophobic domain	• Mast cell degranulation • Th2 type skin inflammation
Phenol-soluble modulins	Keratinocyte damage by cell wall lysis	Release of the alarmins (IL-1α and IL-36α) → Induction of IL-17-producing ϒδT cells and ILC3
Enzymes		
V8 serine protease	Epidermal barrier dysfunction	
Cell wall proteins		
Protein A		TNFR1 activation on keratinocytes
Clumping factor A	Adhesion and internalization into keratinocytes	
Fibronectin binding proteins		
Lipoproteins		Toll-like receptor 2 activation on keratinocytes

ILC3 Type 3 innate lymphoid cells, *TNFR1* Tumor necrosis factor receptor 1

Superantigens also act as allergens and superantigens-specific IgE antibodies induce the degranulation of mast cells and basophils. Enterotoxins can also trigger mast cell degranulation directly via an unknown mechanism and induce Langerhans cell activation and eosinophils recruitment [36, 39]. The findings that the density of superantigens-expressing bacteria and the level of IgE recognizing the superantigens correlate with disease activity of AD suggest a role of *S. aureus*-secreted superantigens in the pathogenesis of AD [40, 41]. *S. aureus* also secretes cytotoxins such as α-, β-, and δ-toxin and phenol-soluble modulins (PSM). On the surface of the epithelial barrier, α-type PSMs (PSMα) induces keratinocyte damage, releasing alarmins, IL-1α and IL-36α from keratinocytes. In a mouse model of *S. aureus* cutaneous infection, induction of IL-17-producing ϒδT cells and type 3 innate lymphoid cells through these alarmins via Myd88 signaling has been shown to be crucial for cutaneous inflammation in response to *S. aureus* [42]. The δ-toxin is also the member of the PSM family and has been shown to trigger mast cell degranulation that is not mediated by IgE cross-linking [43]. In the ovalbumin-sensitized murine AD model, δ-toxin from *S. aureus* has been shown to be important for IgE and IL-4 production, and cutaneous inflammation during *S. aureus* colonization. α-toxin, also known as α-hemolysin that belongs to the pore-forming toxin family has been shown to induce keratinocyte cell death in AD skin [44]. α-hemolysin also contributes to skin barrier disruption by interacting with lipid sphingomyelin and by altering the integrity of E-cadherin [45]. β-toxin from *S. aureus* can also hydrolyze sphingomyelin, thereby disrupting the lipid barrier of the skin [46]. In addition to exotoxins, *S. aureus* secretes many enzymes such as multiple proteases that can facilitate epithelial infection and immune evasion and disrupt the skin barrier. *S. aureus*-derived serine protease V8 and serine-like protease exfoliative toxins have been shown to disrupt the integrity of skin barrier via desmoglein 1 cleavage in corneodesmosomes, which causes abnormal desquamation [47]. *S. aureus* can also stimulate human keratinocytes to increase the activity of endogenous proteases, such as kallikrein (KLK)6, KLK13, and KLK14, that degrade epidermal barrier proteins, desmoglein-1 and filaggrin [48]. The cell wall proteins of *S. aureus*, including clumping factor A, fibronectin-binding proteins, autolysin, and serine aspartate repeat containing protein D facilitate *S. aureus* to adhere and internalize into keratinocytes via binding to each receptor [49]. Protein A has been shown to induce inflammation by binding to Tumor necrosis factor receptor-1. *S. aureus* also activates innate immune responses by activating Toll-like receptor 2 via lipoprotein and NLRP3 inflammasome via hemolysins and bacterial lipoproteins in keratinocytes [50]. These findings suggest that toxins from *S. aureus* infection plays an important role in atopic eczema by disrupting the skin barrier and triggering the innate and acquired immune responses.

Biofilm is one of the virulence factors of many bacteria. By formation of biofilm, microorganisms become resistant to antibiotics and the immune responses. The formation of biofilm of *S. aureus* was identified in AD-affected skin. Staphylococcal biofilms have been shown to inhibit the differentiation of keratinocytes and induce apoptosis and cytokine secretion by keratinocytes [51]. In addition, biofilm of *S. aureus* is thought to occlude the sweat ducts, leading to inflammation and pruritus in AD.

Regulation of *Staphylococcus aureus* Virulence

For survival in the host, many bacteria use a cell–cell communication system called quorum sensing to coordinate population density-dependent changes in behavior. The accessory gene regulator (agr) was identified as a quorum-sensing system in *S. aureus* [52]. Agr senses the local concentration of the self-produced peptides known as autoinducing peptides, allowing *S. aureus* to sense its own population density and translate this information into a specific gene expression pattern [52]. RNAIII is the major effector of agr system. The expression of virulence factors of *S. aureus* such as δ-toxin is known to be controlled by this quorum-sensing agr system [53]. In addition, an autoinducing peptide from Coagulase-negative staphylococci species has been shown to inhibit the agr activity of *S. aureus*, suggesting commensal bacteria can control the colonization and virulence of *S. aureus* [54].

A recent study demonstrated that the inhibition of agr by solonamide B abolished δ-toxin production and reduced skin inflammation in BALB/c mice colonized epicutaneously with *S. aureus*, suggesting that targeting the agr might be an effective strategy to prevent *S. aureus*-induced cutaneous inflammation [55].

The Protective Role of Skin Commensal Bacteria Against Atopic Dermatitis and the Important Role of Early-Life Skin Microbiome in the Development of Atopic Dermatitis

A decreased diversity of microbiome is a characteristic microbial change of both lesional and non-lesional skin of atopic dermatitis (AD), suggesting a protective role of skin commensal bacteria against AD. Recently various mechanisms underlying the beneficial effects of skin commensal bacteria on AD have been revealed.

First, commensal bacteria can regulate innate and acquired immune responses. Defined skin commensal bacteria, in particular Staphylococcus epidermidis, have been shown to induce a commensal-specific IL-17A+ CD8+ T cell response, that enhances innate protection against fungus, while preserving tissue homeostasis. Distinct dendritic cell subsets are suggested to mediate host–commensal interaction in the skin [14]. Commensal bacteria have been demonstrated to inhibit injury-induced skin inflammation via staphylococcal lipoteichoic acid-TLR2-mediated suppression of TLR3 signaling [16]. Staphylococcus epidermidis can increase the induction of antimicrobial peptide (AMP) expression, thereby amplifying the innate immune response of epidermis to pathogenic microorganisms [15]. In addition, several species of commensal bacteria can metabolize glycerol into antimicrobial compounds to inhibit the overgrowth of *S. aureus* [15, 18, 19].

Moreover, a recent study reported that Lactococcus lactis strain plasma elicit IL-17A production from CD8+ T cells via the Toll-like receptor 9 signaling pathway, which in turn, suppresses *S. aureus* burdens and reduces skin inflammation [17].

Coagulase-negative staphylococci that are commensal organisms of human skin including Staphylococcus epidermidis and Staphylococcus hominis are significantly reduced in AD skin. Certain strains of Coagulase-negative staphylococci produce AMP that synergize with a human AMP [15]. Indeed, many challenges of topical probiotics or skin bacterial transplant for the restoration of a healthy skin microbiome in AD patients are ongoing. Based on the beneficial effect of topical application of commensal bacteria, *Roseomonas mucosa* on the AD murine model, first in-human topical microbiome transplantation with Lethally irradiated *Roseomonas mucosa* was performed in AD patients and showed decreased disease severity and *S. aureus* burden [56]. In addition, topical application of selected *Coagulase-negative staphylococci* strains with antimicrobial activity has been demonstrated to decrease *S. aureus* colonization in murine and atopic patients' skin [15]. Future research should be continued on safer ways to restore the commensal bacteria or improve their beneficial effects on AD.

Moreover, recent birth cohort studies demonstrated that skin colonization by *S. aureus* in early-life is positively associated with subsequent AD development, whereas skin colonization by commensal staphylococci such as *S. hominis* in infancy is negatively associated with subsequent AD development, suggesting a beneficial role of early-life skin colonization by commensal staphylococci on AD development [33, 57].

Fungal Infection in AD

Fungi are also the aggravating factors of AD due to the frequent detection of IgE antibodies to fungi *Malassezia* species in patients with AD and to the fact that topical or systemic antifungal therapy is effective in some patients with AD. *Malassezia furfur*, a lipophilic yeast, is considered to be a pathogenic allergen in this form of AD. Head and neck dermatitis is thought to be a variant of atopic dermatitis often seen in young adults. Head and neck is seborrheic area and is prone to colonization by *Malassezia*, a lipophilic yeast. Recent evidences suggest that *Malassezia furfur* is a pathogenic allergen in AD with prominent symptoms in the head and neck. In a recent study that analyzed 173 patients with AD, 49.1% of AD patients were shown to have a specific IgE to *Malassezia*. In addition, more patients with head and neck type AD (58%) had higher levels of specific IgE to Malassezia than non-head and neck type AD patients (42%) [58]. *Malassezia* yeasts except *Malassezia furfur* have been shown to induce proinflammatory cytokines, IL-6, IL-8, and TNF-α in keratinocytes [59]. A recent study demonstrated that *Malassezia* selectively triggers Th17 responses in the skin that is crucial for antifungal immunity but also promotes skin inflammation [60]. Further studies are ongoing on the mechanisms underlying the yeast colonization and AD exacerbation.

Viral Infection in AD

The lesional skin of AD is also susceptible to viral skin infection. In particular, eczema herpeticum, a widespread viral infection caused by herpes simplex virus 1 (HSV-1) in eczematous skin, is one of the acute and severe cutaneous infectious events in AD. An early-onset AD, more severe disease, and high total serum IgE/peripheral eosinophils are known to be the risk factors of eczema herpeticum in AD patients [61, 62]. In addition, topical application of calcineurin inhibitor has been associated with an occurrence of eczema herpeticum in AD [63].

Decreased levels of AMP, such as LL-37 and HBD2 in AD skin may underlie the susceptibility to viral infection, and previous studies have shown that genetic variants in thymic stromal lymphopoietin, signal transducer and activator of transcription 6 (STAT6), Interferon(IFN)-gamma, interferon regulatory factor 2, and IFNGR1 gene are significantly associated with eczema herpeticum in AD patients [64]. These findings suggest that Th2-skewed immune responses and impaired pathway of IFN, a crucial cytokine in the immunity against virus underlie the susceptibility to viral skin infection in AD patients.

Molluscum contagiosum is a common childhood skin infection caused by a poxvirus. In healthy children, molluscum contagiosum is usually self-limiting, whereas, in pediatric patients with AD, infection can be widespread and frequently recurred. The impaired skin barrier function may be associated with frequent and widespread molluscum contagiosum in AD patients. Indeed, a recent study demonstrated that the presence of FLG polymorphisms significantly increased the risk of M contagiosum virus-associated skin infection [65]. Conversely, Molluscum contagiosum virus (MCV) infection is thought to aggravate atopic eczema in pediatric patients with AD. Moreover, MCV infection within the specific localization to the flexural areas in children younger than 3 years of age seems to have the potential to trigger AD in susceptible individuals [66]. The strategies for reinforcement of skin barrier function, such as topical evening primrose oil application might be the preventive method to reduce the MCV-associated skin infection in AD patients.

References

1. Byrd AL, Belkaid Y, Segre JA. The human skin microbiome. Nat Rev Microbiol. 2018;16(3):143–55.
2. Dimitriu PA, Iker B, Malik K, et al. New insights into the intrinsic and extrinsic factors that shape the human skin microbiome. mBio. 2019;10:e00839–19.
3. Grice EA, Kong HH, Conlan S, et al. Topographical and temporal diversity of the human skin microbiome. Science. 2009;324:1190–2.
4. Lai Y, Di Nardo A, Nakatsuji T, et al. Commensal bacteria regulate Toll-like receptor 3-dependent inflammation after skin injury. Nat Med. 2009;15:1377e1382.
5. Bernard JJ, Cowing-Zitron C, Nakatsuji T, et al. Ultraviolet radiation damages self noncoding RNA and is detected by TLR3. Nat Med. 2012;18:1286e1290.
6. Lai Y, Cogen AL, Radek KA, et al. Activation of TLR2 by a small molecule produced by Staphylococcus epidermidis increases antimicrobial defense against bacterial skin infections. J Invest Dermatol. 2010;130:2211e2221.
7. Li D, Lei H, Li Z, Li H, Wang Y, Lai Y. A novel lipopeptide from skin commensal activates TLR2/CD36-p38 MAPK signaling to increase antibacterial defense against bacterial infection. PLoS One. 2013;8:e58288.
8. Naik S, Bouladoux N, Wilhelm C, et al. Compartmentalized control of skin immunity by resident commensals. Science. 2012;337:1115e1119.
9. Naik S, Bouladoux N, Linehan JL, et al. Commensal-dendritic-cell interaction specifies a unique protective skin immune signature. Nature. 2015;520:104e108.
10. Linehan JL, Harrison OJ, Han SJ, et al. Non-classical immunity controls microbiota impact on skin immunity and tissue repair. Cell. 2018;172:784e796.
11. Dominguez-Bello MG, Costello EK, Contreras M, Magris M, et al. Delivery mode shapes the acquisition and structure of the initial microbiota across multiple body habitats in newborns. Proc Natl Acad Sci U S A. 2010;107(26):11971–5.
12. Scharschmidt TC, Vasquez KS, Truong HA, Gearty SV, Pauli ML, Nosbaum A, et al. A wave of regulatory T cells into neonatal skin mediates tolerance to commensal microbes. Immunity. 2015;43:1011–21.
13. Oh J, Byrd AL, Park M, Kong HH, Segre JA. Temporal stability of the human skin microbiome. Cell. 2016;165:854–66.
14. Naik S, Bouladoux N, Linehan JL, Han SJ, Harrison OJ, Wilhelm C, et al. Commensal-dendritic-cell interaction specifies a unique protective skin immune signature. Nature. 2015;520(7545):104–8.
15. Nakatsuji T, Chen TH, Narala S, Chun KA, Two AM, Yun T, et al. Antimicrobials from human skin commensal bacteria protect against *Staphylococcus aureus* and are deficient in atopic dermatitis. Sci Transl Med. 2017;9:378.
16. Lai Y, Di Nardo A, Nakatsuji T, Leichtle A, Yang Y, Cogen AL, et al. Commensal bacteria regulate Toll-like receptor 3-dependent inflammation after skin injury. Nat Med. 2009;15(12):1377–82.
17. Tsuji R, Fujii T, Nakamura Y, Yazawa K, Kanauchi O. *Staphylococcus aureus* epicutaneous infection is suppressed by Lactococcus lactis strain plasma via interleukin 17A elicitation. J Infect Dis. 2019;220(5):892–901.
18. Francuzik W, Franke K, Schumann RR, Heine G, Worm M. Propionibacterium acnes abundance correlates inversely with *Staphylococcus aureus*: data from atopic dermatitis skin microbiome. Acta Derm Venereol. 2018;98(5):490–5.

19. Shu M, Wang Y, Yu J, et al. Fermentation of Propionibacterium acnes, a commensal bacterium in the human skin microbiome, as skin probiotics against methicillin-resistant *Staphylococcus aureus*. PLoS One. 2013;8(2):e55380.
20. Paller AS, Kong HH, Seed P, Naik S, Scharschmidt TC, Gallo RL, et al. The microbiome in patients with atopic dermatitis. J Allergy Clin Immunol. 2019 Jan;143(1):26–35.
21. Kong HH, Oh J, Deming C, et al. Temporal shifts in the skin microbiome associated with disease flares and treatment in children with atopic dermatitis. Genome Res. 2012;22:850–9.
22. Williams MR, Gallo RL. The role of skin microbiome in atopic dermatitis. Curr Allergy Asthma Rep. 2015;11:65.
23. Alekseyenko AV, Perez-Perez GI, De Souza A, et al. Community differentiation of the cutaneous microbiota in psoriasis. Microbiome. 2013;1:31.
24. Murillo N, Raoult D. Skin microbiota: overview and role in the skin diseases acne vulgaris and rosacea. Future Microbiol. 2013;8(2):209–22.
25. Thyssen JP, Kezic S. Causes of epidermal filaggrin reduction and their role in the pathogenesis of atopic dermatitis. J Allergy Clin Immunol. 2014;134(4):792–9.
26. Feuillie C, Vitry P, McAleer MA, Kezic S, Irvine AD, Geoghegan JA, et al. Adhesion of *Staphylococcus aureus* to corneocytes from atopic dermatitis patients is controlled by natural moisturizing factor levels. MBio. 2018;9(4):e01184-18.
27. Melnik B. Disturbances of antimicrobial lipids in atopic dermatitis. J Dtsch Dermatol Ges. 2006;4(2):114–23.
28. Clausen ML, Agner T, Lilje B, Edslev SM, Johannesen TB, Andersen PS. Association of disease severity with skin microbiome and filaggrin gene mutations in adult atopic dermatitis. JAMA Dermatol. 2018;154(3):293–300.
29. Howell MD, Gallo RL, Boguniewicz M, et al. Cytokine milieu of atopic dermatitis skin subverts the innate immune response to vaccinia virus. Immunity. 2006;24:341e348.
30. Cho SH, Strickland I, Boguniewicz M, Leung DY. Fibronectin and fibrinogen contribute to the enhanced binding of *Staphylococcus aureus* to atopic skin. J Allergy Clin Immunol. 2001 Aug;108(2):269–74.
31. Callewaert C, Nakatsuji T, Knight R, Kosciolek T, Vrbanac A, Kotol P, et al. IL-4Rα blockade by dupilumab decreases *Staphylococcus aureus* colonization and increases microbial diversity in atopic dermatitis. J Invest Dermatol. 2020;140(1):191–202.e7.
32. Totté JE, van der Feltz WT, Hennekam M, van Belkum A, van Zuuren EJ, Pasmans SG. Prevalence and odds of *Staphylococcus aureus* carriage in atopic dermatitis: a systematic review and meta-analysis. Br J Dermatol. 2016;175(4):687–95.
33. Meylan P, Lang C, Mermoud S, Johannsen A, Norrenberg S, Hohl D, et al. Skin colonization by *Staphylococcus aureus* precedes the clinical diagnosis of atopic dermatitis in infancy. J Invest Dermatol. 2017;137(12):2497–504.
34. Kobayashi T, Glatz M, Horiuchi K, Kawasaki H, Akiyama H, Kaplan DH, et al. Dysbiosis and *Staphylococcus aureus* colonization drives inflammation in atopic dermatitis. Immunity. 2015;42(4):756–66.
35. Geoghegan JA, Irvine AD, Foster TJ. *Staphylococcus aureus* and atopic dermatitis: a complex and evolving relationship. Trends Microbiol. 2018;26(6):484–97.
36. Spaulding AR, et al. Staphylococcal and streptococcal superantigen exotoxins. Clin Microbiol Rev. 2013;26:422–47.
37. Skov L, Olsen JV, Giorno R, Schlievert PM, Baadsgaard O, Leung DY. Application of Staphylococcal enterotoxin B on normal and atopic skin induces up-regulation of T cells by a superantigen-mediated mechanism. J Allergy Clin Immunol. 2000;105(4):820–6.
38. Niebuhr M, Mamerow D, Heratizadeh A, Satzger I, Werfel T. Staphylococcal α-toxin induces a higher T cell proliferation and interleukin-31 in atopic dermatitis. Int Arch Allergy Immunol. 2011;156(4):412–5.
39. Ono HK, et al. Submucosal mast cells in the gastrointestinal tract are a target of staphylococcal enterotoxin type A. FEMS Immunol Med Microbiol. 2012;64:392–402.
40. Leung DY, et al. Presence of IgE antibodies to staphylococcal exotoxins on the skin of patients with atopic dermatitis. Evidence for a new group of allergens. J Clin Invest. 1993;92:1374–80.
41. Bunikowski R, et al. Prevalence and role of serum IgE antibodies to the *Staphylococcus aureus*-derived superantigens SEA and SEB in children with atopic dermatitis. J Allergy Clin Immunol. 1999;103:119–24.
42. Nakagawa S, Matsumoto M, Katayama Y, Oguma R, Wakabayashi S, Nygaard T, et al. *Staphylococcus aureus* virulent PSMα peptides induce keratinocyte alarmin release to orchestrate IL-17-dependent skin inflammation. Cell Host Microbe. 2017;22(5):667–677.e5.
43. Nakamura Y, Oscherwitz J, Cease KB, Chan SM, Muñoz-Planillo R, Hasegawa M, et al. Staphylococcus δ-toxin induces allergic skin disease by activating mast cells. Nature. 2013;503(7476):397–401.
44. Brauweiler AM, et al. Filaggrin-dependent secretion of sphingomyelinase protects against staphylococcal alpha-toxin induced keratinocyte death. J Allergy Clin Immunol. 2013;131:421–7.
45. Triplett KD, Pokhrel S, Castleman MJ, Daly SM, Elmore BO, Joyner JA, et al. GPER activation protects against epithelial barrier disruption by *Staphylococcus aureus* α-toxin. Sci Rep. 2019;9(1):1343.
46. Otto M. *Staphylococcus aureus* toxins. Curr Opin Microbiol. 2014;17:32–7.
47. Hirasawa Y, et al. *Staphylococcus aureus* extracellular protease causes epidermal barrier dysfunction. J Invest Dermatol. 2010;130:614–7.
48. Williams MR, Nakatsuji T, Sanford JA, Alison F, et al. *Staphylococcus aureus* induces increased serine

protease activity in keratinocytes. J Invest Dermatol. 2017;137(2):377–84.
49. Iwamoto K, Moriwaki M, Miyake R, Hide M. *Staphylococcus aureus* in atopic dermatitis: strain-specific cell wall proteins and skin immunity. Allergol Int. 2019 Jul;68(3):309–15.
50. Iwamoto K, Moriwaki M, Miyake R, Hide M. *Staphylococcus aureus* in atopic dermatitis: strain-specific cell wall proteins and skin immunity. Allergol Int. 2019;68(3):309–15.
51. Gonzalez T, Biagini Myers JM, Herr AB, Khurana Hershey GK. Staphylococcal biofilms in atopic dermatitis. Curr Allergy Asthma Rep. 2017;17(12):81.
52. Wang R, Braughton KR, Kretschmer D, Bach TH, Queck SY, Li M, et al. Identification of novel cytolytic peptides as key virulence determinants for community-associated MRSA. Nat Med. 2007;13(12):1510–4.
53. Janzon L, Löfdahl S, Arvidson S. Identification and nucleotide sequence of the delta-lysin gene, hld, adjacent to the accessory gene regulator (agr) of *Staphylococcus aureus*. Mol Gen Genet. 1989;219:480–5.
54. Williams MR, Costa SK, Zaramela LS, Khalil S, Todd DA, Winter HL, et al. Quorum sensing between bacterial species on the skin protects against epidermal injury in atopic dermatitis. Sci Transl Med. 2019;11(490):eaat8329.
55. Baldry M, Nakamura Y, Nakagawa S, Frees D, Matsue H, Núñez G, et al. Application of an agr-specific antivirulence compound as therapy for *Staphylococcus aureus*-induced inflammatory skin disease. J Infect Dis. 2018;218(6):1009–13.
56. Myles IA, Earland NJ, Anderson ED, Moore IN, Kieh MD, Williams KW, et al. First-in-human topical microbiome transplantation with Roseomonas mucosa for atopic dermatitis. JCI Insight. 2018;3(9):e120608.
57. Kennedy EA, Connolly J, Hourihane JO, Fallon PG, McLean WHI, Murray D, et al. Skin microbiome before development of atopic dermatitis: early colonization with commensal staphylococci at 2 months is associated with a lower risk of atopic dermatitis at 1 year. J Allergy Clin Immunol. 2017;139(1):166–72.
58. Brodská P, Panzner P, Pizinger K, Schmid-Grendelmeier P. IgE-mediated sensitization to malassezia in atopic dermatitis: more common in male patients and in head and neck type. Dermatitis. 2014;25(3):120–6.
59. Thomas DS, Ingham E, Bojar RA, Holland KT. In vitro modulation of human keratinocyte pro- and anti-inflammatory cytokine production by the capsule of Malassezia species. FEMS Immunol Med Microbiol. 2008;54(2):203–14.
60. Sparber F, De Gregorio C, Steckholzer S, Ferreira FM, Dolowschiak T, Ruchti F, et al. The skin commensal yeast malassezia triggers a type 17 response that coordinates anti-fungal immunity and exacerbates skin inflammation. Cell Host Microbe. 2019;25(3):389–403.e6.
61. Beck LA, Boguniewicz M, Hata T, Schneider LC, Hanifin J, Gallo R, Paller AS, Lieff S, Reese J, Zaccaro D, Milgrom H, Barnes KC, Leung DY. Phenotype of atopic dermatitis subjects with a history of eczema herpeticum. J Allergy Clin Immunol. 2009;124(2):260–9.
62. Wollenberg A, Zoch C, Wetzel S, Plewig G, Przybilla B. Predisposing factors and clinical features of eczema herpeticum: a retrospective analysis of 100 cases. J Am Acad Dermatol. 2003;49:198–205.
63. Segura S, Romero D, Carrera C, Iranzo P, Estrach T. Eczema herpeticum during treatment of atopic dermatitis with 1% pimecrolimus cream. Acta Derm Venereol. 2005;85(6):524–5.
64. Ong PY, Leung DY. Bacterial and viral infections in atopic dermatitis: a comprehensive review. Clin Rev Allergy Immunol. 2016;51(3):329–37.
65. Manti S, Amorini M, Cuppari C, Salpietro A, Porcino F, Leonardi S, et al. Filaggrin mutations and Molluscum contagiosum skin infection in patients with atopic dermatitis. Ann Allergy Asthma Immunol. 2017;119(5):446–51.
66. Silverberg NB. Molluscum contagiosum virus infection can trigger atopic dermatitis disease onset or flare. Cutis. 2018;102(3):191–4.

Psychological Stress

Jung U Shin

Introduction

Stress is a normal physiological response to internal or external adverse changes that threaten our body. To overcome these challenges, our body activates physiological systems, which is called *stress response*. While stress is generally considered immunosuppressive, the duration (acute or chronic), intensity, and persistence (intermittent or sustained) of the stressor are important distinguishing factors that modulate *stress response* [1, 2]. Acute stress occurs within a period of minutes to hour, whereas chronic stress persists for days to months [2]. In this chapter, we will review which body system is involved in the stress response, how it is related to the aggravation of atopic dermatitis (AD), and what strategies can be applied to ameliorate stress-induced AD aggravation.

J. U. Shin (✉)
Department of Dermatology, CHA Bundang Medical Center, CHA University, Seongnam, Korea (Republic of)
e-mail: likesomeone@cha.ac.kr

Clinical Evidence of the Psychological Stress-Induced Aggravation in Atopic Dermatitis

Studies reported that AD can be triggered or exacerbated by psychological stress, and emotional factors can change the natural course of the disease [3–6]. For example, Oh et al. [7] demonstrated that AD patients frequently experienced depression, anxiety, and anxiousness and showed lower life quality than healthy controls. Interestingly, these psychological parameters did not correlate with the severity of clinical symptoms but showed a positive correlation with the intensity of pruritus. As a support to the relationship between pruritus and psychological stress, more than 70% of AD patients reported that stressful life events preceded the onset of itching [8]. Increased itch due to psychological stress can activate the vicious itch-scratch cycle, leading to worsening of AD. In another study, stress was the second most prevalent factor that aggravates AD following seasonal variation, affecting 60% of the patients [9]. After a major earthquake in January 1995 in Japan, AD cases were exacerbated in the affected areas compared with the undamaged ones; further statistical analysis suggested that subjective distress is the vital factor responsible for the exacerbation of skin symptoms [10]. As a possible mechanism of AD exacerbation following psychological stress, AD patients demonstrated increasing eosinophil

K. H. Lee et al. (eds.), *Practical Insights into Atopic Dermatitis*,
https://doi.org/10.1007/978-981-15-8159-5_12

counts and IgE in blood in response to stress [11]. Moreover, a higher level of anxiety was correlated with higher serum total IgE levels and Th2-skewed immunity [12].

Psychological stress not only aggravates AD symptoms but also increases offspring's risk for AD when mothers were exposed to stress during pregnancy. A prospective cohort study showed that stress-related maternal factors during pregnancy are associated with childhood eczema during the first 2 years of life [5, 13]. Recently, Isabel et al. [14] demonstrated that maternal adverse life events during the second half of gestation are linked to an increased risk of atopic diseases, such as asthma and eczema of the child. Consistent with these reports, maternal stress contributes to the immune dysfunction in the offspring and cytokine production that would lead to the development of allergic diseases [15, 16]. In addition, it appears that caregiver stress can also increase the risk of AD development after birth. In one study, higher caregiver stress was related to increased total IgE in the serum and enhanced allergen-specific immune responses in AD-predisposed children [17]. In another study, children who experienced stressful life events had a higher risk of developing atopic diseases later in their life [6, 18].

Hypothalamic–Pituitary–Adrenal Axis in Stress Response

To comprehend the *stress response*, it is necessary to understand the hypothalamic–pituitary–adrenal (HPA) axis that initiates the stress response. Upon the activation of the HPA axis, corticotrophin-releasing hormone (CRH) is released from the hypothalamus in a pulsatile pattern. It induces the secretion of proopiomelanocortin-derived peptides, such as adrenocorticotropic hormone (ACTH), alpha-melanocyte-stimulating hormone, and β-endorphin [19] to regulate homeostasis [20]. ACTH and alpha-melanocyte-stimulating hormone directly regulate pigmentation and inflammatory response [21, 22], and β-endorphin shows analgesic and anti-inflammatory properties [23]. As an immune regulator, ACTH has been proposed to increase the production of pro-inflammatory cytokines [interleukin (IL)-1, IL-4, IL-6, IL-18, and tumor necrosis factor (TNF)-α]. At the same time, ACTH stimulates the production of adrenal glucocorticoid (GC) which is mostly known to trigger anti-inflammatory response [19, 24]. GCs have an immunosuppressive effect on pro-inflammatory T cells, activate regulatory T cells and induce tolerogenic dendritic cells (DCs). Increased GCs regulate the transcription of GC response elements of anti-inflammatory genes. Low and high levels of GCs stimulate and inhibit macrophages, respectively. GCs also reduce the number of basophils and decrease the apoptosis rate of neutrophils and eosinophils. Furthermore, GCs inhibit the synthesis and function of cytokines, chemokines, and costimulatory molecules from immune cells and endothelial cells [25]. These pro-inflammatory and anti-inflammatory responses to acute stress aimed to precisely maintain body homeostasis following stressful stimuli.

During chronic stress, the HPA axis response and immune response can be altered. Chronic stress decreases morning cortisol level, but increases baseline cortisol level [26], suggesting an impaired HPA axis homeostasis. Chronic stress induces increased neuroinflammation, altered secretion of pro-inflammatory cytokines and chemokines, increased oxidative stress, and altered tight junction structure [27, 28]. Chronic stress also modulates the secretion of several mediators, such as catecholamine, prolactin, nerve growth factors, and neuropeptides [29, 30]. In addition, sustained stress delays wound healing and impairs skin barrier integrity [31, 32].

In AD patients, the blunted response of the HPA axis has been reported. Cortisol and ACTH responses to a certain stressor were significantly attenuated, whereas basal cortisol and ACTH concentrations were not different between AD patients and healthy controls. This aberrant *stress response* in AD may increase one's susceptibility to allergic inflammation and contribute to stress-related aggravation of AD [11, 33].

Autonomic Nervous System in Stress Response

The autonomic nervous system is composed of the sympathetic, parasympathetic, and enteric subdivisions, affecting physiological response following psychological stress. The autonomic nervous system innervates various tissues and controls involuntary activities. The parasympathetic nervous system participates in the maintenance of homeostasis, whereas the sympathetic nervous system mostly responds to stress stimulus [34]. Skin innervation by the autonomic nervous system is mostly sympathetic and makes up a small proportion of the nerve fibers. These nerves are located at the dermal layer and innervate skin appendages and vasculatures [35, 36].

Altered sympathetic responses have been reported in AD patients. The heart rate was consistently elevated in AD patients compared with healthy controls [37]. Increased very low-frequency component of the power spectrum, which indicates sympathetic activity, in AD patients, suggested an overactive sympathetic response in AD patients [37].

Immune Response in Stress

T Cells

Psychological stress significantly decreases the number of leukocytes and lymphocytes in the blood [38, 39] and impairs lymphocyte function [40]. Several studies have shown that stress response can skew the immune response toward a Th2-dominant response. GCs, an effector regulator of the HPA axis, drive the Th1/Th2 immune balance toward a Th2-dominant response [41–45]. GCs have been found to inhibit the secretion of IL-12 in human monocytes and to enhance the production of IL-4 in CD4+ T cells [41]. Since IL-12 potently enhances the differentiation of naïve T cells to Th1 cells, inhibition of IL-12 can lead to Th2 shift [46]. Furthermore, not only HPA axis factors but also end products of the autonomic nervous system in stress response, i.e., catecholamines, have been shown to drive to a Th2-skewed immune response and to consolidate the effects of GCs [47]. Using a murine model, Iwakabe et al. [48] revealed direct evidence that emotional stress causes an immunity shift toward a Th2-dominant response by strong inhibition of interferon (IFN)-γ production. Parallel to IFN-γ reduction with increased corticosterone levels, reduced activities of cytotoxic T cells, and natural killer (NK) cells were found following emotional stress exposure.

Some studies suggest that stress-induced T cell alteration can be induced by CRH, an initiating hormone following HPA axis activation. Oh and Park et al. [49] revealed that T cells express functional CRH receptors, namely, CRHR1 and CRHR2, and CRH can alter IL-4 and IFN-γ secretion from T cells. In AD patients, the expression of CRHR1 and CRHR2 is downregulated in T cells, and CRH does not alter cytokine expression. However, CRH suppressed the IL-10 secretion from FOXP3-negative regulatory T (Treg) cells in AD patients, suggesting that alteration of Treg cells by CRH might trigger the stress-induced aggravation of AD. Another study demonstrated that DOCK8 is a downstream mediator of CRH-induced dysfunction of Treg cells [50].

Dendritic Cells and Langerhans Cells

DCs are specialized antigen-presenting cells located in the skin, and they can uptake allergens and present it to T cells to initiate an allergic reaction in AD. Lee et al. [51] demonstrated that monocyte-derived DCs (moDCs) express CRHR1 and CRHR2 and that exposure of moDCs to CRH reduces IL-18 level, suggesting that CRH can modulate immune response by directly acting upon moDCs.

Langerhans cells, which are epidermal antigen-presenting cells in the skin, can be affected by psychological stress and stress-related elements. Kleyn et al. [52] reported that psychological stress significantly decreased the density of Langerhans cells in the epidermis. In addition, GCs can affect Langerhans cells by inhibiting their maturation and function. The expressions of maturation markers, such as CD25 and CD205, and costimulatory molecules were inhibited with GCs, and Langerhans cells from GC-treated skin showed significantly impaired antigen-presenting function and migration [53]. Moreover, epinephrine inhibits antigen presentation in epidermal cell preparations and in purified Langerhans cells [54]. Interestingly, the inhibition of beta2-AR impaired the migration of Langerhans cells to the lymph nodes and blunted the allergen sensitization [54].

Other Cells

GCs have also been demonstrated to inhibit monocyte/macrophage differentiation and many of their functions [55] and to decrease NK cell activity [56].

Neurogenic Mediators and Mast Cells

AD patients who were exposed to the acute Trier social stress test showed a decreased number of nerve growth factor (NGF)+ and protein gene product (PGP) 9.5+ nerve fibers and decreased contacts between tryptase+ mast cells and PGP 9.5+ nerve fibers in the AD lesional skin [57]. In another study, video game- or mobile phone-induced stress exposure enhanced allergen-induced skin reaction and increased plasma levels of substance P (SP), vasoactive intestinal peptide, and NGF in AD patients. These results support that psychological stress might be closely correlated with neuro-mast cell interaction to manipulate inflammation and itch sensation in AD skin.

The nerve fibers innervated in the skin are closely located to structural and functional cells, including keratinocytes, fibroblasts, endothelial cells, and immune cell populations [58]. The cutaneous sensory nerve fibers make up most of the skin nerve fibers, and they innervate both the epidermis and dermis. These sensory nerve fibers are responsible for itch and pain as well as touch, thermosensation, and mechanosensation [36, 59]. In addition to sensory function, nervous system-innervated skin is closely related to the immune reaction of the skin. In response to irritants, noxious stimuli, and pathogens, cutaneous sensory nerve fibers release mediators, such as SP, calcitonin gene-related peptide (CGRP), and NGF which induce vasodilation and immune cell recruitment and elicit inflammatory response [60, 61].

Compared with healthy controls, AD patients were reported to have an increased density of cutaneous nerve fibers [62, 63], which may contribute to the severe itch sensation. Plasma levels of NGF and SP were higher in AD patients, and they were positively correlated with disease severity [64–66]. In addition to increased nerve density and neuromediators, researchers observed that skin-innervated nerve fibers are located closely to the immune cells, especially mast cells, in the skin. Both lesional and non-lesional skin in AD patients showed increased SP- and CGRP-positive nerve fibers along with increased mast cell-nerve fiber contacts [67]. In the AD mice model, stress exacerbates clinical and histological AD features via SP-dependent neurogenic inflammation in the skin, and this worsening was abolished in mice lacking neurokinin-1 receptors. In this model, stress shifted the cytokine profile toward Th2 in the skin; however, the number of CD4+ T cells was not altered [68].

Among various immune cells, compelling evidence suggests that mast cell activation plays an important role in stress-induced neuroinflammation. Thus, it is crucial to understand its mediators and their role on neuro–immune interaction in the skin. Mast cells can be the source and target of CRH and other neuropeptides to mediate neuroinflammation [69]. Mast cells express functional CRHR1 and CRHR2 [70]. At the same time, mast cells can produce CRH, suggesting that these cells have both autocrine and paracrine function [71]. Upon the activation of mast cells with CRH and other neuropeptides, mast cells release inflammatory mediators, such as histamine, tryptase, serotonin, prostaglandins, CRH, NGF, IL-1b, TNF-a, IL-8, and IL-33 [69, 72–74]. Inflammatory mediators released by mast cells act on nociceptors in sensory neurons to induce itch sensation and to release neuropeptides, such as SP and neurokinin A. Subsequently, these neuropeptides activate mast cells, creating a vicious cycle. This continuous process leads to increased vascular permeability, chronic pain, itch, inflammation, and neuroinflammation [75].

Compared with healthy controls, AD patients have increased tryptase-positive mast cells and chymase-positive mast cells in both non-lesional and lesional skin [76]. However, the enzyme activity of chymase is decreased in lesional skin compared with that in non-lesional skin [77]. Inactivation of chymase may cause further inflammation by degrading inflammatory mediators, such as IL-6, IL-13, TNF-α, IL-4, IL-5, SP, and vasoactive intestinal peptide [78–80]. In addition to the role of mast cells on inflammatory response, these cells are also related to the skin barrier of AD patients. The number of tryptase-positive and IL-6-positive mast cells was inversely correlated with profilaggrin expression in the AD skin [81].

Based on these previous reports, we can assume that stress-induced neurogenic inflammation and mast cell activation might modulate immune responses to a Th2-skewed response, lead to impaired skin barrier function, and contribute to AD aggravation.

Mast Cell Mediators

Histamine, one of the most well-known mast cell-released mediator, acts on histamine 1 receptor (H1R), H2R, H3R, and H4R in nociceptive C and A-delta nerve fibers. Rosa et al. [82] reviewed the effects of histamine on itch. Histamine induces SP and glutamate secretion from nerve fibers [83], and histamine administration to the nasal mucosa induced the release of CGRP and SP from nerve ending [84]. Although histamine playa a multiple role in the neurogenic inflammation, the administration of oral antihistamines to manage pruritus in AD patients was not satisfactory. Recently, H4R has been revealed as a new target of itch and inflammation in AD, suggesting that combined inhibition of both H1R and H4R can be another treatment strategy in AD patients [85].

Tryptase, another mast cell-released mediator, acts on nerve fibers through proteinase-activated receptor 2 (PAR-2) and increased secretion of neuropeptides, such as SP and CGRP, which consequently induce mast cell activation and release inflammatory mediators [86]. However, no clinically successful inhibitors are yet developed to target tryptase of PAR2.

Mast cells also release NGF that can act on both mast cells and nerve fibers through tropomyosin receptor kinase A (TrkA). The activation of TrkA on mast cells induces further release of histamine and NGF. The expression level of NGF has been shown to be increased in various inflammatory conditions that are associated with mast cell activation [75, 87].

Sphingosine-1-phosphate (S1P) is another mediator that is released from mast cells. S1P acts on S1P1 and S1P2 receptors on mast cells in an autocrine manner. S1P is thought to be important for the migration of mast cells and their recruitment to the inflammatory site [88]. S1P also induced the production and release of cytokines, such as TNF-α, IL-6, and CCL2 [89]. Because of its autocrine activity, it might contribute to sustained activation of mast cells during inflammation.

Psychological Stress and Barrier

Many studies demonstrated the negative effects of psychological stress on the skin barrier function. These studies indicated that psychological stress impairs the recovery of the cutaneous permeability barrier. In rodent models, psychological stress altered skin barrier function, and it was reversed by the administration of sedatives [90, 91]. The mechanism of disrupted skin barrier function under psychological stress was explained by increased endogenous GCs during psychological stress. Inhibition of GCs by receptor antagonist RU486 ameliorated barrier abnormalities induced by psychological stress [91]. In addition, Kao et al. [92] demonstrated the direct effect of GCs on barrier homeostasis, characterized by impaired barrier recovery and disrupted stratum corneum integrity. In another study, higher stress events caused delayed permeability barrier recovery, and it was recovered in a lower stress period [93]. Stress-induced disruption of stratum integrity was also reported by Choi et al. [32] in an insomniac psychological stress model. These clinical deteriorations of skin barrier caused by psychological stress could be explained by decreased epidermal cell proliferation, impaired epidermal differentiation, and decreased production and release of lamellar bodies [32, 92]. Stress-induced barrier disruption was rescued by the topical application of physiologic lipids, indicating that lipid deficiency may contribute to these functional abnormalities [32].

Recently, elevated 11 beta-hydroxysteroid dehydrogenase type 1 (11β-HSD1) with increased cortisol in the stratum corneum was observed under psychological stress. Elevated 11β-HSD1 caused by psychological stress, which leads to increased active cortisol in the skin, can further disrupt skin barrier homeostasis, since cortisol inhibits the differentiation of keratinocytes and decreases cytokine expression. To support this hypothesis, treatment with SSRI recovered skin barrier function [94].

Psychological Intervention

Since psychological stress can aggravate AD symptoms, relieving stress can improve the clinical severity of AD consequently. For this purpose, psychological interventions such as biofeedback, progressive muscle relaxation therapy, massage therapy, and hypnosis have been utilized for AD. Although most of these therapies are limited to case series, they showed significant improvement in eczema severity and itching intensity in AD patients [95].

In a randomized controlled trial, compared with the control subjects, who did not receive psychotherapies, children who received hypnotherapy or biofeedback showed a significant decrease in surface damage and lichenification, but not in affected body area [96]. Stewart et al. [97] demonstrated the beneficial effect of hypnotherapy on both adults and children. Most of the patients showed immediate improvement, and the improvement of clinical symptoms was maintained up to 18 months after the treatment. Progressive muscle relaxation therapy, another therapeutic modality, was also effective to significantly decrease the degree of pruritus and loss of sleep in AD compared with the control group, although no significant changes were found in the serological parameters [98].

Conclusion

Although stress response tends to be immunosuppressive, stress can induce a Th2-skewed immune response and impair barrier function. In this process, the neuro–immune–skin network precisely interacts to regulate immune response in the skin. Although it might be difficult to fully prevent stress-induced AD aggravation because of such complex interaction, clinicians can utilize strategies to block each step in the stress response. Considerable strategies include relieving the stress by psychological intervention, attenuation of Th2 response with biologics, and repair or reinforcement of skin barrier with moisturizer or other topical agents. In the future, inhibition of neurogenic or mast cell-derived mediators could be another possible strategy with further research.

References

1. Busse WW, Kiecolt-Glaser JK, Coe C, Martin RJ, Weiss ST, Parker SR. NHLBI Workshop summary. Stress and asthma. Am J Respir Crit Care Med. 1995;151(1):249–52.
2. Dhabhar FS. Acute stress enhances while chronic stress suppresses skin immunity. The role of stress hormones and leukocyte trafficking. Ann N Y Acad Sci. 2000;917:876–93.
3. Morren MA, Przybilla B, Bamelis M, Heykants B, Reynaers A, Degreef H. Atopic dermatitis: triggering factors. J Am Acad Dermatol. 1994;31(3 Pt 1):467–73.
4. Amano H, Negishi I, Akiyama H, Ishikawa O. Psychological stress can trigger atopic dermatitis in NC/Nga mice: an inhibitory effect of corticotropin-releasing factor. Neuropsychopharmacology. 2008;33(3):566–73.
5. Bockelbrink A, Heinrich J, Schafer I, Zutavern A, Borte M, Herbarth O, et al. Atopic eczema in chil-

dren: another harmful sequel of divorce. Allergy. 2006;61(12):1397–402.
6. Kilpelainen M, Koskenvuo M, Helenius H, Terho EO. Stressful life events promote the manifestation of asthma and atopic diseases. Clin Exp Allergy. 2002;32(2):256–63.
7. Oh SH, Bae BG, Park CO, Noh JY, Park IH, Wu WH, et al. Association of stress with symptoms of atopic dermatitis. Acta Derm Venereol. 2010;90(6):582–8.
8. Faulstich ME, Williamson DA. An overview of atopic dermatitis: toward a bio-behavioural integration. J Psychosom Res. 1985;29(6):647–54.
9. Chu H, Shin JU, Park CO, Lee H, Lee J, Lee KH. Clinical diversity of atopic dermatitis: a review of 5,000 patients at a single institute. Allergy Asthma Immunol Res. 2017;9(2):158–68.
10. Kodama A, Horikawa T, Suzuki T, Ajiki W, Takashima T, Harada S, et al. Effect of stress on atopic dermatitis: investigation in patients after the great hanshin earthquake. J Allergy Clin Immunol. 1999;104(1):173–6.
11. Buske-Kirschbaum A, Gierens A, Hollig H, Hellhammer DH. Stress-induced immunomodulation is altered in patients with atopic dermatitis. J Neuroimmunol. 2002;129(1–2):161–7.
12. Hashizume H, Horibe T, Ohshima A, Ito T, Yagi H, Takigawa M. Anxiety accelerates T-helper 2-tilted immune responses in patients with atopic dermatitis. Br J Dermatol. 2005;152(6):1161–4.
13. Sausenthaler S, Rzehak P, Chen CM, Arck P, Bockelbrink A, Schafer T, et al. Stress-related maternal factors during pregnancy in relation to childhood eczema: results from the LISA Study. J Investig Allergol Clin Immunol. 2009;19(6):481–7.
14. Hartwig IR, Sly PD, Schmidt LA, van Lieshout RJ, Bienenstock J, Holt PG, et al. Prenatal adverse life events increase the risk for atopic diseases in children, which is enhanced in the absence of a maternal atopic predisposition. J Allergy Clin Immunol. 2014;134(1):160–9.
15. Pincus-Knackstedt MK, Joachim RA, Blois SM, Douglas AJ, Orsal AS, Klapp BF, et al. Prenatal stress enhances susceptibility of murine adult offspring toward airway inflammation. J Immunol. 2006;177(12):8484–92.
16. Veru F, Laplante DP, Luheshi G, King S. Prenatal maternal stress exposure and immune function in the offspring. Stress. 2014;17(2):133–48.
17. Wright RJ, Finn P, Contreras JP, Cohen S, Wright RO, Staudenmayer J, et al. Chronic caregiver stress and IgE expression, allergen-induced proliferation, and cytokine profiles in a birth cohort predisposed to atopy. J Allergy Clin Immunol. 2004;113(6):1051–7.
18. Lietzen R, Virtanen P, Kivimaki M, Sillanmaki L, Vahtera J, Koskenvuo M. Stressful life events and the onset of asthma. Eur Respir J. 2011;37(6):1360–5.
19. Elenkov IJ, Chrousos GP. Stress system—organization, physiology and immunoregulation. Neuroimmunomodulation. 2006;13(5–6):257–67.
20. Slominski AT, Zmijewski MA, Zbytek B, Tobin DJ, Theoharides TC, Rivier J. Key role of CRF in the skin stress response system. Endocr Rev. 2013;34(6):827–84.
21. Catania A, Airaghi L, Colombo G, Lipton JM. Alpha-melanocyte-stimulating hormone in normal human physiology and disease states. Trends Endocrinol Metab. 2000;11(8):304–8.
22. Millington GW. Proopiomelanocortin (POMC): the cutaneous roles of its melanocortin products and receptors. Clin Exp Dermatol. 2006;31(3):407–12.
23. Slominski AT, Zmijewski MA, Skobowiat C, Zbytek B, Slominski RM, Steketee JD. Sensing the environment: regulation of local and global homeostasis by the skin's neuroendocrine system. Adv Anat Embryol Cell Biol. 2012;212:v, vii, 1–115.
24. Kim JE, Cho BK, Cho DH, Park HJ. Expression of hypothalamic-pituitary-adrenal axis in common skin diseases: evidence of its association with stress-related disease activity. Acta Derm Venereol. 2013;93(4):387–93.
25. Zen M, Canova M, Campana C, Bettio S, Nalotto L, Rampudda M, et al. The kaleidoscope of glucorticoid effects on immune system. Autoimmun Rev. 2011;10(6):305–10.
26. Stephens MA, Wand G. Stress and the HPA axis: role of glucocorticoids in alcohol dependence. Alcohol Res. 2012;34(4):468–83.
27. Kempuraj D, Selvakumar GP, Thangavel R, Ahmed ME, Zaheer S, Raikwar SP, et al. Mast cell activation in brain injury, stress, and post-traumatic stress disorder and Alzheimer's disease pathogenesis. Front Neurosci. 2017;11:703.
28. Lurie DI. An integrative approach to neuroinflammation in psychiatric disorders and neuropathic pain. J Exp Neurosci. 2018;12:1179069518793639.
29. Paus R, Theoharides TC, Arck PC. Neuroimmunoendocrine circuitry of the 'brain-skin connection'. Trends Immunol. 2006;27(1):32–9.
30. Fukada M, Kaidoh T, Ito A, Yano T, Hayashibara C, Watanabe T. "Green odor" inhalation reduces the skin-barrier disruption induced by chronic restraint stress in rats: physiological and histological examinations. Chem Senses. 2007;32(6):633–9.
31. Aioi A, Okuda M, Matsui M, Tonogaito H, Hamada K. Effect of high population density environment on skin barrier function in mice. J Dermatol Sci. 2001;25(3):189–97.
32. Choi EH, Brown BE, Crumrine D, Chang S, Man MQ, Elias PM, et al. Mechanisms by which psychologic stress alters cutaneous permeability barrier homeostasis and stratum corneum integrity. J Invest Dermatol. 2005;124(3):587–95.
33. Buske-Kirschbaum A, Geiben A, Hollig H, Morschhauser E, Hellhammer D. Altered responsiveness of the hypothalamus-pituitary-adrenal axis and the sympathetic adrenomedullary system to stress in patients with atopic dermatitis. J Clin Endocrinol Metab. 2002;87(9):4245–51.
34. McMahon SB, La Russa F, Bennett DL. Crosstalk between the nociceptive and immune systems

in host defence and disease. Nat Rev Neurosci. 2015;16(7):389–402.
35. Vetrugno R, Liguori R, Cortelli P, Montagna P. Sympathetic skin response: basic mechanisms and clinical applications. Clin Auton research. 2003;13(4):256–70.
36. Laverdet B, Danigo A, Girard D, Magy L, Demiot C, Desmouliere A. Skin innervation: important roles during normal and pathological cutaneous repair. Histol Histopathol. 2015;30(8):875–92.
37. Tran BW, Papoiu AD, Russoniello CV, Wang H, Patel TS, Chan YH, et al. Effect of itch, scratching and mental stress on autonomic nervous system function in atopic dermatitis. Acta Derm Venereol. 2010;90(4):354–61.
38. Dhabhar FS, Miller AH, Stein M, McEwen BS, Spencer RL. Diurnal and acute stress-induced changes in distribution of peripheral blood leukocyte subpopulations. Brain Behav Immun. 1994;8(1):66–79.
39. Dhabhar FS, Miller AH, McEwen BS, Spencer RL. Effects of stress on immune cell distribution. Dynamics and hormonal mechanisms. J Immunol. 1995;154(10):5511–27.
40. Bartrop RW, Luckhurst E, Lazarus L, Kiloh LG, Penny R. Depressed lymphocyte function after bereavement. Lancet. 1977;1(8016):834–6.
41. Blotta MH, DeKruyff RH, Umetsu DT. Corticosteroids inhibit IL-12 production in human monocytes and enhance their capacity to induce IL-4 synthesis in CD4+ lymphocytes. J Immunol. 1997;158(12):5589–95.
42. Daynes RA, Araneo BA. Contrasting effects of glucocorticoids on the capacity of T cells to produce the growth factors interleukin 2 and interleukin 4. Eur J Immunol. 1989;19(12):2319–25.
43. Norbiato G, Bevilacqua M, Vago T, Clerici M. Glucocorticoids and Th-1, Th-2 type cytokines in rheumatoid arthritis, osteoarthritis, asthma, atopic dermatitis and AIDS. Clin Exp Rheumatol. 1997;15(3):315–23.
44. Ramirez F, Fowell DJ, Puklavec M, Simmonds S, Mason D. Glucocorticoids promote a TH2 cytokine response by CD4+ T cells in vitro. J Immunol. 1996;156(7):2406–12.
45. Wilckens T, De Rijk R. Glucocorticoids and immune function: unknown dimensions and new frontiers. Immunol Today. 1997;18(9):418–24.
46. DeKruyff RH, Fang Y, Umetsu DT. Corticosteroids enhance the capacity of macrophages to induce Th2 cytokine synthesis in CD4+ lymphocytes by inhibiting IL-12 production. J Immunol. 1998;160(5):2231–7.
47. Elenkov IJ, Chrousos GP. Stress hormones, Th1/Th2 patterns, Pro/Anti-inflammatory cytokines and susceptibility to disease. Trends Endocrinol Metab. 1999;10(9):359–68.
48. Iwakabe K, Shimada M, Ohta A, Yahata T, Ohmi Y, Habu S, et al. The restraint stress drives a shift in Th1/Th2 balance toward Th2-dominant immunity in mice. Immunol Lett. 1998;62(1):39–43.
49. Oh SH, Park CO, Wu WH, Kim JY, Jin S, Byamba D, et al. Corticotropin-releasing hormone downregulates IL-10 production by adaptive forkhead box protein 3-negative regulatory T cells in patients with atopic dermatitis. J Allergy Clin Immunol. 2012;129(1):151–9.e1-6.
50. Jin S, Shin JU, Noh JY, Kim H, Kim JY, Kim SH, et al. DOCK8: regulator of Treg in response to corticotropin-releasing hormone. Allergy. 2016;71(6):811–9.
51. Lee HJ, Kwon YS, Park CO, Oh SH, Lee JH, Wu WH, et al. Corticotropin-releasing factor decreases IL-18 in the monocyte-derived dendritic cell. Exp Dermatol. 2009;18(3):199–204.
52. Kleyn CE, Schneider L, Saraceno R, Mantovani C, Richards HL, Fortune DG, et al. The effects of acute social stress on epidermal Langerhans' cell frequency and expression of cutaneous neuropeptides. J Invest Dermatol. 2008;128(5):1273–9.
53. Hoetzenecker W, Meingassner JG, Ecker R, Stingl G, Stuetz A, Elbe-Burger A. Corticosteroids but not pimecrolimus affect viability, maturation and immune function of murine epidermal Langerhans cells. J Invest Dermatol. 2004;122(3):673–84.
54. Seiffert K, Hosoi J, Torii H, Ozawa H, Ding W, Campton K, et al. Catecholamines inhibit the antigen-presenting capability of epidermal Langerhans cells. J Immunol. 2002;168(12):6128–35.
55. Baybutt HN, Holsboer F. Inhibition of macrophage differentiation and function by cortisol. Endocrinology. 1990;127(1):476–80.
56. Bateman A, Singh A, Kral T, Solomon S. The immune-hypothalamic-pituitary-adrenal axis. Endocr Rev. 1989;10(1):92–112.
57. Peters EM, Michenko A, Kupfer J, Kummer W, Wiegand S, Niemeier V, et al. Mental stress in atopic dermatitis--neuronal plasticity and the cholinergic system are affected in atopic dermatitis and in response to acute experimental mental stress in a randomized controlled pilot study. PLoS One. 2014;9(12):e113552.
58. Peters EM, Liezmann C, Klapp BF, Kruse J. The neuroimmune connection interferes with tissue regeneration and chronic inflammatory disease in the skin. Ann N Y Acad Sci. 2012;1262:118–26.
59. Schwendinger-Schreck J, Wilson SR, Bautista DM. Interactions between keratinocytes and somatosensory neurons in itch. Handb Exp Pharmacol. 2015;226:177–90.
60. Buddenkotte J, Steinhoff M. Pathophysiology and therapy of pruritus in allergic and atopic diseases. Allergy. 2010;65(7):805–21.
61. Raap U, Kapp A. Neuroimmunological findings in allergic skin diseases. Curr Opin Allergy Clin Immunol. 2005;5(5):419–24.
62. Tobin D, Nabarro G, Baart de la Faille H, van Vloten WA, van der Putte SC, Schuurman HJ. Increased number of immunoreactive nerve fibers in atopic dermatitis. J Allergy Clin Immunol. 1992;90(4 Pt 1):613–22.
63. Urashima R, Mihara M. Cutaneous nerves in atopic dermatitis. A histological, immunohistochemical and electron microscopic study. Virchows Archiv. 1998;432(4):363–70.

64. Hodeib A, El-Samad ZA, Hanafy H, El-Latief AA, El-Bendary A, Abu-Raya A. Nerve growth factor, neuropeptides and cutaneous nerves in atopic dermatitis. Indian J Dermatol. 2010;55(2):135–9.
65. Toyoda M, Nakamura M, Makino T, Hino T, Kagoura M, Morohashi M. Nerve growth factor and substance P are useful plasma markers of disease activity in atopic dermatitis. Br J Dermatol. 2002;147(1):71–9.
66. Wang IJ, Hsieh WS, Guo YL, Jee SH, Hsieh CJ, Hwang YH, et al. Neuro-mediators as predictors of paediatric atopic dermatitis. Clin Exp Allergy. 2008;38(8):1302–8.
67. Jarvikallio A, Harvima IT, Naukkarinen A. Mast cells, nerves and neuropeptides in atopic dermatitis and nummular eczema. Arch Dermatol Res. 2003;295(1):2–7.
68. Pavlovic S, Daniltchenko M, Tobin DJ, Hagen E, Hunt SP, Klapp BF, et al. Further exploring the brain-skin connection: stress worsens dermatitis via substance P-dependent neurogenic inflammation in mice. J Invest Dermatol. 2008;128(2):434–46.
69. Kempuraj D, Mentor S, Thangavel R, Ahmed ME, Selvakumar GP, Raikwar SP, et al. Mast cells in stress, pain, blood-brain barrier, neuroinflammation and Alzheimer's disease. Front Cell Neurosci. 2019;13:54.
70. Cao J, Papadopoulou N, Kempuraj D, Boucher WS, Sugimoto K, Cetrulo CL, et al. Human mast cells express corticotropin-releasing hormone (CRH) receptors and CRH leads to selective secretion of vascular endothelial growth factor. J Immunol. 2005;174(12):7665–75.
71. Kempuraj D, Papadopoulou NG, Lytinas M, Huang M, Kandere-Grzybowska K, Madhappan B, et al. Corticotropin-releasing hormone and its structurally related urocortin are synthesized and secreted by human mast cells. Endocrinology. 2004;145(1):43–8.
72. Schwartz LB. Tryptase, a mediator of human mast cells. J Allergy Clin Immunol. 1990;86(4 Pt 2):594–8.
73. Levy D, Kainz V, Burstein R, Strassman AM. Mast cell degranulation distinctly activates trigemino-cervical and lumbosacral pain pathways and elicits widespread tactile pain hypersensitivity. Brain Behav Immun. 2012;26(2):311–7.
74. Kempuraj D, Thangavel R, Selvakumar GP, Zaheer S, Ahmed ME, Raikwar SP, et al. Brain and peripheral atypical inflammatory mediators potentiate neuroinflammation and neurodegeneration. Front Cell Neurosci. 2017;11:216.
75. Gupta K, Harvima IT. Mast cell-neural interactions contribute to pain and itch. Immunol Rev. 2018;282(1):168–87.
76. Jarvikallio A, Naukkarinen A, Harvima IT, Aalto ML, Horsmanheimo M. Quantitative analysis of tryptase- and chymase-containing mast cells in atopic dermatitis and nummular eczema. Br J Dermatol. 1997;136(6):871–7.
77. Ilves T, Harvima IT. Decrease in chymase activity is associated with increase in IL-6 expression in mast cells in atopic dermatitis. Acta Derm Venereol. 2015;95(4):411–6.
78. Franconi GM, Graf PD, Lazarus SC, Nadel JA, Caughey GH. Mast cell tryptase and chymase reverse airway smooth muscle relaxation induced by vasoactive intestinal peptide in the ferret. J Pharmacol Exp Ther. 1989;248(3):947–51.
79. Tunon de Lara JM, Okayama Y, McEuen AR, Heusser CH, Church MK, Walls AF. Release and inactivation of interleukin-4 by mast cells. Ann N Y Acad Sci. 1994;725:50–8.
80. Zhao W, Oskeritzian CA, Pozez AL, Schwartz LB. Cytokine production by skin-derived mast cells: endogenous proteases are responsible for degradation of cytokines. J Immunol. 2005;175(4):2635–42.
81. Ilves T, Tiitu V, Suttle MM, Saarinen JV, Harvima IT. Epidermal expression of filaggrin/profilaggrin is decreased in atopic dermatitis: reverse association with mast cell tryptase and IL-6 but not with clinical severity. Dermatitis. 2015;26(6):260–7.
82. Rosa AC, Fantozzi R. The role of histamine in neurogenic inflammation. Br J Pharmacol. 2013;170(1):38–45.
83. Riedel W, Neeck G. Nociception, pain, and antinociception: current concepts. Z Rheumatol. 2001;60(6):404–15.
84. Tani E, Senba E, Kokumai S, Masuyama K, Ishikawa T, Tohyama M. Histamine application to the nasal mucosa induces release of calcitonin gene-related peptide and substance P from peripheral terminals of trigeminal ganglion: a morphological study in the guinea pig. Neurosci Lett. 1990;112(1):1–6.
85. Ohsawa Y, Hirasawa N. The role of histamine H1 and H4 receptors in atopic dermatitis: from basic research to clinical study. Allergol Int. 2014;63(4):533–42.
86. Steinhoff M, Vergnolle N, Young SH, Tognetto M, Amadesi S, Ennes HS, et al. Agonists of proteinase-activated receptor 2 induce inflammation by a neurogenic mechanism. Nat Med. 2000;6(2):151–8.
87. Skaper SD. Nerve growth factor: a neuroimmune crosstalk mediator for all seasons. Immunology. 2017;151(1):1–15.
88. Jolly PS, Bektas M, Olivera A, Gonzalez-Espinosa C, Proia RL, Rivera J, et al. Transactivation of sphingosine-1-phosphate receptors by FcepsilonRI triggering is required for normal mast cell degranulation and chemotaxis. J Exp Med. 2004;199(7):959–70.
89. Oskeritzian CA, Alvarez SE, Hait NC, Price MM, Milstien S, Spiegel S. Distinct roles of sphingosine kinases 1 and 2 in human mast-cell functions. Blood. 2008;111(8):4193–200.
90. Denda M, Tsuchiya T, Hosoi J, Koyama J. Immobilization-induced and crowded environment-induced stress delay barrier recovery in murine skin. Br J Dermatol. 1998;138(5):780–5.
91. Denda M, Tsuchiya T, Elias PM, Feingold KR. Stress alters cutaneous permeability barrier homeostasis. Am J Physiol Regul Integr Comp Physiol. 2000;278(2):R367–72.

92. Kao JS, Fluhr JW, Man MQ, Fowler AJ, Hachem JP, Crumrine D, et al. Short-term glucocorticoid treatment compromises both permeability barrier homeostasis and stratum corneum integrity: inhibition of epidermal lipid synthesis accounts for functional abnormalities. J Invest Dermatol. 2003;120(3):456–64.
93. Garg A, Chren MM, Sands LP, Matsui MS, Marenus KD, Feingold KR, et al. Psychological stress perturbs epidermal permeability barrier homeostasis: implications for the pathogenesis of stress-associated skin disorders. Arch Dermatol. 2001;137(1):53–9.
94. Choe SJ, Kim D, Kim EJ, Ahn JS, Choi EJ, Son ED, et al. Psychological stress deteriorates skin barrier function by activating 11beta-hydroxysteroid dehydrogenase 1 and the HPA Axis. Sci Rep. 2018;8(1):6334.
95. Chida Y, Steptoe A, Hirakawa N, Sudo N, Kubo C. The effects of psychological intervention on atopic dermatitis. A systematic review and meta-analysis. Int Arch Allergy Immunol. 2007;144(1):1–9.
96. Ersser SJ, Cowdell F, Latter S, Gardiner E, Flohr C, Thompson AR, et al. Psychological and educational interventions for atopic eczema in children. Cochrane Database Syst Rev. 2014;2014(1):Cd004054.
97. Stewart AC, Thomas SE. Hypnotherapy as a treatment for atopic dermatitis in adults and children. Br J Dermatol. 1995;132(5):778–83.
98. Bae BG, Oh SH, Park CO, Noh S, Noh JY, Kim KR, et al. Progressive muscle relaxation therapy for atopic dermatitis: objective assessment of efficacy. Acta Derm Venereol. 2012;92(1):57–61.

Endophenotype and Biomarker

Kwang Hoon Lee and Chang Ook Park

Introduction

Atopic dermatitis (AD) is the most common chronic inflammatory skin disease [1], which causes severe itching and semipermanent changes in the skin, which places a great socioeconomic burden on the AD patient [2, 3]. Another major factor in the economic burden on AD patients is the lack of adequate medications to control the symptoms of dermatitis in the long term periods [4]. The difficulty in developing systemic medications for atopic dermatitis is originated from the clinical phenotypes and endotypes of atopic dermatitis are very diverse and difficult to describe in a unified model. In this respect, various studies have been conducted on the effects of IgE-mediated sensitivity, food allergy, and microbiome on the clinical phenotypes of atopic dermatitis [5, 6]. Despite these ongoing studies, many attempts to classify patients with AD based on clinical characteristics and specific markers might not accurately reflect the diversity of pathophysiology of AD.

Our understanding of AD has dramatically deepened over the last few decades by many studies to understand pathophysiology in terms of immunology, barrier function, and allergology. In addition, the genetic and epidemiological studies of AD have revealed the new aspects about the persistence of AD [7, 8], along with the natural history of AD [9, 10] represented by atopic march [11]. Many leading studies have broadened the understanding of immunological mechanisms leading to chronic inflammation and key genetic predisposition to epidermal barrier dysfunction [12–14]. In parallel, various hypotheses have been demonstrated for the effects of IgE-mediated sensitivity and contact sensitivity on AD [15, 16].

Clinicians and researchers coping with AD are clearly aware that the clinical phenotype of AD is extremely diverse, but most AD treatments have been developed and used under the concept of treating all phenotypes in one way. The concept of using specialized treatments (e.g., precision medicine) by classifying AD according to the clinical phenotypes or genetic endotypes is still ignored [17, 18].

In line with the recent understanding of the immunological and genetic pathogenesis of AD, the classical treatment methods will be replaced in the way of using different treatment methods according to specific clinical phenotypes and genetic endotypes represented by precision medicine. In particular, it is important to develop reliable biomarkers that can help clinicians select

K. H. Lee (✉) · C. O. Park
Department of Dermatology, Cutaneous Biology Research Institute, Yonsei University College of Medicine, Seoul, Korea (Republic of)
e-mail: kwanglee@yuhs.ac

K. H. Lee et al. (eds.), *Practical Insights into Atopic Dermatitis*,
https://doi.org/10.1007/978-981-15-8159-5_13

more patient-specific treatments to enable differentiated access to AD patients. This precise approach will open up new horizons for AD treatment in a variety of aspects, including the prevention of AD, the appropriate choice of various systemic therapies, and the timing of drug transitions [19–22].

Endophenotypes and Biomarkers: Implement to Achieve Personalized Medicine in AD

Since the completion of the human genome mapping in the 2000s, the rapid development of high output bioinformatics techniques, commonly referred to as Omics, has increased the genetic understanding of diseases with complex pathophysiology such as AD [23, 24]. As a result, the understanding of genetic complexity based on existing clinical subtype classifications has increased, making it difficult to keep up with the increasing rate of biological information that enables to presume the prevention, diagnosis, and prognosis of AD [25]. By identifying the molecular pathways involved in pathophysiology based on genetic background, the therapeutic goals that can be applied to specific subgroups of patients who were previously classified by only clinical subtype are being identified [26], and this fact leads to a new definition of endophenotypes of AD. Ultimately, the novel stratification of AD by emerging endophenotypes allows a more appropriate definition of AD subgroups, which makes it easier to predict response to specific therapies [27] or to analyze risk–benefit ratio. It also helps to avoid unnecessary side effects in subgroups of patients who are unlikely to respond to a specific treatment modality.

Biomarker is the most important factor to classify AD endophenotype and enable personalized medicine on AD. Recent advancement of research in omics, such as proteomics, genomics, and so forth, has led to progressive results that have led to a better understanding of the pathophysiology of complex diseases with a wide variety of clinical phenotypes, such as AD. These techniques will drive the emergence of new biomarkers that can classify AD patients based on endophenotype [28]. Of course, the discovery of new biomarkers and the clinical and genetic classification by those new criteria are important, but it is also essential to validate their sensitivity and specificity so that newly discovered biomarkers can be used in clinical practice [29]. This requires bioinformatics based on clinical subtypes that are detailed and statistically appropriately classified, and bioinformatic tools need to be able to process large amounts of data using complex algorithms. As a result, systemic biologics implement, along with high-quality bioinformatics and information about clinical subtypes, are the three elements needed to develop and validate new biomarkers [30, 31].

Clinical Heterogeneity of AD

AD constitutes a complex clinical phenotype with a wide range of individual symptoms, and the resulting clinical phenotype is characterized under a single diagnosis of AD. This diagnostic approach necessarily involves clinical heterogeneity and reflects complicated pathophysiology in the aspect of diverse genetic and immunological factors of AD. In addition, clinical heterogeneity confers a wide range of therapeutic responses to classical AD treatments, which may result in risks for patients who are not expected to respond appropriately to specific treatment modality which is effective but may cause serious side effects [32]. As described above, the ultimate goal of precision medicine is to deliver the right medication to the right patient at the right time, and the biomarker is an essential element of precision medicine. Along with the growing understanding of epigenetic and genetic backgrounds that make pathophysiological understanding of AD difficult, the fact that various prophylactic, therapeutic, and prognostic biomarkers are being discovered will lead to the classification of heterogeneous clinical phenotype of AD into more obvious and homogenous phenotypes.

In this context, AD is expected to be redefined by molecular classification methods based on biomarkers. As the understanding level of biochemical and immunological pathways as well as genetic and epigenetic information increases, various clinical information such as dietary habits, lifestyles, and exposure to external environmental factors are integrated to convert the treatment paradigm from disease remission toward a prophylactic approach of AD. Current approaches to precision medicine require an understanding of the interactions of various key factors facing different challenges, of which clinically meaningful biomarkers are essential success factors [33]. The establishment of reliable biomarkers that can be applied clinically will help to reclassify the endophenotype of AD to assist in maximizing the efficacy while minimizing the side effects of specific treatment modalities.

Classic Clinical Phenotypes of AD

Traditionally, enormous attempts have been made to classify AD based on clinical subtype (Table 1). Despite these attempts, it is clearly recognized that AD is a kind of syndrome and is diagnosed as a sum of symptoms, thus there is a limitation in the classification according to the clinical characteristics that are simply visible by physical examination and laboratory blood tests. However, the ongoing research on the establishment of the endophenotype of AD through the defining of biomarkers is based on the traditional classification of clinical phenotypes, which is surely suggest that the understanding of traditional stratification of clinical phenotype of AD is essential.

Table 1 The classic classification of AD phenotype [34]

• Acute vs. chronic AD
• Associated with ichthyosis, keratosis pilaris, palmar hyperlinearity, early-onset, severe and persistent eczema (FLG null genotype)
• Intrinsic vs. extrinsic AD
• Phenotypes according to age of onset
• Morphological variants
– Nummular eczema
– Atopic prurigo
– Lichen planus-like
– Pityriasis alba
• Localized variants
– Hand eczema
– Juvenile palmar and plantar dermatitis
– Eyelid dermatitis
– Cheilitis
– Nipple dermatitis
– Periorificial dermatitis

Acute AD Versus Chronic AD

AD is classified as acute and chronic, according to the duration of eczema lesions. Acute AD lesions are represented by erythema, microvesicles, exudates, and crust formation. Eczema lesions of chronic AD are characterized by dry, erythematous lesions with slight scaling. If the skin lesions are constantly scratched due to extreme itching sensation, the vicious cycle of itching–scratching is repeated, resulting in a leather-like skin, which is called lichenification. Sudden increase of exudate with acute exacerbation of erythema and itching in patients with chronic AD should be suspected of staphylococcal infection or herpes virus infection. Patients with moderate to severe AD typically show severe dryness of the non-lesional skin along with chronic lichenified lesions in the flexural area, relatively pale face with hyperpigmentation on the area around the orbit and the neck. Since AD is a chronic recurrent eczematous disease, acute and chronic eczema lesions are often presented at the same time. Depending on the clinical presentation, the choice of appropriate treatment options, e.g., short-term oral steroids in acute phenotypes, in case of suspicion of bacterial and viral infections, oral antibiotics, or oral antiviral drugs may be used.

AD Associated with Ichthyosis (Filaggrin Mutation)

Impairment of epidermal barrier function in the pathogenesis of AD plays a major role along with immunological mechanisms. Impaired epidermal barrier function causes skin dryness and facilitates transdermal penetration of external allergens and irritants, finally causing persistent inflammation. This occurs when the proteinase activity in the skin is unbalanced, which results in the reduced amount of ceramide and unsaturated fatty acids, and the expression of structural proteins changes. The decreased expression of filaggrins together with involucrin and loricrin are well known structural proteins which are involved in impaired skin barrier function. The fact that filaggrin mutation plays a key role in the development of AD was a cornerstone in the study of AD pathogenesis [35].

Filaggrin mutations are the cause of Ichthyosis vulgaris, which is characterized by dry, rough fish-like skin. Over the past few years, various studies on the association between filaggrin mutations and AD have led to the recognition of filaggrin as the strongest genetic factor affecting susceptibility to AD. In animal model experiments with filaggrin mutations, low or no filaggrin expression was found to facilitate skin inflammation and transdermal penetration of allergens, which lead to the allergic reactions centered on Th2 immune responses and high serum IgE levels. More severe and persistent eczema occurs in AD patients with filaggrin mutations, especially in early-onset AD patients, which persist until adulthood [36, 37]. In addition, filaggrin mutations are associated with ichthyosis, keratosis pilaris, and palmar hyperlinearity, increased incidence of other atopic diseases (e.g., atopic asthma, food allergy, which are constituents of so-called "Atopic march" with atopic dermatitis), and eczema herpeticum [34, 38].

Intrinsic AD Versus Extrinsic AD

The majority of AD patients have high serum and skin IgE levels for food and inhalant allergens, and/or simultaneously have a personal or family history of allergic rhinitis and allergic asthma. On the other hand, some patients have a single AD phenotype without specific atopy features. Based on this fact, Brunello Wuthrich proposed to divide AD into extrinsic AD and intrinsic AD, based on the model of Rackeman's classification of asthma [39]. Extrinsic AD is also called as IgE-associated AD, allergic AD, and intrinsic AD is called as non-allergic AD, atopiform dermatitis [40]. Clinically, those two phenotypes are indistinguishable from one another (Table 2).

The main difference between extrinsic and intrinsic AD is the presence or absence of a Th2 immune response. In patients with extrinsic AD, Th2 type immune responses that secrete IL-4, IL-13, and IL-5 occur throughout the whole body

Table 2 Comparison between extrinsic AD with intrinsic AD [34]

	Extrinsic	Intrinsic
Frequency	50–93%	7–50%
Age	Earlier (<20 years)	Later (>20 years)
Sex	M = F	F > M
Clinical presentation Family history Disease duration	Similar	
Skin dryness	Yes	Yes
Skin hyperactivity	Yes	Yes
Histology	Similar	
Airway atopic disease (allergic asthma, allergic rhinitis)	Yes	No
High serum IgE	Yes	No
Allergen-specific IgE	increased	Not increased
Exacerbation by allergens	Yes	No
Lesional skin IFN-γ	Similarly increased	
Peripheral eosinophils	Highly elevated	Mild to moderately increased
ECP level	Highly elevated	Normal to mild elevated
T cells circulating peripheral blood		
HLA-DR	Similar	
IL-4, IL-5	Similar	
CD23+ B cells	+++	+
Skin resident T cells		
IL-5	+++	+
IL-4, IL-13	+++	+
High affinity IgE receptor (FcεRI/II) expression ratio in epidermal dendritic cells	>1.5	<0.56

and skin [41], resulting in elevated eosinophil levels and elevated eosinophilic cationic protein (ECP) levels [42]. In addition, high-affinity IgE receptors are expressed in epidermal dendritic cells of an extrinsic AD patient. The difference between these two types may not run parallel lines throughout the disease course. Intrinsic AD can be changed to extrinsic AD as the course of the disease progresses or as a result of IgE production for a particular allergen, but conversion of extrinsic AD to intrinsic AD rarely occurs. The proportion of the two clinical phenotypes varies slightly depending on the population surveyed. It is known that between 7 and 50% of patients have an intrinsic AD phenotype [40]. Studies on the association between severity and atopic characteristics of AD show a statistically significant relationship between the number of antigens which is shown to be positive in the skin prick test, the specificity of IgE antibodies, the serum IgE levels, and the severity of AD. Although IgE measurements correlate strongly with the severity of AD, excluding specific IgE measurements from Hanifin and Rajka diagnostic criteria does not affect the sensitivity and specificity [42]. The lack of significant difference in clinical presentation between intrinsic AD and extrinsic AD, and the fact that specific IgE measurements do not significantly affect the diagnosis of AD, raise the question of whether measurement of IgE antibody is essential for the development of AD. However, high IgE levels can affect the frequency and intensity of acute exacerbations of AD and serve as a predictor of the associated presence of allergic rhinitis and allergic asthma in AD patients.

Phenotypes According to Age of Onset

In addition to various blood test results and clinical presentations, the classification of clinical phenotypes of AD using the onset of AD development has also been attempted. This classification suggests a comprehensive understanding of the epidemiologic aspects of AD and is based on a deep understanding of the natural clinical course of AD. In addition, immunological pathophysiology may be different depending on the age of onset. Thus, the classification of clinical phenotypes by age of onset may identify patients who are most at risk of developing persistent inflammation due to AD. This enables early termination of chronic dermatitis of AD using an early targeted approach. In the past, AD was recognized as a disease occurring in childhood, and by the age of 10, more than half of the patients were thought to have a definite remission. However, according to the results of recent epidemiological studies, the concept that AD can last a patient's lifetime is being introduced.

To date, many cohort studies and retrospective epidemiological studies have revealed six clinical phenotypes by age of onset. This classification of phenotypes is based on the concept that each phenotype according to the age of onset is affected by exposure to various external environmental factors that have a different susceptibility to a specific phenotype. Studies supporting this assumption have been shown to prevent AD which might be developed in the first year after birth if maternal animal contact is present [43], while eating habits during the first year after birth are associated with AD after the first year of birth [44, 45].

Six phenotypes by age of onset is composed of "very early onset," "early onset," "childhood onset," "adolescent onset," "adult onset," and "very late onset." Those classifications are well described in Fig. 1.

Very early onset (between 3 months and 2 years) accounts for 60–80% of all forms of AD by several epidemiologic studies. Many of the patients in this type can reach complete remission before age 2 years. Patients in other portion, observed at about 40%, have an AD that persists beyond the age of two and are most at risk for transition to "atopic march" which is represented by respiratory allergies.

Early onset (between 2 and 6 years) also has a high risk of having a chronic disease course. Childhood onset (between 6 and 14 years) is a relatively small-sized phenotype, accounting for about 10% of all AD patients. Little is known about disease progression, the possibility of having atopic features, and respiratory allergies.

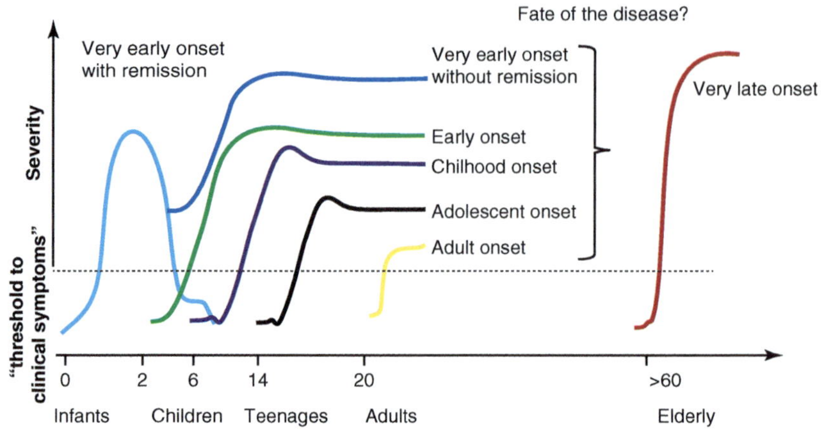

Fig. 1 The classification of clinical phenotype by age of onset [46, 47]

Adolescent onset (between 14 and 18 years) is the smallest phenotype of the six clinical phenotypes which is classified by age of onset, comprising less than 10% of patients. It is one of the subgroups where epidemiological studies are needed to define features along with the childhood onset phenotype.

Adult onset (between 20 and 60 years) accounts for about 20% of all AD patients, and attention is focused on the fact that most patients are women and have relatively mild symptoms. In addition, sensitization to external allergens is very limited and serum IgE levels are observed to be normal.

Very late onset (over 60 years) is more recently defined than the other five phenotypes and is increasingly recognized according to the global aging trend [48]. This phenotype can be further divided into two subgroups. The first case is a recurrence of AD who has had AD before but has remained in remission for a long time, and the second case is the first development of chronic recurrent eczema lesion after 60 years of age who had never AD before [49]. Older AD patients have relatively severe symptoms and have higher serum IgE levels. To date, due to the recognition that AD is a disease of infancy, no suitable diagnostic criteria for diagnosing older AD patients have been established.

Phenotypes According to the Typical Clinical Features by Age

AD has a characteristic distribution of eczematous lesions according to the age of the patient [50]. To date, at least four age-specific patterns have been defined, which consists of infantile, childhood, adolescent/adult, and elderly [51]. In general, acute eczematous lesions prevail in the infantile pattern, chronic eczematous lesions represented by lichenification caused by continuous scratching appear in the later age group, sometimes with a more nodular clinical form, similar in appearance to prurigo nodularis. The distribution of lesions and the pattern of lesions differ by age group, but severe itching is a common feature in all clinical forms except at the very beginning of AD.

Infantile AD (between 3 months and 2 years) is represented by small eczematous papules from the second month after birth, which form edematous papules and vesicles on both cheeks. They also merge with each other to form larger plaques, with considerable amounts of exudate or accompanied by crust. In addition, the scalp may be severely accompanied by severe scales, which is named "cradle cap." In addition, eczematous lesions occur on the scalp, neck, extensor surface of the extremities, and torso, whereas the diaper area is not involved. What should not be overlooked is that the very early stage of AD is very difficult to diagnose, while the characteristic lesional distribution of AD appears several weeks after the onset.

In childhood AD (between 2 and 12 years), the proportion of acute eczematous lesions, which accounted for the majority of infantile AD, is reduced, and the proportion of chronic eczematous lesions with some lichenification is increased. The areas where the lesions are mainly distributed are the popliteal fossa and antecubital fossa, which is also called "flexural eczema," and eczematous lesions also appear around the mouth (e.g., periorificial eczema). Relatively often, nummular plaques appear on the hands and wrists with oozing and crusting, which can be classified as "nummular subtype." Compared to infantile AD, xerosis becomes more severe.

Adolescent/Adult AD (between 12 and 60 years) tend to be confined to typical areas such as the head, neck, and flexural areas. In addition, in adults, it may develop into chronic hand eczema, a form of more localized AD. Female patients are more vulnerable to have periorbital eczema than male patients. Patients who have been suffering from long-term eczema due to poorly managed AD show systemic erythematous lesions rather than localized eczematous lesions.

AD in the elderly (over 60 years) is one of the clinical phenotypes of AD that have been relatively undervalued to date. This clinical form shows severe and extensive eczematous lesions, even erythrodermic features, and is characterized by severe itching. Sometimes, unlike adult AD, the eczematous lesions do not involve the flexural areas. This particular phenotype requires analysis for precise diagnostic criteria for accurate diagnosis. Differential diagnosis of elderly AD should take into account the disease which may appear as erythrodermic features, such as allergic contact dermatitis and cutaneous T cell lymphoma, which can be accompanied by severe itching.

Phenotypes According to the Severity of AD

AD includes a very broad spectrum of severity, from very mild to very severe phenotypes. In addition to the classical diagnostic criteria, a proven scoring system such as SCORAD (SCORing Atopic Dermatitis) or EASI (Eczema Area and Severity Index) can be used to define the severity that distinguishes between mild, moderate, and severe phenotypes. SCORAD is a scoring system developed in 1993 and widely used to assess the severity of atopic dermatitis. SCORAD includes the range of skin lesions based on Wallace's "rule of nine," and the objective criteria which consist of erythema, papules/edema, crusting/oozing, erosions, lichenification, dry skin (e.g., xerosis). Subjective patient-oriented evaluation indicators such as severity of pruritus and sleep disturbance due to itching sensation are also included [52]. EASI is a scoring system developed in 2001, similar to the modified PASI used to assess the severity of psoriasis. EASI excluded subjective score scales from SCORAD but included the assessment of the extent of lesions by dividing them into head and neck, trunk, upper limbs, and lower limbs, and the assessment criteria of individual lesions consisting of four types: erythema, papules/edema, lichenification, and excoriation so that EASI has the advantage of simpler measurements compared to SCORAD [53].

Nowadays, in order to make the various scoring systems to be consistent, an indicator like Fig. 2 is presented. The consistency of those scoring systems is thought to be useful for comparing primary and secondary endpoints in different clinical studies, particularly in integrating the results of different trials such as systemic review and meta-analysis. There is still a lot of debate about which scoring system is the easiest to measure in a clinical setting and accurately assessing the patient's current disease status, and it is a hot topic in the era of biologics.

Phenotypes According to Ethnicity

Until the turn of the twentieth century, the differences in clinical phenotypes of AD according to

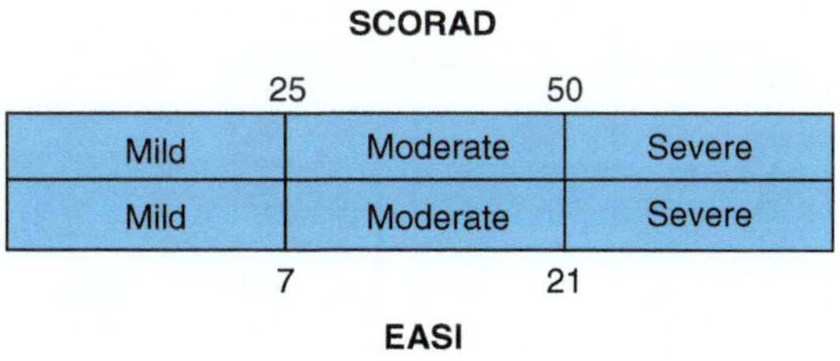

Fig. 2 The classification of clinical phenotype by severity [46, 53]

variable ethnicity and regional distribution of patients have been overlooked. Recently, however, it has been discovered that there are different clinical and molecular phenotypes on behalf of ethnicity. For example, when comparing the transcriptomic profiles between white AD patients and Asian AD patients, the composition of cytokines and pathophysiology involved in chronic inflammation is different from each other, according to previous white patient-centered studies [54]. And another study which compared the genomic profiling and immunohistochemistry on lesional and non-lesional skin between European/American (EA) and Asian patients, the Asian AD phenotype presents (even in the presence of increased IgE levels) a blended phenotype between that of EA patients with AD and those with psoriasis, including increased epidermal hyperplasia, parakeratosis, higher Th17 activation, and a strong Th2 component [55] (Fig. 3). In addition, the expression of potent Th17 cells has been observed in skin lesions in Japanese and Korean AD patients. Th17-driven skin inflammation, which is characteristically observed in Asian AD patients, reflects a more clinically pronounced lichenification, with profound epidermal hyperplasia in the skin lesions of Asian AD patients [54]. Those studies suggest that there may be various clinical phenotypes depending on the difference in ethnicities.

On the other hand, it has recently been reported that the clinical phenotype of AD seen in African American patients differs from that of Caucasian patients [56]. In addition, differences in gene levels have also been suggested, filaggrin deficiency, which is frequently observed in white AD patients, is rarely observed in other race patients, suggesting that there may be differences in the pathogenesis of AD [57]. Given the recent pathophysiological differences among diverse ethnicities, ongoing epidemiologic studies will suggest clinical phenotypes for different ethnicities, which implies that pathophysiology underlying chronic dermatitis may be different according to ethnicities and regional patient distribution. This is supported by the fact that hotspots for filaggrin mutations differ in whites and Asians [58]. In the end, as the differences in gene levels and clinical phenotypes are identified according to race, there is a possibility that some modifications should be made for various races by modifying the diagnosis criteria of AD which are widely used. Ultimately, in developing a variety of biologics that target specific cytokines in recent years, differences in molecular pathogenesis due to ethnic differences should be considered.

Definition of Biomarkers and Their Clinical Application

The term "biomarker" encompasses both normal biological mechanisms and pathological processes, and refers to the measurement and evaluation of all indicators that reflect the interaction between a specific biological system and the chemical, physical, and biological environment.

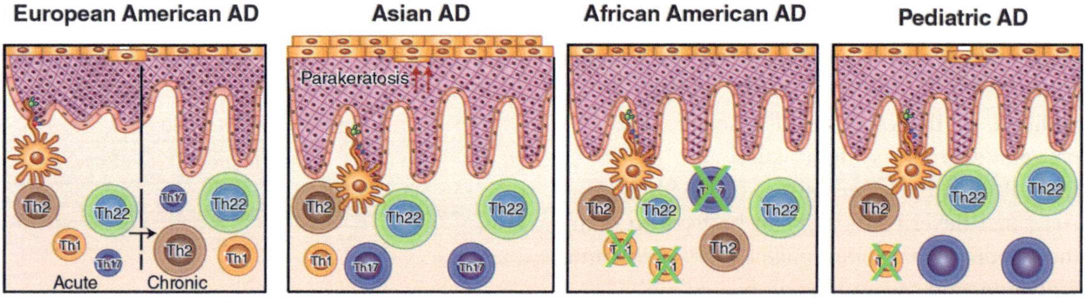

Fig. 3 AD endophenotypes. Greater expression of Th17-related cytokines is related to epidermal hyperplasia and parakeratosis in the skin of Asian patients with AD [54]

In the literature, there are two main definitions: the WHO (World Health Organization) definition and the definitions from NIH biomarkers definition working group. WHO defines biomarkers as "any substance, structure or process that can be measured in the body or its products and influence or predict the incidence of outcome or disease. Biomarkers can be classified into markers of exposure, effect and susceptibility" [59]. In addition, NIH defines biomarker as "a characteristic that is objectively measured and evaluated as an indicator of normal biological processes, pathogenic processes, or pharmacologic responses to a therapeutic intervention" [60]. These two definitions have overlapping meanings and different meanings; however, they recognize biomarkers as indicators of predictive value for specific biological operations. As a result, there is a wide range of indicators that can be used as biomarkers, such as genetics, imaging modalities, metabolites, proteins, lipids, epigenetics. In recent years, not only biomarkers widely used such as single genes or single blood test indexes, but also a wide range of "omics" data are being studied as biomarkers, such as proteomics, transcriptomics, epigenomics, metabonomics, and nutrigenomics The development of a large data set that incorporates the relevant factors will be an important framework for the establishment of endophenotypes of AD and even for personalized medical approaches [61].

Endophenotype is defined as a measurable element that cannot be observed without specific help, among various molecular or genetic factors between disease and genotype [62]. This means that endophenotype is a specific combination of all kinds of biomarkers that can be measured between clinical phenotype and genotype. Previously used biomarkers have limitations that reflect only one scene of the particular disease course (e.g., snapshot approach), while biological markers which are called endophenotype reflect the interaction between the external environment and biological systems, as well as biological data from patients with certain diseases. AD is characterized by chronic course of skin inflammation, the clinical phenotype changes with the age of the patient, and the interaction with external allergens which contributes significantly to the pathophysiological mechanism, so the endophenotype is more suitable to follow the chronic disease course of AD because it can act as a more continuous and predictive biomarker. Eventually, endophenotype could be used for future therapeutic approaches and even for preventive purposes.

In the near future, a large set of data representing clinical phenotypes, genotypes, and endophenotypes will enable AD patients to be individually defined and to predict the most effective treatments, the most appropriate preventive and therapeutic strategies [63]. The most interfering factor in finding such biomarkers in AD is screening out the various biomarkers which are spurted out nowadays, looking for the biomarkers that will serve as the most beneficial and surrogate markers. In addition, since the biomarker plays an important role in continuously measuring and reflecting the trend of change in specific diseases, the measurement method should be easy and have high reproducibility. For example, using mass spectrometry to measure the activity of a specific molecule or cytokine on the skin is very expensive, time-consuming, and very complex and difficult to measure, so this method is not an efficient way to continuously obtain the biological information. On the other hand, using PCA (Principal component analysis) might be an inexpensive, simple, easy-to-measure method which is suitable for performing the biomarker's original functions.

Based on the definitions of the WHO and NIH biomarkers definitions group mentioned above, biomarkers can be divided into two categories according to their purpose of use and the nature of the mechanism to be reflected. The first category, Selection/Stratification biomarkers, is used to select specific patients or to classify patient groups. The second category, Monitoring biomarkers, is used to monitor the clinical response to specific treatments and interventions. The first category can be further subdivided into four subclasses, including screening biomarkers and diagnostic biomarkers, and also including prognostic biomarkers and predictive biomarkers. Prognostic biomarkers play a role in predicting

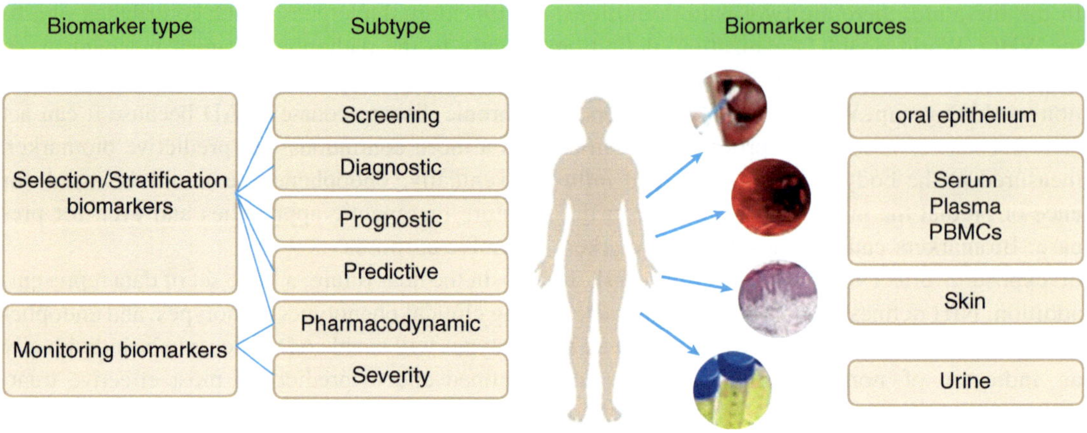

Fig. 4 Biomarker types and subtypes [64]

disease course or patient risk for clinical endpoints such as hospitalization or death [65]. Predictive biomarkers serve to select a group of patients that are most likely to be effective for a particular disease or to select a group of patients who are likely to experience a particular side effect. The second category includes measurement of the disease severity, serves as a pivotal endpoint in clinical trials, and also includes pharmacodynamic biomarkers (Fig. 4).

The Need for Biomarkers in Atopic Dermatitis

Biomarkers for the Classification of Phenotypes and Figuring Out the Disease Heterogeneity

AD has a broad spectrum of phenotypes depending on the clinical features and the natural course of the disease [47, 66, 67]. As mentioned in the previous chapter, considerable attempts have been made to classify clinical phenotypes according to the scoring system, age of onset, distribution of lesions by age, and ethnicity. However, these attempts did not generally reflect the Th2 driven immunological pathways underlying AD. For example, the classification of clinical phenotypes into intrinsic AD and extrinsic AD through serum IgE levels suggested higher expression of genes associated with Th2 immune responses in extrinsic type AD patients with elevated serum IgE levels, but recent studies have shown that the expression of Th2-related genes are similar between intrinsic AD and extrinsic AD [68]. This fact indicates that those two clinical phenotypes show differences in single blood test results, but the underlying pathogenesis is likely to overlap each other. Accordingly, the establishment of endophenotype through the development of new biomarkers will help to classify the AD patient subgroup reflecting the underlying pathogenesis.

For most patients with AD, topical steroid agents or oral medications such as cyclosporin A or methotrexate for nonspecific immunosuppression are still the mainstay of treatment. Many studies are underway, but the link between treatment efficacy of oral immunosuppressant and clinical phenotypes has not been established. Recently, with the development of biologics targeting specific cytokines such as dupilumab or lebrikizumab, it is important to classify AD patients through specific immune pathways which is polarized in a certain individual and to find out which biologics can achieve the maximum therapeutic effect.

Biomarkers for Prediction of Treatment Response

Severe, treatment-resistant AD patients do not respond well to topical treatments and are currently being treated with several systemic immunosuppressive agents. Most immunosuppressive drugs are used off-label except for cyclosporin, and only cyclosporin is registered as an AD treatment drug in European nations. If there is no therapeutic response by cyclosporin, then substitutional agents such as methotrexate, azathioprine (AZA), and mycophenolic acid (MPA) are mainly used as off-labels. These systemic immunosuppressive agents may of course be accompanied by side effects from broad systemic immune suppression, but the most worrying part of patients and clinicians is that treatment failure rate is quite high as 40–50% [69–71]. On behalf of this background, it is urgent to develop biomarkers that can predict treatment response to systemic immunosuppressants, but there are no biomarkers that can be used in the clinical situation.

Biomarkers based on pharmacogenetics and therapeutic drug monitoring (TDM) can help to balance the response and adverse reactions to systemic immunosuppressive therapy. Pharmacogenetic biomarkers can be used to determine the presence or absence of a response to a particular immunosuppressive agent, as well as to help to maintain the appropriate drug dose by minimizing side effects [72, 73].

Biomarkers that predict therapeutic response may also be useful in the introduction of new, targeted therapies. It is already known that serum biomarkers can predict the therapeutic response of allergic asthma to targeted therapies. For example, asthma patients with high serum periostin levels have been shown to have a higher therapeutic response to lebrikizumab, an anti-IL-13 antibody [74]. Periostin is an extracellular matrix protein that is increased in expression by Th2-induced IL-4 and IL-3, which is a hallmark immune response of asthma and AD. This suggests that the Th2 immune response is more active in patients with high periostin and that periostin can be used to evaluate treatment response as well as explaining the pathophysiological mechanism of the disease. Asthma is also a disease with a wide range of clinical phenotypes, such as AD, and because it shares many common features with AD, biomarkers that predict the response to new biologics can be expected to play an important role in the treatment of AD. Biomarkers for predicting treatment response will be useful not only for clinical use but also for the development of biologics in the clinical studies. Numerous drugs fail to demonstrate their effectiveness for the development of a single biologics, whereas the possibility that these drugs may have efficacy for a particular subgroup of patients cannot be ruled out. Eventually, biomarkers that can predict the response of developing biologics will allow a large number of targeted therapies to be used again in clinical settings.

Biomarkers for Objective Measurement of AD Severity

To date, over 20 different scoring systems with their own structure has been developed and used to assess the severity of AD, but there is no single gold standard [9]. According to a recent systematic review, various scoring systems have been used in AD-related clinical trials, but only 27% of the scoring systems had evidence that is published before the specific clinical trial [11]. In addition, according to a retrospective study on the reliability and validity of the 20 most commonly used scoring systems, only three scoring systems (e.g., EASI, SCORAD, and Three Item Severity Score) were proved as appropriate severity evaluating tools [9]. In the absence of appropriate severity outcome measures, the Harmonizing Outcome Measurements in Eczema (HOME) initiative, which includes a large number of AD specialists, has been formed to provide a core severity outcome measure which is validated to improve the comparability of different clinical trials [75]. The HOME initiative evaluated 16 outcome measures and found that only two indicators, EASI and objective SCORAD index, had adequate reliability and validity [10]. In particular, EASI excelled other outcome measures in terms of validity, responsiveness, and consistency among observers, so that EASI was thought to be a most favored scoring system for clinical trials by consensus which was consisted of patients, clinicians, nurses, and pharmaceutical industry representatives [10]. Nevertheless, it remains controversial which of the EASI and SCORAD scoring systems should be preferred [76]. Compared to EASI, SCORAD assesses subjective symptoms as well as objective indicators, allowing for a better measure of patient's quality of life compared to EASI. In spite of this discussion, scoring methods such as EASI and SCORAD have considerable disadvantages such as significant observer bias and inconsistencies that may occur as the evaluator changes. Therefore, it is necessary to develop reliable and objective severity biomarkers, and through this biomarker, both objective and subjective aspects of AD might be evaluated simultaneously. In addition, the use of biomarkers in clinical trials as surrogate endpoints will increase the comparability between different clinical trials and make meta-analysis easier.

Current Candidate Biomarkers of AD

While studies on classical clinical phenotypes have been progressing so far, research on the definition of endophenotype through the development of biomarkers is just beginning. As a result, there is no endophenotype defined for AD yet, but a considerable number of biomarkers have been developed and are awaiting verification of their validity and reliability for clinical use. It should be emphasized that none of the various biomarkers mentioned in the section below have been proven reliable for use in the clinical setting. Rather than remembering individual biomarkers below, it is important to understand the context in which the development of the biomarkers is taking place. In near future, the biomarkers described in sections "Screening Biomarkers", "Diagnostic Biomarkers", "Severity Biomarkers", "Predictive and Prognostic Biomarkers", "Pharmacodynamic Biomarkers", and "Monitoring Biomarkers" may define new endophenotype and present new therapeutic paradigms in the biologics era. Current candidates of biomarkers for various purposes are listed in Table 3

Table 3 Current candidate biomarkers in AD [46, 64]

Subtype of biomarker	Candidate biomarkers
Screening	Filaggrin gene mutation, SPINK5, Cord blood IgE level, Infantile LT-α, FcεRI-β genotypes, TSLP, TARC/CCL17, TEWL
Diagnostic	None
Severity	TARC/CCL17, MDC/CCL22, CTACK/CCL27, PARC/CCL18, IL-31, IL-33, IL-22, IL-18, IL-16, soluble IL-2 receptor, LL-37, Periostin, BDNF, Specific IgE to *Malassezia* species
Prognostic	Filaggrin gene mutation, Serum total IgE, Indoleamine 2,3-dioxygenase-1, Specific IgE to *Malassezia* species
Predict comorbidities (for viral complications)	TSLP, IL-33, IDO
Predictive (potential to be used)	Serum total IgE level, filaggrin gene mutation, TEWL
Pharmacodynamic	CYP3A4/CYP3A5 for cyclosporine A UGT1A9 for mycophenolic acid Thiopurine methyltransferase, 6-thioguanine nucleotides, 6-6-methylmercaptopurine ribonucleotides for azathioprine
Monitoring	
Serum	TARC, CTACK, sE-selectin, Macrophage-derived chemokine, Lactate dehydrogenase (LDH), IL-18
Skin	Transcriptome changes
Pruritus	IL-31, wearable measurements

Screening Biomarkers

Given the natural history of early childhood and childhood AD, screening biomarkers can be used to identify susceptible individuals with AD. Recent cohort studies have shown that early treatment, such as moisturizer application, to newborns with a family history of AD may at least slow the emergence of AD [77, 78].

Therefore, the concept of the usage of screening biomarkers to identify the patients with high risk for developing AD is widely accepted to detect the occurrence of AD in advance and prevent the transition to a chronic vicious cycle of AD. In the end, it is important to find out which biomarkers, or combinations of biomarkers, can adequately select individuals that will benefit from early intervention. In this respect, it has recently been reported that measuring TEWL can function as a simple, noninvasive screening biomarker [79].

To date, many genome-wide studies have identified candidate genes that are closely associated with the development of AD. Among them, the filaggrin gene has been shown to be associated with AD by solid evidence from numerous studies [80]. Filaggrin gene mutations have been observed in about 30% of AD patients, but AD does not occur in every individual with filaggrin gene mutation [81]. However, screening for mutations in genes encoding epidermal structural proteins, such as filaggrin, could be used to detect subjects at high risk of AD or to detect the development of concomitant respiratory allergy (e.g., allergic march) [82, 83]. To date, genotyping of a particular individual has been carried out through a complicated and expensive process. Nevertheless, in the near future, gene mutation profiles will be available for AD screening as the latest genotyping technologies, such as Next-Generation Sequencing (NGS), have been developed and applied to the clinical field.

Genes thought to be useful as screening biomarkers for AD as filaggrin-like epidermal proteins include serine protease inhibitor Kazal-type 5 (SPINK5) and thymic stromal lymphopoietin (TSLP) [84, 85]. In addition, childhood lymphotoxin-alpha levels, FceR1-beta genotype during pregnancy, and elevated cord blood IgE levels have been shown to be associated with childhood AD [86], suggesting that they may function as screening biomarkers for AD.

Diagnostic Biomarkers

Since AD is mainly diagnosed through clinical findings, there is no biomarker to confirm the diagnosis of AD for now. Although standardized clinical features of AD in infancy, childhood, and adolescence are used as diagnostic criteria, infants under 3 months old and senile AD, as mentioned in the previous chapter, are difficult to diagnose because their clinical features are different from the classical ones. While studies on diagnostic biomarkers for both subtypes are ongoing, no candidates have emerged yet [87, 88].

Severity Biomarkers

Most of the biomarkers introduced in the literature to date are focused on reflecting the severity of AD or response to treatment. Of the various severity biomarkers, thymus and activation-regulated chemokine (CCL17), macrophage-derived chemokine (CCL22), cutaneous T-cell-attracting chemokine (CCL27), IL-31, IL-33, IL-22, LL37, IL-18, IL-16, pulmonary and activation-regulated chemokine (CCL18), periostin, and the soluble IL-2 receptor and brain-derived neurotrophic factor are highly valued for their potential for clinical use [89–97].

In addition, it has been suggested that sensitization to commensal yeast in the skin, such as *Malassezia*, has been linked to disease activity in AD, so that the sensitization status on behalf of specific IgE to *Malassezia* might be a possible severity biomarker [98]. In addition, sensitization to self-proteins has been considered to cause AD that is different from the classic AD clinical phenotype, contributing to various clinical phenotypes of AD, and the sensitization to *Malassezia* might reflect this autoimmunity in AD [99–101]. Nevertheless, the value of biomarkers of the kind mentioned above is differently accepted in clinical trials and in clinical practice, since the clinical effects of specific treatments to AD are most accurately assessed through visual examinations by clinicians and patients.

Predictive and Prognostic Biomarkers

Biologics for specific cytokines, which play an important role in the pathogenesis of AD, have received a great deal of attention, but there are no clear strategies for using biologics [102, 103]. Accordingly, attempts to develop biomarkers to predict therapeutic responses are just beginning to take off. However, the recent accumulation of evidences suggests that the molecular mechanisms that cause chronic skin inflammation differ according to ethnicity (Caucasus vs. Asian) or age (adults vs. children). So, the importance of developing biomarkers for predicting treatment response is widely recognized. For example, T cell differentiation to Th22 is more apparent in adult AD skin than children [104, 105], whereas skin lesion of children shows dominant Th2, Th9, and Th17 immune responses. This fact suggests that biologics targeting Th2, such as dupilumab, are likely to be more effective in children than adults. Similarly, the dominant Th17 immune response in Asians compared to the Caucasus gives justification for attempting biologics targeting Th17 immune response, which is primarily used in psoriasis.

In addition to tracking the response to specific treatments, biomarkers that provide information about the compliance of patients for specific treatments may also be useful in the clinical setting. The classification of endophenotypes according to these biomarkers can help to establish specific treatment strategies by collecting "omics" data such as transcriptome from blood tissues that reflect the systemic immune response and skin tissues that reflect the skin immune response. Given the high costs of biologics that are being developed recently, this approach will reduce medical costs and the economic burden on AD patients.

Since AD has a chronic and relapsing natural history, biomarkers that predict prognosis such as disease persistence and recurrence potential are the most desired and necessary types of biomarkers among other types of biomarkers. In addition, due to the chronic nature of the disease, AD has various complications such as viral infections, bacterial infections, and various accompanying diseases such as allergic asthma, allergic rhinitis. So, it is important to monitor and prevent those complications and comorbidities by trafficking the specific biomarkers.

Given the fact that the clinical phenotype of AD is very heterogeneous, it can be inferred that there is a group of patients who are likely to be accompanied by the complications and comorbidities mentioned above. Prognostic biomarkers can provide crucial information about the fate of AD in childhood AD patients, including whether or not there is complete remission before adolescence and the development of respiratory allergies such as allergic asthma. It also prevents them by predicting the risk of serious complications, such as bacterial infections or eczema herpeticum [106, 107]. Considering the recent senile AD phenotype and the fact that AD is a lifelong disease due to systemic immune response [36, 37], the prognostic biomarker might be very useful in predicting natural history of AD in particular individual and preventing serious complications [108].

Pharmacodynamic Biomarkers

Although various biologics have been developed recently, systemic immunosuppressive agents such as cyclosporine have been widely used in patients with moderate to severe AD. However, as there is no biomarker for therapeutic response to biologics, no biomarker for monitoring the response to classical systemic immunosuppressants is used clinically. As a result, pharmacogenetic studies are being conducted to select patients who respond to a specific drug, and the association between pharmacodynamics, pharmacokinetics, efficacy, safety, and specific gene variation has been suggested [109]. The most commonly observed genetic variations are single nucleotide polymorphisms (SNPs), copy number variation, and insertion/deletion of specific genes, all of which have the potential to be used as pharmacodynamic biomarkers [72, 73].

In vivo metabolism and bioavailability of cyclosporine are mainly determined by isoenzymes of CYP3A4 and CYP3A5 [110]. Therefore, as further studies progress, gene tests for CYP3A4 and CYP3A5 might be useful to predict serum cyclosporine levels and determine the efficacy of the drug on a specific subject. Similarly, mycophenolate acid (MPA) is known to have their efficacy only in about half of the patients who are administered the medication

[69, 71], and it is one of the immunosuppressive agents that can be most helpful in selecting a group of patients who can benefit from MPA administration through pharmacogenetic biomarkers. MPA is mainly metabolized by UGT1A9, and the presence of SNPs in the promoter region of UGT1A9 and the blood levels of MPA are correlated with each other [111, 112]. Accordingly, the SNPs of UGT1A9 of AD patients might be used as a pharmacodynamic biomarker that can help prevent the unnecessary administration of MPA for patients who are ineffective or make clinicians to increase the drug dose for patients who are expected to have low drug concentrations, thereby supporting proper drug utilization. Azathioprine (AZA) is also known to have efficacy in about half of patients treated similarly to MPA, and in particular, the drug is often discontinued even though it is effective due to serious side effects [69]. Studies from Crohn's disease or ulcerative colitis have shown that genetic variations of thiopurine methyltransferase affects the metabolism of AZA [113]. Therefore, by examining the gene status of thiopurine methyltransferase before starting medication, subjects with high risk of side effects may be selected. In addition, blood concentrations of 6-thioguanine nucleotides and 6-methylmercaptopurine ribonucleotides, which are metabolites of AZA, can be used as biomarkers to predict the risk of side effects such as bone marrow toxicity or liver toxicity [113].

The pharmacodynamics biomarkers mentioned above are just candidates for use in the clinical field, along with other biomarker types. Pharmacodynamic biomarkers that are easy to measure and reliable to be used have not yet been proposed, but biomarkers for classic systemic immunosuppressants are expected to be introduced into the clinical field following the introduction of personalized medicine concepts.

Monitoring Biomarkers

AD is a skin disease characterized by heterogeneous clinical phenotypes and pathophysiology. However, AD with various clinical phenotypes share the clinical features; chronicity and tendency of recurrence. Accordingly, various monitoring biomarkers have been proposed to identify disease activity in the natural course of individual AD patients.

Among various monitoring biomarkers, serum total IgE levels are one of the most frequently measured serological markers in the clinical settings and clinical trials [114]. Although serum total IgE levels tend to be elevated in patients with high disease activity, baseline serum total IgE levels are normal in intrinsic AD patients. This implies that serum total IgE levels are not appropriate for monitoring disease activity and disease severity. In particular, a recent meta-analysis study shows that the relationship between serum total IgE level and disease activity is very weak, increasing the demand for new monitoring biomarkers [114].

In addition to serum total IgE levels, biomarkers reported to measure disease activity include eosinophilic cationic protein (ECP), IL-2 receptor, and thymus and activation-regulated chemokine (TARC/CCL17) [115–117]. Among them, TARC is currently the most reliable and effective biomarker. According to a recent meta-analysis, the pooled correlation coefficient of the longitudinal randomized trials was 0.6 (95% confidence interval, 0.48–0.70) and the pooled correlation coefficient of the cross-sectional studies was 0.64 (95% confidence interval, 0.57–0.70) [114]. Monitoring biomarkers that are likely to be used in clinical settings other than TARC in this meta-analysis include serum cutaneous T cell-attracting chemokine (CTACK), serum sE-selectin, serum macrophage-derived chemokine, serum lactate dehydrogenase (LDH), and serum IL-18 [118–122].

Although TARC has been shown to be strongly associated with disease activity in AD, serum TARC levels between patients with the same severity score show different values each other [20]. Differences in TARC levels between individuals are thought to be the result of heterogeneous pathogenetic mechanisms that are involved in AD. According to a recent pilot study which includes 17 patients with AD, when using a biomarker panel consisting of TARC, pulmonary- and activation-regulated chemokine (PARC),

IL-22 and soluble IL-2R, the six area/six sign AD severity score showed a high correlation coefficient of 0.86 [123]. This suggests that a biomarker panel might be a reasonable method to follow disease activity in diseases in which factors are intricately intertwined like AD.

Although serological samples are easy to use as biomarkers because they are easy to collect, test, and interpret, most of the important information about the pathogenesis of AD is present in skin lesions. A study by the Emma–Guttman group found that changes in skin transcriptome were observed following Narrow Band Ultraviolet B (NBUVB), cyclosporine administration, and dupilumab treatment [124–126]. These studies provide a prototype of biomarker panel for monitoring disease activity and severity, and treatment response to various biologics to be developed in the future.

An essential component of the severity assessment of AD is chronic, extreme pruritus. Pruritus might cause sleep disturbances and poor daily life functions, which greatly reduces the quality of life of AD patients and increases the severity of skin lesions by the itching–scratching vicious cycle. Although various questionnaires are used in clinical trials and real-world settings to measure the itch and subsequent deterioration in the patient's quality of life, there is no method for objectively measuring the itch with high reproducibility. Against this background, IL-31, which is recently known to be associated with pruritus in AD, is expected to be used as a biomarker for pruritus. Several studies have been reported on the correlation between disease activity and serum IL-31 levels [127], but the correlation with itching has not been studied yet, so further studies are needed to determine the correlation between pruritus and serum IL-31 level. In addition to serological markers, recent attempts have been made to measure scratching behaviors which reflect the severity of pruritus through wearable devices, which might be used as biomarkers for pruritus [128].

Conclusions and Future Perspectives

Although AD is not a life-threatening disorder, its unique chronic and recurrent characteristics and extreme pruritus increase the quality of life of the patient as well as socioeconomic burden. There is a growing understanding of the various pathomechanisms of AD, but the same guidelines are used under a single diagnosis in a real clinical setting. This approach does not take into account the clinical phenotype of AD at all, and instead of predicting the patient's response to a particular treatment, the "one-size-fits-all" approach is still prevalent. This imposes an unnecessary cost on patients who will not respond to certain treatments, while also causing serious side effects that patients do not have to be suffered, thereby increasing patients' frustration to AD treatment. In particular, this approach reveals limitations in the early onset AD, which is the cornerstone of transition to other allergic diseases.

In this background, the challenge of defining biomarkers as an aid to diagnosis and establishing endophenotypes is essential in the era of personalized medicine represented by the establishment of new treatment strategies and preventive approaches. Currently, various serological tests have been proposed as candidates for biomarkers, but a number of new trials have been made, including the establishment of completely new biomarkers and biomarker panels following the development of "omics" data. In the near future, AD patients will be classified into different endophenotypes by biomarkers from serum, skin tissue, and genetic variation, as well as biomarker panels that combine various types of biomarkers. This will provide a fundamental foundation for personalized medicine in line with the recent biologics era and for advances in the understanding of heterogeneous pathogenesis of AD.

References

1. Eyerich K, Novak N. Immunology of atopic eczema: overcoming the Th1/Th2 paradigm. Allergy. 2013;68(8):974–82.
2. Boyman O, Kaegi C, Akdis M, Bavbek S, Bossios A, Chatzipetrou A, et al. EAACI IG Biologicals task force paper on the use of biologic agents in allergic disorders. Allergy. 2015;70(7):727–54.
3. Williams H, Stewart A, von Mutius E, Cookson W, Anderson HR. Is eczema really on the increase worldwide? J Allergy Clin Immunol. 2008;121(4):947–54.e15.
4. Deckers IA, McLean S, Linssen S, Mommers M, van Schayck CP, Sheikh A. Investigating international time trends in the incidence and prevalence of atopic

eczema 1990–2010: a systematic review of epidemiological studies. PLoS One. 2012;7(7):e39803.
5. Simpson EL, Bieber T, Eckert L, Wu R, Ardeleanu M, Graham NM, et al. Patient burden of moderate to severe atopic dermatitis (AD): insights from a phase 2b clinical trial of dupilumab in adults. J Am Acad Dermatol. 2016;74(3):491–8.
6. Zuberbier T, Lotvall J, Simoens S, Subramanian SV, Church MK. Economic burden of inadequate management of allergic diseases in the European Union: a GA(2) LEN review. Allergy. 2014;69(10):1275–9.
7. Chalmers JR, Simpson E, Apfelbacher CJ, Thomas KS, von Kobyletzki L, Schmitt J, et al. Report from the fourth international consensus meeting to harmonize core outcome measures for atopic eczema/dermatitis clinical trials (HOME initiative). Br J Dermatol. 2016;175(1):69–79.
8. Charman CR, Venn AJ, Williams HC. Measurement of body surface area involvement in atopic eczema: an impossible task? Br J Dermatol. 1999;140(1):109–11.
9. Schmitt J, Langan S, Williams HC. What are the best outcome measurements for atopic eczema? A systematic review. J Allergy Clin Immunol. 2007;120(6):1389–98.
10. Schmitt J, Spuls PI, Thomas KS, Simpson E, Furue M, Deckert S, et al. The harmonising outcome measures for eczema (home) statement to assess clinical signs of atopic eczema in trials. J Allergy Clin Immunol. 2014;134(4):800–7.
11. Charman C, Chambers C, Williams H. Measuring atopic dermatitis severity in randomized controlled clinical trials: what exactly are we measuring? J Investig Dermatol. 2003;120(6):932–41.
12. Kakinuma T, Nakamura K, Wakugawa M, Mitsui H, Tada Y, Saeki H, et al. Thymus and activation-regulated chemokine in atopic dermatitis: serum thymus and activation-regulated chemokine level is closely related with disease activity. J Allergy Clin Immunol. 2001;107(3):535–41.
13. Zhao CY, Tran AQ, Lazo-Dizon JP, Kim J, Daniel BS, Venugopal SS, et al. A pilot comparison study of four clinician-rated atopic dermatitis severity scales. Br J Dermatol. 2015;173(2):488–97.
14. Zheng X, Nakamura K, Furukawa H, Nishibu A, Takahashi M, Tojo M, et al. Demonstration of TARC and CCR4 mRNA expression and distribution using in situ RT-PCR in the lesional skin of atopic dermatitis. J Dermatol. 2003;30(1):26–32.
15. Imai T, Nagira M, Takagi S, Kakizaki M, Nishimura M, Wang J, et al. Selective recruitment of CCR4-bearing Th2 cells toward antigen-presenting cells by the CC chemokines thymus and activation-regulated chemokine and macrophage-derived chemokine. Int Immunol. 1999;11(1):81–8.
16. Kayserova J, Capkova S, Skalicka A, Vernerova E, Polouckova A, Malinova V, et al. Serum immunoglobulin free light chains in severe forms of atopic dermatitis. Scand J Immunol. 2010;71(4):312–6.
17. Rijnierse A, Redegeld FA, Blokhuis BR, Van der Heijden MW, Te Velde AA, Pronk I, et al. Ig-free light chains play a crucial role in murine mast cell-dependent colitis and are associated with human inflammatory bowel diseases. J Immunol. 2010;185(1):653–9.
18. Schouten B, van Esch BC, van Thuijl AO, Blokhuis BR, Groot Kormelink T, Hofman GA, et al. Contribution of IgE and immunoglobulin free light chain in the allergic reaction to cow's milk proteins. J Allergy Clin Immunol. 2010;125(6):1308–14.
19. Kraneveld AD, Kool M, van Houwelingen AH, Roholl P, Solomon A, Postma DS, et al. Elicitation of allergic asthma by immunoglobulin free light chains. Proc Natl Acad Sci U S A. 2005;102(5):1578–83.
20. Landheer J, de Bruin-Weller M, Boonacker C, Hijnen D, Bruijnzeel-Koomen C, Rockmann H. Utility of serum thymus and activation-regulated chemokine as a biomarker for monitoring of atopic dermatitis severity. J Am Acad Dermatol. 2014;71(6):1160–6.
21. Pivarcsi A, Gombert M, Dieu-Nosjean MC, Lauerma A, Kubitza R, Meller S, et al. CC chemokine ligand 18, an atopic dermatitis-associated and dendritic cell-derived chemokine, is regulated by staphylococcal products and allergen exposure. J Immunol. 2004;173(9):5810–7.
22. Redegeld FA, van der Heijden MW, Kool M, Heijdra BM, Garssen J, Kraneveld AD, et al. Immunoglobulin-free light chains elicit immediate hypersensitivity-like responses. Nat Med. 2002;8(7):694–701.
23. Broder S, Venter JC. Whole genomes: the foundation of new biology and medicine. Curr Opin Biotechnol. 2000;11(6):581–5.
24. Ocana A, Pandiella A. Personalized therapies in the cancer "omics" era. Mol Cancer. 2010;9:202.
25. Chen R, Snyder M. Promise of personalized omics to precision medicine. Wiley Interdiscip Rev Syst Biol Med. 2013;5(1):73–82.
26. Bieber T, Broich K. [Personalised medicine. Aims and challenges]. Bundesgesundheitsblatt Gesundheitsforschung Gesundheitsschutz. 2013;56(11):1468–72.
27. Dorfman R, Khayat Z, Sieminowski T, Golden B, Lyons R. Application of personalized medicine to chronic disease: a feasibility assessment. Clin Transl Med. 2013;2(1):16.
28. Bieber T. Stratified medicine: a new challenge for academia, industry, regulators and patients. Future Med. 2013; https://doi.org/10.2217/9781780843186.
29. Olson JE, Bielinski SJ, Ryu E, Winkler EM, Takahashi PY, Pathak J, et al. Biobanks and personalized medicine. Clin Genet. 2014;86(1):50–5.
30. Fernald GH, Capriotti E, Daneshjou R, Karczewski KJ, Altman RB. Bioinformatics challenges for personalized medicine. Bioinformatics. 2011;27(13):1741–8.
31. Suh KS, Sarojini S, Youssif M, Nalley K, Milinovikj N, Elloumi F, et al. Tissue banking, bioinformatics, and electronic medical records: the front-end requirements for personalized medicine. J Oncol. 2013;2013:368751.
32. Momper JD, Wagner JA. Therapeutic drug monitoring as a component of personalized medicine:

applications in pediatric drug development. Clin Pharmacol Ther. 2014;95(2):138–40.
33. Kesselheim AS, Shiu N. The evolving role of biomarker patents in personalized medicine. Clin Pharmacol Ther. 2014;95(2):127–9.
34. Pugliarello S, Cozzi A, Gisondi P, Girolomoni G. Phenotypes of atopic dermatitis. J Deutsch Dermatol Ges. 2011;9(1):12–20.
35. Dharmage SC, Lowe AJ, Matheson MC, Burgess JA, Allen KJ, Abramson MJ. Atopic dermatitis and the atopic march revisited. Allergy. 2014;69(1):17–27.
36. Margolis JS, Abuabara K, Bilker W, Hoffstad O, Margolis DJ. Persistence of mild to moderate atopic dermatitis. JAMA Dermatol. 2014;150(6):593–600.
37. Mortz CG, Andersen KE, Dellgren C, Barington T, Bindslev-Jensen C. Atopic dermatitis from adolescence to adulthood in the TOACS cohort: prevalence, persistence and comorbidities. Allergy. 2015;70(7):836–45.
38. Leung DY, Guttman-Yassky E. Deciphering the complexities of atopic dermatitis: shifting paradigms in treatment approaches. J Allergy Clin Immunol. 2014;134(4):769–79.
39. Wuthrich B. [Atopic dermatitis]. Ther Umsch Rev Ther. 1989;46(9):633–40.
40. Bos JD, Brenninkmeijer EE, Schram ME, Middelkamp-Hup MA, Spuls PI, Smitt JH. Atopic eczema or atopiform dermatitis. Exp Dermatol. 2010;19(4):325–31.
41. Akdis CA, Akdis M. Immunological differences between intrinsic and extrinsic types of atopic dermatitis. Clin Exp Allergy. 2003;33(12):1618–21.
42. Flohr C, Johansson SG, Wahlgren CF, Williams H. How atopic is atopic dermatitis? J Allergy Clin Immunol. 2004;114(1):150–8.
43. Roduit C, Wohlgensinger J, Frei R, Bitter S, Bieli C, Loeliger S, et al. Prenatal animal contact and gene expression of innate immunity receptors at birth are associated with atopic dermatitis. J Allergy Clin Immunol. 2011;127(1):179–85, 185.e1.
44. Roduit C, Frei R, Depner M, Schaub B, Loss G, Genuneit J, et al. Increased food diversity in the first year of life is inversely associated with allergic diseases. J Allergy Clin Immunol. 2014;133(4):1056–64.
45. Roduit C, Frei R, Loss G, Buchele G, Weber J, Depner M, et al. Development of atopic dermatitis according to age of onset and association with early-life exposures. J Allergy Clin Immunol. 2012;130(1):130–6.e5.
46. Bieber T, D'Erme AM, Akdis CA, Traidl-Hoffmann C, Lauener R, Schappi G, et al. Clinical phenotypes and endophenotypes of atopic dermatitis: where are we, and where should we go? J Allergy Clin Immunol. 2017;139(4s):S58–s64.
47. Garmhausen D, Hagemann T, Bieber T, Dimitriou I, Fimmers R, Diepgen T, et al. Characterization of different courses of atopic dermatitis in adolescent and adult patients. Allergy. 2013;68(4):498–506.
48. Tanei R, Katsuoka K. Clinical analyses of atopic dermatitis in the aged. J Dermatol. 2008;35(9):562–9.
49. Tanei R, Hasegawa Y. Atopic dermatitis in older adults: a viewpoint from geriatric dermatology. Geriatr Gerontol Int. 2016;16(Suppl 1):75–86.
50. Weidinger S, Novak N. Atopic dermatitis. Lancet. 2016;387(10023):1109–22.
51. Bolognia J, Jorizzo J, Schaffer J, Callen J, Cerroni L, Heymann W, et al. Bolognia textbook of dermatology. Spain: Mosby Elsevier; 2012.
52. Severity scoring of atopic dermatitis: the SCORAD index. Consensus Report of the European Task Force on Atopic Dermatitis. Dermatology. 1993;186(1):23–31.
53. Hanifin JM, Thurston M, Omoto M, Cherill R, Tofte SJ, Graeber M. The eczema area and severity index (EASI): assessment of reliability in atopic dermatitis. EASI Evaluator Group. Exp Dermatol. 2001;10(1):11–8.
54. Czarnowicki T, He H, Krueger JG, Guttman-Yassky E. Atopic dermatitis endotypes and implications for targeted therapeutics. J Allergy Clin Immunol. 2019;143(1):1–11.
55. Wen HC, Czarnowicki T, Noda S, Malik K, Pavel AB, Nakajima S, et al. Serum from Asian patients with atopic dermatitis is characterized by TH2/TH22 activation, which is highly correlated with nonlesional skin measures. J Allergy Clin Immunol. 2018;142(1):324–8.e11.
56. Torrelo A. Atopic dermatitis in different skin types. What is to know? J Eur Acad Dermatol Venereol. 2014;28(Suppl 3):2–4.
57. Thawer-Esmail F, Jakasa I, Todd G, Wen Y, Brown SJ, Kroboth K, et al. South African amaXhosa patients with atopic dermatitis have decreased levels of filaggrin breakdown products but no loss-of-function mutations in filaggrin. J Allergy Clin Immunol. 2014;133(1):280–2.e1-2.
58. Park J, Jekarl DW, Kim Y, Kim J, Kim M, Park YM. Novel FLG null mutations in Korean patients with atopic dermatitis and comparison of the mutational spectra in Asian populations. J Dermatol. 2015;42(9):867–73.
59. World Health Organization and International Programme on Chemical Safety. Biomarkers in risk assessment: validity and validation, 2001. 2018.
60. Biomarkers Definitions Working Group. Biomarkers and surrogate endpoints: preferred definitions and conceptual framework. Clin Pharmacol Ther. 2001;69(3):89–95.
61. Schneider MV, Orchard S. Omics technologies, data and bioinformatics principles. Methods Mol Biol. 2011;719:3–30.
62. Gottesman II, Gould TD. The endophenotype concept in psychiatry: etymology and strategic intentions. Am J Psychiatry. 2003;160(4):636–45.
63. Bousquet J, Anto JM, Sterk PJ, Adcock IM, Chung KF, Roca J, et al. Systems medicine and integrated care to combat chronic noncommunicable diseases. Genome Med. 2011;3(7):43.
64. Thijs JL, de Bruin-Weller MS, Hijnen D. Current and future biomarkers in atopic dermatitis. Immunol Allergy Clin N Am. 2017;37(1):51–61.

65. Kramer F, Dinh W. Molecular and digital biomarker supported decision making in clinical studies in cardiovascular indications. Arch Pharm. 2016;349(6):399–409.
66. Bieber T. Atopic dermatitis 2.0: from the clinical phenotype to the molecular taxonomy and stratified medicine. Allergy. 2012;67(12):1475–82.
67. Guttman-Yassky E, Dhingra N, Leung DY. New era of biologic therapeutics in atopic dermatitis. Expert Opin Biol Ther. 2013;13(4):549–61.
68. Suarez-Farinas M, Dhingra N, Gittler J, Shemer A, Cardinale I, de Guzman Strong C, et al. Intrinsic atopic dermatitis shows similar TH2 and higher TH17 immune activation compared with extrinsic atopic dermatitis. J Allergy Clin Immunol. 2013;132(2):361–70.
69. van der Schaft J, Politiek K, van den Reek JM, Kievit W, de Jong EM, Bruijnzeel-Koomen CA, et al. Drug survival for azathioprine and enteric-coated mycophenolate sodium in a long-term daily practice cohort of adult patients with atopic dermatitis. Br J Dermatol. 2016;175(1):199–202.
70. Politiek K, van der Schaft J, Coenraads PJ, de Bruin-Weller MS, Schuttelaar ML. Drug survival for methotrexate in a daily practice cohort of adult patients with severe atopic dermatitis. Br J Dermatol. 2016;174(1):201–3.
71. Garritsen FM, Roekevisch E, van der Schaft J, Deinum J, Spuls PI, de Bruin-Weller MS. Ten years experience with oral immunosuppressive treatment in adult patients with atopic dermatitis in two academic centres. J Eur Acad Dermatol Venereol. 2015;29(10):1905–12.
72. Crews KR, Hicks JK, Pui CH, Relling MV, Evans WE. Pharmacogenomics and individualized medicine: translating science into practice. Clin Pharmacol Ther. 2012;92(4):467–75.
73. Ventola CL. The role of pharmacogenomic biomarkers in predicting and improving drug response: part 2: challenges impeding clinical implementation. P T. 2013;38(10):624–7.
74. Corren J, Lemanske RF, Hanania NA, Korenblat PE, Parsey MV, Arron JR, et al. Lebrikizumab treatment in adults with asthma. N Engl J Med. 2011;365(12):1088–98.
75. Schmitt J, Williams H, Group HD. Harmonising outcome measures for eczema (HOME). Report from the first international consensus meeting (HOME 1), 24 July 2010, Munich, Germany. Br J Dermatol. 2010;163(6):1166–8.
76. Flohr C. Third time coming HOME: not just EASI. Br J Dermatol. 2014;171(6):1287–8.
77. Horimukai K, Morita K, Narita M, Kondo M, Kitazawa H, Nozaki M, et al. Application of moisturizer to neonates prevents development of atopic dermatitis. J Allergy Clin Immunol. 2014;134(4):824–30.e6.
78. Simpson EL, Chalmers JR, Hanifin JM, Thomas KS, Cork MJ, McLean WH, et al. Emollient enhancement of the skin barrier from birth offers effective atopic dermatitis prevention. J Allergy Clin Immunol. 2014;134(4):818–23.
79. Kelleher MM, Dunn-Galvin A, Gray C, Murray DM, Kiely M, Kenny L, et al. Skin barrier impairment at birth predicts food allergy at 2 years of age. J Allergy Clin Immunol. 2016;137(4):1111–6.e8.
80. Kezic S, O'Regan GM, Yau N, Sandilands A, Chen H, Campbell LE, et al. Levels of filaggrin degradation products are influenced by both filaggrin genotype and atopic dermatitis severity. Allergy. 2011;66(7):934–40.
81. Weidinger S, O'Sullivan M, Illig T, Baurecht H, Depner M, Rodriguez E, et al. Filaggrin mutations, atopic eczema, hay fever, and asthma in children. J Allergy Clin Immunol. 2008;121(5):1203–9.e1.
82. McAleer MA, Irvine AD. The multifunctional role of filaggrin in allergic skin disease. J Allergy Clin Immunol. 2013;131(2):280–91.
83. Bager P, Wohlfahrt J, Boyd H, Thyssen JP, Melbye M. The role of filaggrin mutations during pregnancy and postpartum: atopic dermatitis and genital skin diseases. Allergy. 2016;71(5):724–7.
84. Kim J, Kim BE, Lee J, Han Y, Jun HY, Kim H, et al. Epidermal thymic stromal lymphopoietin predicts the development of atopic dermatitis during infancy. J Allergy Clin Immunol. 2016;137(4):1282–5.e4.
85. Namkung JH, Lee JE, Kim E, Byun JY, Kim S, Shin ES, et al. Hint for association of single nucleotide polymorphisms and haplotype in SPINK5 gene with atopic dermatitis in Koreans. Exp Dermatol. 2010;19(12):1048–53.
86. Wen HJ, Wang YJ, Lin YC, Chang CC, Shieh CC, Lung FW, et al. Prediction of atopic dermatitis in 2-yr-old children by cord blood IgE, genetic polymorphisms in cytokine genes, and maternal mentality during pregnancy. Pediatr Allergy Immunol. 2011;22(7):695–703.
87. Quaranta M, Knapp B, Garzorz N, Mattii M, Pullabhatla V, Pennino D, et al. Intraindividual genome expression analysis reveals a specific molecular signature of psoriasis and eczema. Sci Transl Med. 2014;6(244):244ra90.
88. Hawro T, Lehmann S, Altrichter S, Fluhr JW, Zuberbier T, Church MK, et al. Skin provocation tests may help to diagnose atopic dermatitis. Allergy. 2016;71(12):1745–52.
89. Kou K, Aihara M, Matsunaga T, Chen H, Taguri M, Morita S, et al. Association of serum interleukin-18 and other biomarkers with disease severity in adults with atopic dermatitis. Arch Dermatol Res. 2012;304(4):305–12.
90. Folster-Holst R, Papakonstantinou E, Rudrich U, Buchner M, Pite H, Gehring M, et al. Childhood atopic dermatitis-Brain-derived neurotrophic factor correlates with serum eosinophil cationic protein and disease severity. Allergy. 2016;71(7):1062–5.
91. Leung TF, Ching KW, Kong AP, Wong GW, Chan JC, Hon KL. Circulating LL-37 is a biomarker for eczema severity in children. J Eur Acad Dermatol Venereol. 2012;26(4):518–22.

92. Hon KL, Ching GK, Ng PC, Leung TF. Exploring CCL18, eczema severity and atopy. Pediatr Allergy Immunol. 2011;22(7):704–7.
93. Mansouri Y, Guttman-Yassky E. Immune pathways in atopic dermatitis, and definition of biomarkers through broad and targeted therapeutics. J Clin Med. 2015;4(5):858–73.
94. Rabenhorst A, Hartmann K. Interleukin-31: a novel diagnostic marker of allergic diseases. Curr Allergy Asthma Rep. 2014;14(4):423.
95. Thijs JL, van Seggelen W, Bruijnzeel-Koomen C, de Bruin-Weller M, Hijnen D. New developments in biomarkers for atopic dermatitis. J Clin Med. 2015;4(3):479–87.
96. Kou K, Okawa T, Yamaguchi Y, Ono J, Inoue Y, Kohno M, et al. Periostin levels correlate with disease severity and chronicity in patients with atopic dermatitis. Br J Dermatol. 2014;171(2):283–91.
97. Nygaard U, Hvid M, Johansen C, Buchner M, Folster-Holst R, Deleuran M, et al. TSLP, IL-31, IL-33 and sST2 are new biomarkers in endophenotypic profiling of adult and childhood atopic dermatitis. J Eur Acad Dermatol Venereol. 2016;30(11):1930–8.
98. Glatz M, Buchner M, von Bartenwerffer W, Schmid-Grendelmeier P, Worm M, Hedderich J, et al. Malassezia spp.-specific immunoglobulin E level is a marker for severity of atopic dermatitis in adults. Acta Derm Venereol. 2015;95(2):191–6.
99. Mothes N, Niggemann B, Jenneck C, Hagemann T, Weidinger S, Bieber T, et al. The cradle of IgE autoreactivity in atopic eczema lies in early infancy. J Allergy Clin Immunol. 2005;116(3):706–9.
100. Tang TS, Bieber T, Williams HC. Does "autoreactivity" play a role in atopic dermatitis? J Allergy Clin Immunol. 2012;129(5):1209–15.e2.
101. Altrichter S, Kriehuber E, Moser J, Valenta R, Kopp T, Stingl G. Serum IgE autoantibodies target keratinocytes in patients with atopic dermatitis. J Investig Dermatol. 2008;128(9):2232–9.
102. Howell MD, Parker ML, Mustelin T, Ranade K. Past, present, and future for biologic intervention in atopic dermatitis. Allergy. 2015;70(8):887–96.
103. Simpson EL, Bieber T, Guttman-Yassky E, Beck LA, Blauvelt A, Cork MJ, et al. Two phase 3 trials of dupilumab versus placebo in atopic dermatitis. N Engl J Med. 2016;375(24):2335–48.
104. Czarnowicki T, Esaki H, Gonzalez J, Malajian D, Shemer A, Noda S, et al. Early pediatric atopic dermatitis shows only a cutaneous lymphocyte antigen (CLA)(+) TH2/TH1 cell imbalance, whereas adults acquire CLA(+) TH22/TC22 cell subsets. J Allergy Clin Immunol. 2015;136(4):941–51.e3.
105. Esaki H, Brunner PM, Renert-Yuval Y, Czarnowicki T, Huynh T, Tran G, et al. Early-onset pediatric atopic dermatitis is TH2 but also TH17 polarized in skin. J Allergy Clin Immunol. 2016;138(6):1639–51.
106. Staudacher A, Hinz T, Novak N, von Bubnoff D, Bieber T. Exaggerated IDO1 expression and activity in Langerhans cells from patients with atopic dermatitis upon viral stimulation: a potential predictive biomarker for high risk of Eczema herpeticum. Allergy. 2015;70(11):1432–9.
107. Oyoshi MK, Venturelli N, Geha RS. Thymic stromal lymphopoietin and IL-33 promote skin inflammation and vaccinia virus replication in a mouse model of atopic dermatitis. J Allergy Clin Immunol. 2016;138(1):283–6.
108. Schmitt J, Schwarz K, Baurecht H, Hotze M, Folster-Holst R, Rodriguez E, et al. Atopic dermatitis is associated with an increased risk for rheumatoid arthritis and inflammatory bowel disease, and a decreased risk for type 1 diabetes. J Allergy Clin Immunol. 2016;137(1):130–6.
109. Nebert DW. Pharmacogenetics and pharmacogenomics: why is this relevant to the clinical geneticist? Clin Genet. 1999;56(4):247–58.
110. de Jonge H, Naesens M, Kuypers DR. New insights into the pharmacokinetics and pharmacodynamics of the calcineurin inhibitors and mycophenolic acid: possible consequences for therapeutic drug monitoring in solid organ transplantation. Ther Drug Monit. 2009;31(4):416–35.
111. van Schaik RH, van Agteren M, de Fijter JW, Hartmann A, Schmidt J, Budde K, et al. UGT1A9 -275T>A/-2152C>T polymorphisms correlate with low MPA exposure and acute rejection in MMF/tacrolimus-treated kidney transplant patients. Clin Pharmacol Ther. 2009;86(3):319–27.
112. Kuypers DR, Naesens M, Vermeire S, Vanrenterghem Y. The impact of uridine diphosphate-glucuronosyltransferase 1A9 (UGT1A9) gene promoter region single-nucleotide polymorphisms T-275A and C-2152T on early mycophenolic acid dose-interval exposure in de novo renal allograft recipients. Clin Pharmacol Ther. 2005;78(4):351–61.
113. Bloomfeld RS, Bickston SJ, Levine ME, Carroll S. Thiopurine methyltransferase activity is correlated with azathioprine metabolite levels in patients with inflammatory bowel disease in clinical gastroenterology practice. J Appl Res. 2006;6(4):282–8.
114. Thijs J, Krastev T, Weidinger S, Buckens CF, de Bruin-Weller M, Bruijnzeel-Koomen C, et al. Biomarkers for atopic dermatitis: a systematic review and meta-analysis. Curr Opin Allergy Clin Immunol. 2015;15(5):453–60.
115. Kägi M, Joller-Jemelka H, Wüthrich B. Correlation of eosinophils, eosinophil cationic protein and soluble lnterleukin-2 receptor with the clinical activity of atopic dermatitis. Dermatology. 1992;185(2):88–92.
116. Czech W, Krutmann J, Schöpf E, Kapp A. Serum eosinophil cationic protein (ECP) is a sensitive measure for disease activity in atopic dermatitis. Br J Dermatol. 1992;126(4):351–5.
117. Kakinuma T, Sugaya M, Nakamura K, Kaneko F, Wakugawa M, Matsushima K, et al. Thymus and activation-regulated chemokine (TARC/CCL17) in mycosis fungoides: serum TARC levels reflect the disease activity of mycosis fungoides. J Am Acad Dermatol. 2003;48(1):23–30.

118. Morishima Y, Kawashima H, Takekuma K, Hoshika A. Changes in serum lactate dehydrogenase activity in children with atopic dermatitis. Pediatr Int. 2010;52(2):171–4.
119. Morita H, Kitano Y, Kawasaki N. Elevation of serum-soluble E-selectin in atopic dermatitis. J Dermatol Sci. 1995;10(2):145–50.
120. Kakinuma T, Saeki H, Tsunemi Y, Fujita H, Asano N, Mitsui H, et al. Increased serum cutaneous T cell-attracting chemokine (CCL27) levels in patients with atopic dermatitis and psoriasis vulgaris. J Allergy Clin Immunol. 2003;111(3):592–7.
121. Leung TF, Ma KC, Hon KL, Lam CW, Wan H, Li CY, et al. Serum concentration of macrophage-derived chemokine may be a useful inflammatory marker for assessing severity of atopic dermatitis in infants and young children. Pediatr Allergy Immunol. 2003;14(4):296–301.
122. Yoshizawa Y, Nomaguchi H, Izaki S, Kitamura K. Serum cytokine levels in atopic dermatitis. Clin Exp Dermatol. 2002;27(3):225–9.
123. Thijs JL, Nierkens S, Herath A, Bruijnzeel-Koomen C, Knol EF, Giovannone B, et al. A panel of biomarkers for disease severity in atopic dermatitis. Clin Exp Allergy. 2015;45(3):698–701.
124. Khattri S, Shemer A, Rozenblit M, Dhingra N, Czarnowicki T, Finney R, et al. Cyclosporine in patients with atopic dermatitis modulates activated inflammatory pathways and reverses epidermal pathology. J Allergy Clin Immunol. 2014;133(6):1626–34.
125. Hamilton JD, Suárez-Fariñas M, Dhingra N, Cardinale I, Li X, Kostic A, et al. Dupilumab improves the molecular signature in skin of patients with moderate-to-severe atopic dermatitis. J Allergy Clin Immunol. 2014;134(6):1293–300.
126. Tintle S, Shemer A, Suárez-Fariñas M, Fujita H, Gilleaudeau P, Sullivan-Whalen M, et al. Reversal of atopic dermatitis with narrow-band UVB phototherapy and biomarkers for therapeutic response. J Allergy Clin Immunol. 2011;128(3):583–93.e4.
127. Raap U, Wichmann K, Bruder M, Ständer S, Wedi B, Kapp A, et al. Correlation of IL-31 serum levels with severity of atopic dermatitis. J Allergy Clin Immunol. 2008;122(2):421–3.
128. Ebata T, Iwasaki S, Kamide R, Niimura M. Use of a wrist activity monitor for the measurement of nocturnal scratching in patients with atopic dermatitis. Br J Dermatol. 2001;144(2):305–9.

Part VI

Management

Topical Treatment

Seung-Phil Hong

Topical Corticosteroids

Introduction

Since hydrocortisone was first developed in the early 1950s, topical corticosteroid (TCS) was produced in various potencies and formulations and is the most widely used basic topical treatment modality to date. Side effects became more prominent with increased usage in the 1960s and 1970s due to its outstanding effects. Some patients have steroid phobia due to the concerns expressed through media reports about the hazards [1, 2]. However, TCS is a double-edged sword that is very cost-effective and has the potential for various physiological side effects. It is associated with paradoxical safety as it can be used for pregnant women and infants, who are not permitted to use new topical drugs, due to clinical experience of over 60 years. Therefore, doctors should pay particular attention to steroids in order to prevent abuse and ensure that patients adhere to proper usage.

S.-P. Hong (✉)
Department of Dermatology, Yonsei University Wonju College of Medicine, Wonju, Korea (Republic of)
e-mail: hongsp@yonsei.ac.kr

Action Mechanism

Among the various effects of corticosteroids, four pharmacological effects are largely suggested as topical preparations, and they are not separated from each other, but are organically connected to show overall and diverse effects [3–5].

Anti-inflammation

It can suppress the production of phospholipase A2, which is involved in the production of prostaglandins and leukotrienes, and the transcription factors associated with inflammatory reactions such as NF-κB and AP-1. It can also suppress secretion of inflammatory cytokine (IL-1) of keratinocytes.

Immunosuppression

It inhibits the activity and proliferation of almost all inflammatory cells. It reduces T cell proliferation and induces apoptosis through inhibition of IL-2 secreted from lymphocytes. It inhibits the chemoattraction of neutrophils and interferes with the functions of endothelial cells, granulocytes, mast cells, and fibroblasts. A reduction in Langerhans cells has also been observed.

Vasoconstriction

This remains to be further elucidated, however, it suppresses the secretion of vasodilators (e.g., histamine, prostaglandins), which reduce erythema and

K. H. Lee et al. (eds.), *Practical Insights into Atopic Dermatitis*,
https://doi.org/10.1007/978-981-15-8159-5_14

are associated with an anti-inflammatory action. In particular, when topical steroids are applied to normal skin, steroid potency is determined on 4–7 stages depending on the extent and duration of skin paleness caused by vasoconstriction [6].

Anti-proliferation

TCS inhibits DNA synthesis and mitosis in several cells. In particular, Keratinocyte proliferation is decreased, fibroblasts activity and collagen synthesis are suppressed. The proliferation of various immune cells is also inhibited in response to anti-inflammatory and immunosuppressive effects.

Classification and Formulation

The choice of formulation of corticosteroids is important as its potency can vary depending on the formulation even same ingredients and concentrations are used. Ointments become more potent than creams or lotions. Patients are generally not aware that the potency differs according to compositional and formulation-specific, and can be mistaken for determining the strength by concentration only, so providing them the potency information at the clinic is crucial to avoid overdosing [7].

Efficacy of TCS in Atopic Dermatitis

TCS has proven its efficacy through decades of clinical data and experience, but the following should be considered when treating with TCS [8]: risk of side effects due to long-term use, many pediatric patients, common in sensitive areas such as faces and flexural areas, and the presence of alternative anti-inflammatory topical drugs such as topical calcineurin inhibitor. TCS improves acute active and chronic lichenificated lesions of atopic dermatitis and effectively reduces the accompanying itching [9]. It is also effective in preventing recurrence.

How to Choose TCS According to the Potency and Place of Treatment on the Body?

The Considerations of Drug Choice

Before prescribing TCS treatment, factors that influence its effectiveness and the risk of adverse effects must be considered. The results of comparative studies between TCSs are very limited and no standard agents of TCS have been established. Therefore, it should be decided in consideration of various clinical factors such as the patient's age, severity, area, and the skin condition of the lesion, the personal experience of the doctor, and the skin barrier condition.

Choice According to Drug Potency and Application Site

The number of grades varies according to country and generally divides the efficacy of TCS into 4–7 classes (Table 1). In general, in the case of acute flare lesions, it is recommended to select a high-potency TCS for a short period of use, and if the lesion is controlled to some extent, it is recommended to reduce the intensity or dose. Chronic areas with lichenification require the application of more potent TCSs for a longer period [12]. However, super-potent TCSs are not recommended for atopic dermatitis treatment, especially not in children [13]. Additionally, it is recommended to use low potency in areas where skin such as face/perineum/groin is more prone to side effects. Differences in effects may occur depending on body parts due to the thickness of the stratum corneum and epidermis, the degree of sealing or wetness of the skin, the distribution of pores, and the difference in blood supply. However, since the skin barrier in atopic dermatitis patients is often severely damaged, it should be considered that even an anatomical region with low absorption maybe 2–10 times more than normal skin.

Table 1 Grading based on the potency of topical corticosteroids [10, 11]

Potency	Generic name
Class 1 (superpotent)	Betamethasone dipropionate 0.05% Clobetasol propionate 0.05% Halobetasol propionate 0.05% Diflorasone diacetate 0.05%
Class 2 (potent)	Betamethasone dipropionate 0.05% Mometasone furoate 0.1% Halcinonide 0.1% Fluocinonide 0.05% Diflorasone diacetate 0.05% Desoximetasone 0.25% Desoximetasone 0.05%
Class 3 (potent, upper mid-strength)	Amcinonide 0.1% Betamethasone dipropionate 0.05% Betamethasone valerate 0.1% Fluticasone propionate 0.005% Diflorasone diacetate 0.05%
Class 4 (mid-strength)	Mometasone furoate 0.1% Methylprednisolone aceponate 0.1% Triamcinolone acetonide 0.1% Betamethasone valerate 0.12% Fluocinolone acetonide 0.025% Hydrocortisone valerate 0.2% Prednicarbate 0.25%
Class 5 (lower mid-strength)	Fluticasone propionate 0.05% Betamethasone dipropionate 0.05% Triamcinolone acetonide 0.1% Hydrocortisone butyrate 0.1% Hydrocortisone valerate 0.2% Fluocinolone acetonide 0.025% Betamethasone valerate 0.05% Prednicarbate 0.25%
Class 6 (mild strength)	Alclometasone dipropionate 0.05% Desonide 0.05% Triamcinolone acetonide 0.025%
Class 7 (least potent)	Hydrocortisone 2.5%, 1% Dexamethasone 0.1% Flumethasone pivalate 0.02% Flucortin butylester 0.75% Prednisolone acetate Prednisolone valeroacetate Hydrocortisone butyrate propionate

How to Apply TCS for Atopic Dermatitis?

During the acute exacerbation period, two strategies can be used: a method of intensively using high-potency TCS briefly and gradually tapering it, or a method of gradually increasing treatment intensity depending on the patients' tolerance and treatment response while using lower potency TCS for a long time [9, 14]. A low potency drug is applied to the face and neck as much as possible, but in case of severe exacerbation, an intermediate potency may be applied for short periods (3–5) days [12]. Topical treatment should always be applied on hydrated skin, especially when using ointments [13]. Hence, TCSs can be used together with moisturizers, but their application on inflamed areas of the skin is recommended approximately 15 min prior to using moisturizer if the TCS is an ointment; if it is a cream, it can be applied after the emollient [12, 15]. To prevent withdrawal rebound, dose tapering may be necessary. Either switching to a less potent corticosteroid, or keeping a more potent one while reducing the frequency of application (intermittent regimen) [13]. Also, to stabilize the disease and prevent flares, early anti-inflammation treatment (TCS) with continuous emollient skin care is crucial [13].

Despite the efficacy and precautions of using TCS, if the efficacy of TCS does not reach the expected level in patients with atopic dermatitis, it is necessary to first check whether the drug has insufficient strength or the patient's compliance is low. Sometimes the occurrence of bacterial super-infection or allergic reaction to TCS should be considered. On skin with co-existent infections, TCSs have been widely used along with systemic or topical antibiotics [10]. However, no additional benefit was observed compared to TCS alone [16].

Amount, Frequency, and Duration of Application

Amount Unit of Application

The fingertip unit (FTU) is commonly suggested, as it has been found that the amount of TCS from the distal skin crease to the tip of an adult patient's index finger is equivalent to approximately 0.5 g TCS. Using 1 FTU of TCS, applying the amount on the surface area two palms (2% of body surface area) of the patient is appropriate (Fig. 1) [17]. To avoid systemic and local side effects, potent TCSs can be used in the following amounts: 15 g/month in infants, 30 g/month in children, and 60–90 g/month in adults. Children have a greater risk of developing systemic side-effects, since they have a relatively greater body surface area-to-weight ratio and a higher systemic absorption [10]. Therefore, for infants and children, the elderly, or pregnant women, the use of mild-to-moderate TCSs can be recommended rather than more potent varieties of TCSs [10].

Frequency and Duration of Application

It is commonly applied twice a day. Some high-intensity or newly developed medications may be applied once a day [12, 13]. During periods of flare-up, TCSs are applied for 3–5 days until AD is controlled and for up to 2 weeks in moderate and severe atopic dermatitis. Generally, for most topical TCSs, regardless of potency, application once or twice per day for 2–4 weeks is recommended [8, 12, 18].

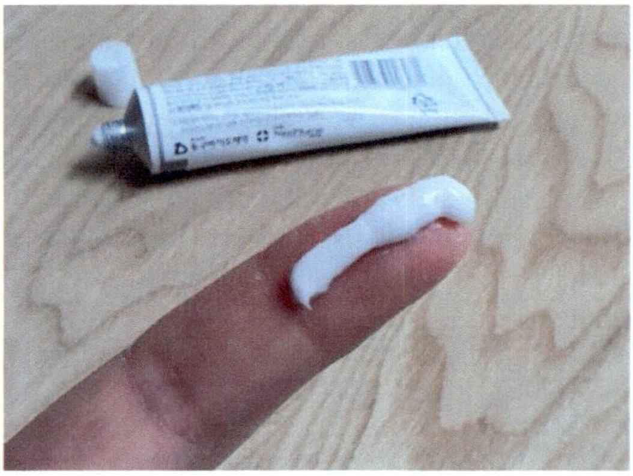

Fig. 1 One Finger-Tip Unit: 1 FTU

After acute lesions have stabilized, the moisturizer is used alone for maintenance and TCS is re-applied only for recurrences. However, in recent years, as evidence for proactive treatment has accumulated, intermittent use of TCS twice a week on frequently recurring sites has become widespread in the clinical practice, even in cases where inflammatory lesions have improved [19].

Special Application Method of TCS

Simple Occlusive Dressing

If occlusive dressing with plastic vinyl or bandage after applying TCS is used in less sensitive skin areas and for brief periods of time, the effect can be increased by several tens of times or more, and increase its efficacy and speed up lesion resolution [13]. However, long-term use is not recommended due to increasing the risk of side effects.

Wet Wrap Therapy

It is similar to the previous occlusion therapy, but it is a method of diluting the drug and obtaining hydrating effects by adding a moisturizer or applying wet dressing, but it is not a standardized treatment method [13, 20]. It can be applied when there is a poorly treated area. Especially, patients with acute, oozing, and erosive lesions and children sometimes do not tolerate standard topical application and so may first be treated with "wet wraps" until the oozing stops [13]. In the case of acute exacerbation, it can be performed once a day for 2–14 days (average 3–7 days) to induce rapid stabilization. This therapy can be modified variably according to the patient's situation [21, 22]. However, when implemented at home, training and patient compliance are important, and when performed at the hospital, professionally trained nursing staff should performing the methods.

Proactive Treatment

Proactive therapy is defined as a combination of predefined, long-term, anti-inflammatory treatment applied usually twice a week to previously affected areas of skin in combination with liberal use of emollients on the entire body and a predefined appointment schedule for clinical examinations [13]. In other words, as a treatment strategy to avoid redness by applying an external treatment twice a week to the skin area where recurrence is frequent, anti-relapse can be expected along with daily moisturizer applications [12, 23].

Even though the duration of the proactive management is usually adapted to the severity and persistence of the disease, topical steroids (fluticasone or methylprednisolone aceponate) on the proactive approach are usually applied only for a very limited period of time and for a maximum of up to 16 weeks [24].

Use of TCS in Children

TCI has no long-term safety in infants under the age of 2 years, so only TCS can be used in infant patients, which is not controlled by a moisturizer. This is the paradoxical safety of TCSs, as mentioned earlier. For children, weak efficacy TCS is effective even for a short period of time, and for such short-term use there is no need to worry about side effects [25]. However, it should be noted that, because children have a large body surface area and relatively low ability to metabolize steroids relative to body weight, systemic effects may be exhibited by topical application alone. In particular, it should be noted that when applied to a diaper area, an occlusive effect may be exhibited.

In the case of atopic dermatitis in children, although it is the child suffering from the disease and it is the caregiver who decides and performs treatment, it is difficult to implement a treatment level according to the patient's symptom level. Therefore, it is often necessary to confirm drug compliance, as it is not used as prescribed by the caregiver's steroid rejection.

Use of TCS in Pregnant Women and the Elderly

A significant association of fetal growth restriction with maternal exposure to potent/very potent topical corticosteroids was observed, but not with mild/moderate topical corticosteroids [26]. Therefore, mild/moderate TCSs are recommended during pregnancy, because of the associated risk of fetal growth restriction with the potent/very potent TCSs. However, recent studies have reported that there is no connection between TCS use and abnormal pregnancy outcomes such as birth defects, premature birth, and stillbirth. Most TCSs have been classified as FDA pregnancy category C, so caution is required. However, short-term or intermittent use of low-to-medium potency of TCS is unlikely to be a problem in pregnant women because there is more safety evidence for TCS than TCI in pregnant women.

Adverse Reactions

The predisposing factors for cutaneous and systemic adverse effects are long-term therapy, use of high-potency, application to highly permeable and/or large areas, occlusion, poor skin integrity, systemic diseases, and younger or older age [12].

Local Adverse Reactions

Local side effects are more common than systemic reactions. The major adverse reactions are telangiectasia, purpura or bruising, stretch marks, skin ulcers, rebound flares due to atrophy and weakening of the epidermal and dermal tissues, and TCS may cause iatrogenic skin diseases such as acne-like eruption, hypertrichosis, and color change. On the face, especially, rosacea-like disease with persistent erythema, so-called "red face syndrome" or "corticosteroid addiction syndrome," often develops in the setting of long-term inappropriate use of potent TCS [13].

It can also be more vulnerable to various secondary infections and uncommonly causes allergic contact dermatitis to the drug itself. In particular, this contact sensitization may be obscured by the original skin lesions, so contact sensitization should be considered whenever there is worsening or failure of skin lesions to respond to application of TCSs. Since TCIs can cross-react with each other, recognizing a group of TCIs that possibly cross-react can help in the selection of alternative drugs when an allergic reaction to is suspected. Allergic contact dermatitis caused by tixocortol pivalate has been reported the most, and TCSs can be divided into several groups depending on whether cross-reactivity is possible [27, 28]. Based on the structural properties of corticosteroids and related research reports, the groups capable of inducing cross-reaction are divided into the following groups with representative drugs (Table 2): (1) Group A (hydrocortisone type), (2) Group B (triamcinolone acetonide type), (3) Group C (betamethasone type), (4) Group D1 (betamethasone type, and (5) Group D2 (methylprednisolone aceponate type).

There are also concerns that it increases the risk of cataracts and glaucoma when applied around the eye area, but the application even over longer periods of time was reported not to be associated with the development of glaucoma or cataracts [29].

Systemic Adverse Reactions

Topically applied corticosteroids can be absorbed back into the body through the skin. When used in small amounts in a small area, it does not cause problems related to systemic reabsorption, but can be increased if high potent drug or occlusive therapy is applied. As a result, iatrogenic Cushing's syndrome, hypothalamic–pituitary–adrenal axis suppression, bone density reduction, bone necrosis, cataracts, glaucoma, hypertension, and growth inhibition in children may be induced [13, 30, 31].

Table 2 Classification according to the cross-reactivity of TCS (modified from [27])

Class	Cross-reaction with other class	Representative drugs
Class A (Hydrocortisone type)	Class D2	Hydrocortisone Hydrocortisone acetate Methylprednisolone Prednisolone *Tixocortol pivalate (Patch test drug)*
Class B (Triamcinolone acetonide type)	Budesonide: Class D2	Amcinonide *Budesonide (Patch test drug)* Desonide Fluocinonide Halcinonide *Triamcinolone acetonide (Patch test drug)* Triamcinolone diacetate
Class C (Betamethasone type)		Clocortonlone pivalate Desoxymethasone
Class D1 (Betamethasone dipropionate type)		Alcometasone dipropionate Betamethasone Dipropionate Betamethasone valerate Clobetasone butyrate *Clobetasone propionate (Patch test drug)* Diflorasone diacetate Fluticasone propionate Mometasone furoate
Class D2 (Methylprednisolone aceponate type)	Class A	Clobetasone butyrate *Hydrocortisone-17-butyrate (Patch test drug)* Hydrocortisone valerate Methylprednisolone Aceponate prednicarbate

Concerns Surrounding TCS Adverse Effects

Due to concerns about adverse effects of TCS, non-compliance was found in about one quarter (24%) of outpatients [1]. The main concerns were skin thinning and systemic absorption delaying growth and development in children. As a result, education of patients or caregivers to address such fears is crucial to ensure patients compliance in the treatment of AD [8, 9]. Correct application, sufficient dose, the use or absence of an occlusive dressing, the prior condition of the skin, and the anatomical area of application determine the absorption of TCSs should be considered to minimize TCS-related adverse effects [8].

Topical Calcineurin Inhibitors

Introduction

Corticosteroids have been the most commonly used drugs to normalize immunological abnormalities and alleviate inflammatory symptoms over the past 60 years, but they have a major drawback. They can cause various systemic or local side effects when abused over a prolonged period of time. Therefore, TCS is inadequate for long-term use and for the prevention of worsening symptoms in patients with frequent relapses and long-lasting lesions. Hence, Topical Calcineurin Inhibitor (TCI) was developed as a new immunomodulator that supplemented the shortcomings of TCSs in the late 1990s and became one of the main topical drugs for the treatment of atopic dermatitis. As numerous clinical results have accumulated, it is considered to be the only substitute for TCS, and it is reported to have an effect on almost all inflammatory skin diseases treated with TCS such as psoriasis, vitiligo, seborrheic dermatitis, and lichen planus, in addition to atopic dermatitis.

Types and Origins of TCI

Cyclosporine, a calcineurin inhibitor that is frequently used as a systemic immunomodulator, has a large molecular weight and does not permeate the skin, and has poor skin affinity, so it was not effective as topical preparation. Later, tacrolimus and pimecrolimus, new drugs that resolved these issues, were developed. Tacrolimus was isolated from the fungus-like bacterium *Streptomyces tsukubaensis*. Pimecrolimus is a semi-synthetic derivative of ascomycin, an antifungal compound extracted from *Streptomyces hygroscopicus var. ascomyceticus*.

Mechanism of Action [32, 33]

The mechanism of action of tacrolimus and pimecrolimus is the same, and they bind to the cytosolic receptor immunophilin (FK binding protein-12 or macrophilin-12) and become complex in immune cells, such as T cell. The complex inhibits calcineurin, which allows the translocation of NF-AT into the nucleus through dephosphorylation of NF-AT (nuclear factor of activated T cells transcription factor) [33]. As a result, the transcription factor NF-AT is inactivated and the production of inflammatory cytokines such as IL-2, IL-4, IL-8, TNF-, IFN-γ, and GM-CSF in T cells is suppressed, resulting in immunosuppression (Fig. 2). In addition to T cells, they also act on immune-related cells such as keratinocytes, Langerhans cells, Mast cells, and eosinophils, resulting in overall inflammatory and immunomodulatory effects.

Application in Atopic Dermatitis

Both tacrolimus and pimecrolimus are indicated as second-line treatments for AD that is not controlled with TCSs, when there is a significant risk of adverse effects due to their application, or when they are contraindicated [12]. The overall effect is better for tacrolimus than for pimecrolimus, hence, tacrolimus ointment is used in moderate or severe patients over 2 years of age, and pimecrolimus cream is used in mild or moderate patients. Instead of treating acute flares with TCI, initial treatment with topical corticosteroids before switching to TCI should be considered. Usually, it is used continuously until the lesion

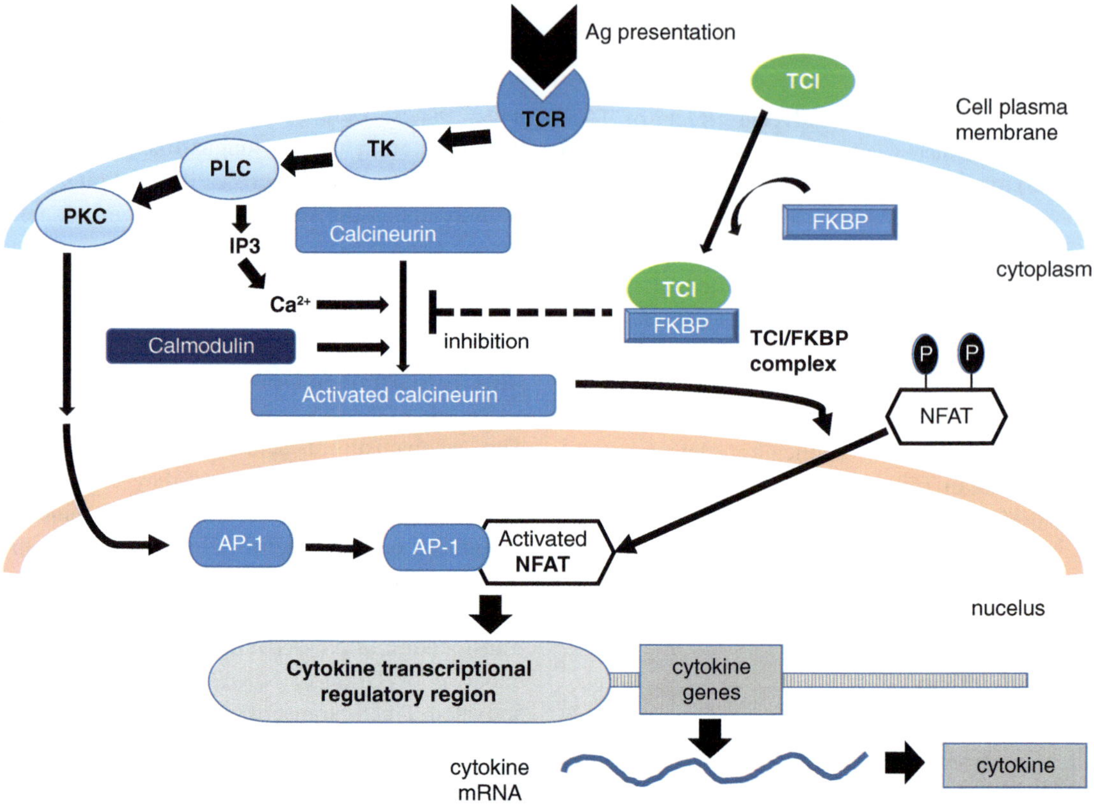

Fig. 2 Mechanism of action for tacrolimus (modified from [33]). It has an immunosuppressive effect by blocking cytokine production such as IL-2 at the transcription level by suppressing calcineurin, which dephosphorylates the nuclear factor of activated T cells (NF-aT) by combining with cytosolic receptor immunophilin (FK binding protein-12). The mechanism of action for tacrolimus and pimecrolimus is the same. *Ag* antigen, *TCR* T cell receptor, *FKBP* FK506-binding protein, *NFAT* nuclear factor of activated T cells, *PKC* protein kinase C, *PLC* phospholipase C, *TCI* topical calcineurin inhibitor, *TK* tyrosine kinase

disappears, and then it is used as a sustained maintenance therapy or as a proactive treatment that expects to suppress recurrence by applying 2–3 times a week, like TCS. TCIs are specifically indicated in sensitive skin areas (face, skinfolds, anogenital region) [12, 15]. There is no medical evidence yet that TCIs cause malignancies in humans, and it is known to be safe, even for usage in children [34].

Tacrolimus

Tacrolimus is available at the following concentrations with ointment formulation: 0.1% for adults and 0.03% for children. To compare the success rates of the TCIs tacrolimus and pimecrolimus in treating atopic dermatitis, a meta-analysis through early clinical trials was reported [35]. Tacrolimus reduced EASI scores by 65.6% after 1 month and 73.0% after 3 months; pimecrolimus reduced the scores by 61.5% after 1 month, 60.3% after 6 months, and 61.9% after 12 months. When the differences in EASI score reductions were compared between the active drug and the placebo. The success rate for tacrolimus was 51.5% higher than that of placebo after 1 month and for pimecrolimus it was 45.9% higher after 1 month, 24.9% after 6 months, and 16.1% after 12 months. In a further study conducted in children, significantly more patients achieved a clinical improvement of 90% or higher with 0.03% or 0.1% tacrolimus ointment compared to the group receiving the vehicle [36].

Treating sensitive body areas such as the face with TCIs while treating other affected body areas with a TCS may be a useful and cost-effective strategy rather than the simultaneous combination of TCSs with TCIs at the same site [13]. However, combined therapy with TCSs (0.25% desoximetasone) and 0.1% tacrolimus have been reported to be more effective and present similar levels of adverse effects compared to the single treatment group [12, 37]. Additionally, the pruritus and burning sensations associated with the application of tacrolimus were lower in the combined therapy group. In patients with severe atopic dermatitis, TCS is initially used to reduce inflammation quickly, followed by TCS being tapered gradually. Following which, there is a strategy to turn it into a tacrolimus ointment and apply it steadily. In children, 0.03% is mainly used, but when 0.1% is used, the effect may be better without a significant increase in the risk.

As a result of long-term use, it was reported to be effective and safe even when used in children (over 2 years of age) and adults at 0.1% concentration twice a day for up to 4 years [38]. The results were consistent with that of another long-term use study [39]. In summary, tacrolimus ointment can be used for long-term use in patients with moderate-to-severe atopic dermatitis.

The favorable effects of wet wrap dressing using TCI can be expected, however, there is a lack of studies demonstrating this [40].

Pimecrolimus

Pimecrolimus is available with a 1% cream vehicle. It should be applied for mild-to-moderate atopic dermatitis in children over 2 years of age and adults [41]. In a clinical study conducted at the time of drug development, within 3 weeks of topical therapy with 1% pimecrolimus cream twice daily, a mean reduction of 71.9% in the Atopic Dermatitis Severity Index (ADSI) score was observed at the actively treated test sites compared with a mean reduction of 10.3% at the placebo-treated test sites [42]. Furthermore, it can reduce itching and erythema 48 h after starting treatment, reduce the number of flares compared to a conventional therapy and consequently reduce or eliminate the need for corticosteroid treatment [43, 44].

In 2005, the results of the Petite Study, a study comparing efficacy and safety for 5 years by dividing it into two treatment groups (1% pimecrolimus vs. low-to-medium potency TCSs) in approximately 2400 infants, reported that long-term management with pimecrolimus or topical corticosteroids was safe without any effects on the developing immune system, and showed that both treatments had a rapid onset of action with >50% of patients achieving treatment success by week 3 and pimecrolimus had similar efficacy to topical corticosteroids [45].

Recently, a new treatment algorithm has been proposed, which recommended pimecrolimus as a first-line therapy when developing first signs and symptoms of the disease in patients with mild-to-moderate atopic dermatitis [41]. Pimecrolimus is also recommended for mild-to-moderate AD after initial treatment with a TCS. After resolution of lesions, maintenance treatment with pimecrolimus may effectively prevent subsequent disease flares.

Efficacy Comparison Among TCIs and TCSs

The efficacy of 0.1% tacrolimus ointment was similar to that of 0.1% hydrocortisone butyrate ointment [46] after 3-week treatment, and superior to fluticasone 0.005% ointment [47] in the treatment of adult patients with moderate-to-severe atopic dermatitis. Tacrolimus was found to be as effective as class III–V topical corticosteroids for atopic dermatitis of the trunk and extremities, and more effective than low-potency class VI or VII corticosteroids for AD of the face or neck [48]. Long-term treatment (≥3 months) is significantly more efficacious than a corticosteroid regimen [49]. In the case of children with moderate-to-severe atopic dermatitis, tacrolimus, 0.03% and 0.1%, was significantly more effective than 1% hydrocortisone acetate, and 0.1% tacrolimus was more effective than 0.03% tacrolimus [50]. However, in actual clinical experience, since the effect of tacrolimus appears later than TCSs and there is an initial burning/irritation pattern, it is used as a maintenance therapy after stabilizing to some degree with TCS treatment. Moreover, the cost-effectiveness of first-line treatment with TCIs has not been conclusively demonstrated [13].

Pimecrolimus was less effective than both, tacrolimus and low-potency topical corticosteroids for moderate-to-severe AD [48]. In the clinical studies comparing the efficacy and safety of tacrolimus ointment and pimecrolimus creams in adults and pediatric patients, with mild to very severe atopic dermatitis, it was demonstrated that tacrolimus ointment is more effective and has a faster onset of action than pimecrolimus cream in both adults and children with atopic dermatitis. Furthermore, their safety profiles were similar [51, 52]. In 2015, a systematic review showed that tacrolimus 0.1% was better than low-potency corticosteroids, pimecrolimus 1%, and tacrolimus 0.03% [53]. Specifically, people treated with tacrolimus 0.1% were almost twice as likely to improve compared to patients treated with pimecrolimus 1%. Tacrolimus 0.03% was superior-to-mild corticosteroids and pimecrolimus. However, when comparing both dose tacrolimus 0.1 and 0.3% to moderate-to-potent corticosteroids, results were equivocal [53]. In terms of safety, two calcineurin inhibitors (pimecrolimus and tacrolimus) showed the same overall incidence of adverse events, but with a small difference in the frequency of local effects [53].

Due to the difference in effect, tacrolimus can be used in more severe atopic dermatitis, and pimecrolimus is applied in less severe groups. However, the formulation of pimecrolimus is a cream formulation, which has a non-negligible advantage that the adherence of patients is better because it is less greasy and easier to apply than the ointment formulation tacrolimus [52]. It is also known that pimecrolimus induces a relatively rapid efficacy response when applied to mild atopic dermatitis lesions. Therefore, clinicians should select the proper drug with the highest treatment efficiency and the adherence based on the patient's skin condition and discomfort.

Proactive Treatment with TCIs

Proactive approach, which prevents recurrence by topically applying an anti-inflammatory drug for 2–3 times a week after the lesion was stabilized, can be applied with TCIs. The basis for proactive treatment is the idea that the inflammatory cells or antigen-presenting cells remain at the site where the flare develops frequently are still active, so the symptoms will recur easily when exposed to the causative factor. In other words, reactivation can be suppressed by applying intermittent TCI to lesions in preclinical condition.

Indeed, clinical results of single TCI's long-term (more than 6–10 years) 2-week intermittent treatment showed significant improvement in clinical symptoms, decreased treatment, reduced viral infection, and improved atopic respiratory symptoms. In addition, no malignant tumors were observed [54]. Moreover, when compared to twice weekly 0.1% tacrolimus proactive treatment with vehicle ointment for 12 months in approximately 230 atopic dermatitis adults, proactive tacrolimus 0.1% ointment application significantly reduced the number of disease exacerbations requiring substantial therapeutic intervention (median difference: 2) and increased the time to first disease exacerbations (median 142 vs. 15 days). The adverse event profile was similar for the two treatment approaches [55]. The same study design with 0.3% tacrolimus proactive treatment in children showed similar efficacy, in which 0.3% tacrolimus proactive treatment delayed the relapse period by 7 times compared to when only acute lesions were treated with 0.03% tacrolimus ointment (median: 173 vs. 38 days) [56]. However, meta-analysis, which is based on vehicle-controlled trials comparing the efficacy of proactive treatment with tacrolimus, fluticasone propionate, and methylprednisolone, showed that topical fluticasone propionate (RR 0.46) may be more efficacious to prevent disease flares than topical tacrolimus (RR 0.78) [19]. However, there are not many clinical trials that will prove the effectiveness of proactive treatment with pimecrolimus, hence it is currently not recommended.

Pharmacokinetics

Tacrolimus

In adults with atopic dermatitis after topical application of tacrolimus 0.1% ointment twice daily for 2 weeks, systemic tacrolimus absorption after tacrolimus ointment application was low and highly variable, with 31% of samples below the quantification limit (0.025 ng/mL) and 94% below 1 ng/mL [57]. The pharmacokinetic investigation results on 2-week 0.1% tacrolimus treatment in children with moderate-to-severe atopic dermatitis showed that 92% of the assayed blood samples contained tacrolimus concentrations below 1 ng/mL, with 17% of samples below the lower limit of quantification (0.025 ng/mL) [58].

Therefore, even though most of the patients showed impaired skin barrier function, even when topical application of tacrolimus ointment, the blood concentration does not reach 5 ng/mL (the toxic concentration) in more than 90% of patients [59]. Similar results were found in children. As a result, systemic accumulation may not occur even after prolonged use, since tacrolimus ointment was decomposed and not detected in the blood in the time when the eczema lesions improve after applications of tacrolimus ointment [60].

Meanwhile, due to this low absorption efficiency, the emollients are recommended to be applied at least half an hour later to avoid interference with the cutaneous absorption [12].

Pimecrolimus

In a 3-week clinical study for adolescent and adult patients with moderate-to-severe atopic dermatitis treated with 1% pimecrolimus cream, most enrolled patients had blood levels below the limit of quantification and the highest single blood level of pimecrolimus measured in any patient was 1.37 ng/mL [61]. In another pharmacokinetic study conducted in children, 97% of patients after 1% pimecrolimus cream treatment did not exceed 2.0 ng/mL in blood [62]. Therefore, 1% pimecrolimus cream also has a low systemic absorption rate, so the risk of systemic toxicity appears to be low.

Adverse Reactions

Topical calcineurin inhibitors (TCIs), tacrolimus and pimecrolimus, have been available for 1–2 decades and are not associated with atrophy or increased percutaneous absorption after prolonged use, and have a much lower potential for systemic effects. It is favorable that skin atrophy caused by long-term use of TCSs does not appear when TCI is used. In addition, viral infections such as eczema herpeticum have been reported in some cases, but overall results showed that it does not increase the risk of skin infections and does not affect vaccinations in children [13, 49, 63, 64]. If local herpes infection occurs, TCI treatment should be discontinued until the infection is cured.

Also, less data is available for children under 2 years of age, pregnant women, and lactating women, so it is not recommended for use as a treatment for these yet.

Tacrolimus

Most of the side effects are local skin reactions including burning sensations, pruritus, folliculitis (acneform eruption), and increased risk of skin infection. The most common adverse events that occur with tacrolimus ointment treatment are transient application-site reactions, such as burning or pruritus. It starts about 5 min after each application and may last up to 1 h, but intensity and duration gradually subside within a few days. These complications are related to disease severity, and decrease in frequency over time as AD improves [65]. The sentence Application site-burning or prutitus reaction is observed in 40–50% in adults and in 20–30% in children. It appears at the beginning of treatment and continues to be applied, which tends to decrease with time. The burning sensation is due to neurotransmitters release (such as substance P) by the drug from the nerve endings. It is known that a rapid secretion and subsequent deficiency of substance P after continuous application explain why the burning sensation occurs and sequentially disappear naturally. As a method to help alleviate the burning sensation, it is recommended to store the TCI tube in a cold place prior to use, alternate with TCS, apply it with a moisturizer, or take oral aspirin in severe cases.

Tachyphylaxis also does not occur during long-term application, and the response of delayed hypersensitivity is not affected.

Pimecrolimus

The most common side effects are burning sensations, pruritus, as in tacrolimus, but the incidence is lower than tacrolimus, which is about 15% in adults and 10% in children. It is a temporary symptom that appears within 1–3 days of application and disappears over time. Another report found that the safety and tolerance of 1% pimecrolimus in children aged 3–23 months has been reviewed for 2 years, with no reports of malignancy or signs of immunosuppression, nevertheless, application in children under the age of 2 years is not recommended [34]. No serious side effects or cumulative effects of long-term applications have been reported.

Risk of Malignancy

In 2006, the United States Food and Drug Administration (US FDA) issued a warning regarding a theoretical risk of malignancy (especially skin cancer and lymphoma) based on their mode of action, the results of animal studies, and case reports, and the effects of systemic tacrolimus [66]. Fortunately, however, systemic absorption of tacrolimus and pimecrolimus, when applied topically, is very low, with blood concentrations being below the level of quantification in most patients [65]. Also, evidence has shown that the use of TCIs does not increase the risk of skin cancer or lymphoma is increasing [60]. There is no evidence of systemic accumulation in patients with moderate-to-severe atopic dermatitis and extensive disease, up to date.

Although there is no evidence of an increase in the incidence of skin tumors due to combined action of long-term application of TCI and exposure to ultraviolet lights, it is recommended to avoid the combination of UV treatment and TCI and to use sunscreen.

Topical Phosphodiesterase 4 Inhibitors (Topical Crisaborole and Others)

Among different phosphodiesterases (PDEs), PDE-4 inactivates cyclic adenosine monophosphate (cAMP), thus increasing the production of pro-inflammatory prostaglandins and cytokines, and is expressed in immune cells, as well as in keratinocytes and fibroblasts, and is more active in patients with AD [9, 12]. Specifically, elevated levels of cAMP result in further activation of protein kinase A and inhibition of nuclear factor κB (NF-κB) and nuclear factor of activated T-cells (NFAT) signaling pathways [67]. Crisaborole deceases through suppression of pro-inflammatory cytokines, including IL-2, IL-5, IFN-γ, and TNF-α. Therefore, many clinical trials have been attempted to suppress PDE-4 for the treatment of inflammatory skin diseases.

Among the newer advances, Crisaborole was actually approved in the United States for the treatment of mild-to-moderate atopic dermatitis in AD in patients ≥2 years of age in 2016. In a recent study, crisaborole 2% ointment (twice daily) was shown to have encouraging results in children and adults with atopic dermatitis, demonstrating early and continued decrease in pruritus, which improves quality of life and reduces the potential risk of infection and scarring [67–70]. The small size of the crisaborole molecule allows for effective skin penetration, while its quick metabolism in the bloodstream limits systemic exposure, which is associated with the long-term use of topical corticosteroids and TCIs [69]. However, since there are less results of comparative studies with other TCSs and TCIs, further studies comparing crisaborole against others are needed to establish its role in the treatment paradigm for mild-to-moderate AD, as well as its utility in children <2 years of age.

The majority of reported adverse events include burning or stinging at the site of application without serious adverse events [67, 71]. Of these adverse events, 77.6% of patients experienced resolution within 1 day of onset. And a long-term safety study with crisaborole 2% ointment demonstrated efficacy, safety, and good tolerance [68].

Other topical PDE4 inhibitors with high selectivity for PDE4 are also under investigation. Topical OPA-15406 twice daily for 4 weeks demonstrated a higher incidence of success in the Investigator Global Assessment score compared with the vehicle group in a phase II, randomized, double-blind, vehicle-controlled, study each in adult or child (2–14 years old) with atopic dermatitis [72, 73]. So, further phase III studies are expecting ongoing now.

Novel Topical Therapy

Beyond topical phosphodiesterase 4 inhibitors, Other class, novel, topical, and nonsteroidal agents are also being investigated. They include Janus kinase (JAK) inhibitors [74, 75], aryl hydrocarbon receptor (AhR) modulating agents [76], and topical TRPV1 antagonist [77, 78]. These drugs have also shown positive effects in a phase II study. However, until actual commercialization, more studies are required to validate these findings.

Moisturizers

The management of atopic dermatitis, unlike other inflammatory diseases, requires restoring the skin barrier defects and dry skin due to primary epidermal barrier dysfunction such as filaggrin mutation and SC intercellular lipid abnormalities. Continuous moisturizer use can prevent dry skin and exacerbation of inflammation, which is crucial for atopic dermatitis and is recommended as a basic treatment [10]. Moisturizers are also effective in the relief of atopic pruritus. Moisturizing agents that are helpful for patients with atopic dermatitis can be largely divided into two groups: the physiological lipid mixture group, which can effectively supplement the poor barrier components of the stratum corneum, and the active ingredients containing group, which can reduce inflammatory reaction.

Physiologic Lipid Mixture (Barrier Cream)

A moisturizing agent that implements the molar ratio of ceramide—cholesterol: free fatty acid showing the optimal barrier function recovery effect is called a physiologic lipid mixture or barrier cream. The mixing ratio of ceramide, cholesterol, and free fatty acids is known to be the most effective 3: 1: 1 molar ratio, and 1: 1: 1 is also known to be effective [79, 80]. Some moisturizers based on these theories have been approved by the US FDA as treatment materials for improving symptoms of atopic dermatitis [81]. In addition, a number of moisturizers that use synthetic pseudoceramides or some of which include a ceramide precursor, or an enhancer capable of ceramide synthesis, have been marketed. These physiological lipid compound moisturizers are also known to reduce barrier function disruption by TCSs, so it will be more valuable if it is found that it may prevent side effects such as epidermal atrophy caused by corticosteroid ointments [82].

Functional Moisturizer with Anti-inflammatory and Anti-bacterial Properties

Previously, it was described about a ceramide-based physiological lipid compound moisturizer. However, it is not always necessary to use physiological lipid mixture. There is also moisturizer group that specializes in atopic dermatitis by attenuating inflammation with anti-inflammatory materials. For example, "Atopiclair" (Sinclair Pharm. Ltd., Surrey, UK), which has been approved by the US FDA. Licorice components Glycyrrhetinic acid, Vitis vinifera (grapevine) extract, and telmesteine were used as the main active ingredients to improve skin barrier function and improve atopic dermatitis symptoms through anti-inflammatory/anti-pruritic effects [83]. Other moisturizers claim to have anti-inflammatory effects, including ingredients such as palmitoylethanolamide (PEA), white tobacco extract, defensamide, and pandulatin A. However, even if the anti-inflammatory and anti-bacterial effects were confirmed through basic research of the individual ingredients, there is insufficient clinical evidence for the effect of cosmetic formulations in which each active ingredient is added in small amounts and mixed with each other. Nevertheless, the notion that the action of a moisturizing agent not only restores barrier function through hydration and emollient, but also affects epidermal lipid metabolism or differentiation, can be used to control inflammation and immune responses and to treat skin diseases, is quite an attractive feature. Therefore, it is necessary to study whether functional moisturizers act on properly in atopic dermatitis.

Recommendation of Moisturizer Application

The type and function of the moisturizer are also important, but how to apply it and how to use it for controlling symptoms in atopic dermatitis patients [84]. The main guidelines for its use, such as the timing, frequency, and amount of application of the moisturizer, are summarized as follows.

For body creams, it is recommended to apply it at least 3 times a day repeatedly since at least 50% of the first applied dose is removed after 8 h in an experimental environment without daily activities, but it is not easy to apply it twice or more a day in real life. Regarding the amount of moisturizer applied, the 2012 European Atopic Dermatology Treatment Guidelines recommend using approximately 500 g/week for adults and 250 g/week for children [15]. The minimum amount in adults is 250 g/week [13]. The FTU method can be also applied to the amount of moisturizer. Even though skin can look normal, since the abnormality of the skin barrier function is observed in the non-lesion skin of patients with atopic dermatitis, the use of a moisturizer should be continued. Moisturizers should be applied at least twice a day even when there are no lesions on the skin, and it is recommended to apply a sufficient amount 4–5 times a day when lesions occur or dry skin is observed. It seems to be more important to use the correct amount frequently and consistently, even with common moisturizers, than to use expensive barrier cream moisturizers.

A moisturizer can be usually applied without prior washing, but if sweat or contaminants get on your skin, it is better to wash and apply it. Immediately after bathing, tap the skin with a towel to dry, then apply a moisturizer within 3 min.

In the areas of inflammation where the stratum corneum of the skin is damaged, even if a moisturizer is applied, it is ineffective. Therefore, it must be co-treated with the prescribed treatment, and emollients should be steadily applied as a basic treatment regardless of flare-up status in order to obtain steroid-sparing effects and reduce the frequency of acute episodes [13].

The choice of moisturizer may vary depending on the season and body area it is being applied to. For patients who are sensitive to oily formulations, moist lotion types are good in the summer, and cream or ointment formulations may be used in the fall or winter.

Early interventions to repair skin barrier problems of atopic skin with the use of appropriate soaps, or moisturizers may be useful in delaying the progression of disease [85] (See more in the prevention section).

The use of pure oil products such as coconut oil instead of emulsions will dry out the skin, increases the trans-epidermal water loss, and is therefore not recommended [13]. Most moisturizers are made of mixtures of humectants and occludents, and other oils, so it may be more effective to use the product rather than a single oil.

What Is the Best Moisturizer?

Moisturizers containing physiological lipid compounds or anti-inflammatory substances improve functionality and are relatively expensive compared to conventional moisturizers Theoretically, a better effect can be expected because it is suitable for a vulnerable skin barrier of patients with atopic dermatitis, but there are not many products that have been verified through a randomized controlled trial with a high level of evidence, and the cost-effectiveness should be considered. You may think that clinical trials for verification are not meaningful for a moisturizer, a type of cosmetic, but you should check whether it is verified from the perspective of the patient who purchases it or of the dermatologist who recommends it.

In fact, studies comparing the use of US FDA approved barrier creams and general moisturizers to improve symptoms in atopic dermatitis patients did not reveal any significant difference in cost-effectiveness [86]. Although the results of clinical studies showing the effectiveness of cosmeceutical moisturizers for atopic dermatitis are presented, more researches with high evidence level are needed. It would be best to apply any moisturizer frequently. Theoretically, a product that contains natural moisturizing factors and ceramides (physiologic lipid mixture) and is hypoallergenic, less-irritated, fragrance-free, non-comedogenic, and as sustainable as possible may be ideal. The ideal requirements for a moisturizer are summarized in Table 3.

Table 3 Ideal conditions of moisturizer for atopic dermatitis skin

Abnormal findings in atopic dermatitis	Condition to solve the problem
Increased skin surface pH	Acidic pH
Decreased stratum corneum lipids (especially ceramide)	Supplementation with physiological lipid mixture
abnormal lipid lamellar structure	Structure that helps to form the stratum corneum lipid layer
Reduced natural moisturizing factor	Supplementation of natural moisturizing factors
Increased skin penetration of allergens/irritants/pathogens	Defensive occlusion to prevent penetration
A vicious cycle of itching and scratching	Anti-pruritic/anti-inflammatory effect
Dry and cracked skin	Excellent sustainability of moisturizing effect
Skin sensitive to cosmetics	Minimal ingredients and excellent formulation

Bathing

Bathing also has a good function of cleansing the skin and directly moisturizing it, but excessive bathing can reduce the lipids in the skin and dry it. The use of excess soap dries the skin, but washing with water alone does not remove enough bacteria or contaminants, so proper soap is required. Weak acidic hypoallergenic liquid or syndet soap is recommended [87].

To wash out pathogenic microorganisms, crusts, and environmental pollutants from the skin, gentle and careful cleansing is necessary for atopic dermatitis patients. It is not recommended to irritate the skin with a harsh towel. The dehydration of the stratum corneum can be also reduced by taking a short bath in lukewarm water (27–30 °C) for as little as 5–10 min, and applying bath oil for the last step [13].

Adding antiseptics (such as sodium hypochlorite) or salts to the bathwater may be an additional useful option because of bacterial count inhibiting activities or removing the dead keratin material, respectively [13, 88, 89]. Sodium hypochlorite baths (bleach bath) were reported to improve atopic dermatitis [90], or may help at least a reduction in TCS and antibiotic usage [91]. Salt baths may also be useful especially in heavily impetiginized or ichthyotic skin [13, 92].

As a final step, moisturizers are preferentially applied directly after a bath or a shower following gentle drying when the skin is still slightly humid [13, 93, 94].

Conclusion

Topical treatments are the fundamentals of atopic dermatitis treatment. Atopic dermatitis is a chronic inflammatory skin disease and requires a long-term treatment strategy, hence a proactive strategy to suppress recurrence/flaring is being widely used. With the recent development of new mechanisms of anti-inflammatory topical agents and biologics, there is a greater hope to avoid

TCS. Even so, the concurrent use of moisturizers and skin care to improve the underlying skin barrier function should be continued.

References

1. Charman CR, Morris AD, Williams HC. Topical corticosteroid phobia in patients with atopic eczema. Br J Dermatol. 2000;142(5):931–6.
2. Li AW, Yin ES, Antaya RJ. Topical corticosteroid phobia in atopic dermatitis: a systematic review. JAMA Dermatol. 2017;153(10):1036–42.
3. Krakowski AC, Dohil MA. Topical therapy in pediatric atopic dermatitis. Semin Cutan Med Surg. 2008;27(2):161–7.
4. Norris DA. Mechanisms of action of topical therapies and the rationale for combination therapy. J Am Acad Dermatol. 2005;53(1 Suppl 1):S17–25.
5. Ahluwalia A. Topical glucocorticoids and the skin—mechanisms of action: an update. Mediat Inflamm. 1998;7(3):183–93.
6. Watson W, Kapur S. Atopic dermatitis. Allergy Asthma Clin Immunol. 2011;7(Suppl 1):S4.
7. Wollenberg A, Oranje A, Deleuran M, Simon D, Szalai Z, Kunz B, et al. ETFAD/EADV Eczema task force 2015 position paper on diagnosis and treatment of atopic dermatitis in adult and paediatric patients. J Eur Acad Dermatol Venereol. 2016;30(5):729–47.
8. Eichenfield LF, Tom WL, Berger TG, Krol A, Paller AS, Schwarzenberger K, et al. Guidelines of care for the management of atopic dermatitis: section 2. Management and treatment of atopic dermatitis with topical therapies. J Am Acad Dermatol. 2014;71(1):116–32.
9. Udkoff J, Waldman A, Ahluwalia J, Borok J, Eichenfield LF. Current and emerging topical therapies for atopic dermatitis. Clin Dermatol. 2017;35(4):375–82.
10. Kim JE, Kim HJ, Lew BL, Lee KH, Hong SP, Jang YH, et al. Consensus guidelines for the treatment of atopic dermatitis in Korea (part I): general management and topical treatment. Ann Dermatol. 2015;27(5):563–77.
11. Ference JD, Last AR. Choosing topical corticosteroids. Am Fam Physician. 2009;79(2):135–40.
12. Sala-Cunill A, Lazaro M, Herraez L, Quinones MD, Moro-Moro M, Sanchez I, et al. Basic skin care and topical therapies for atopic dermatitis: essential approaches and beyond. J Investig Allergol Clin Immunol. 2018;28(6):379–91.
13. Wollenberg A, Barbarot S, Bieber T, Christen-Zaech S, Deleuran M, Fink-Wagner A, et al. Consensus-based European guidelines for treatment of atopic eczema (atopic dermatitis) in adults and children: part I. J Eur Acad Dermatol Venereol. 2018;32(5):657–82.
14. Thomas KS, Armstrong S, Avery A, Po AL, O'Neill C, Young S, et al. Randomised controlled trial of short bursts of a potent topical corticosteroid versus prolonged use of a mild preparation for children with mild or moderate atopic eczema. BMJ. 2002;324(7340):768.
15. Ring J, Alomar A, Bieber T, Deleuran M, Fink-Wagner A, Gelmetti C, et al. Guidelines for treatment of atopic eczema (atopic dermatitis) part I. J Eur Acad Dermatol Venereol. 2012;26(8):1045–60.
16. Birnie AJ, Bath-Hextall FJ, Ravenscroft JC, Williams HC. Interventions to reduce Staphylococcus aureus in the management of atopic eczema. Cochrane Database Syst Rev. 2008;3:CD003871.
17. Long CC, Finlay AY. The finger-tip unit—a new practical measure. Clin Exp Dermatol. 1991;16(6):444–7.
18. Tadicherla S, Ross K, Shenefelt PD, Fenske NA. Topical corticosteroids in dermatology. J Drugs Dermatol. 2009;8(12):1093–105.
19. Schmitt J, von Kobyletzki L, Svensson A, Apfelbacher C. Efficacy and tolerability of proactive treatment with topical corticosteroids and calcineurin inhibitors for atopic eczema: systematic review and meta-analysis of randomized controlled trials. Br J Dermatol. 2011;164(2):415–28.
20. Goodyear HM, Spowart K, Harper JI. 'Wet-wrap' dressings for the treatment of atopic eczema in children. Br J Dermatol. 1991;125(6):604.
21. Devillers AC, Oranje AP. Efficacy and safety of 'wet-wrap' dressings as an intervention treatment in children with severe and/or refractory atopic dermatitis: a critical review of the literature. Br J Dermatol. 2006;154(4):579–85.
22. Devillers AC, Oranje AP. Wet-wrap treatment in children with atopic dermatitis: a practical guideline. Pediatr Dermatol. 2012;29(1):24–7.
23. Berth-Jones J, Damstra RJ, Golsch S, Livden JK, Van Hooteghem O, Allegra F, et al. Twice weekly fluticasone propionate added to emollient maintenance treatment to reduce risk of relapse in atopic dermatitis: randomised, double blind, parallel group study. BMJ. 2003;326(7403):1367.
24. Wollenberg A, Ehmann LM. Long term treatment concepts and proactive therapy for atopic eczema. Ann Dermatol. 2012;24(3):253–60.
25. Morley KW, Dinulos JG. Update on topical glucocorticoid use in children. Curr Opin Pediatr. 2012;24(1):121–8.
26. Chi CC, Kirtschig G, Aberer W, Gabbud JP, Lipozencic J, Karpati S, et al. Evidence-based (S3) guideline on topical corticosteroids in pregnancy. Br J Dermatol. 2011;165(5):943–52.
27. Jacob SE, Steele T. Corticosteroid classes: a quick reference guide including patch test substances and cross-reactivity. J Am Acad Dermatol. 2006;54(4):723–7.
28. English JS. Corticosteroid-induced contact dermatitis: a pragmatic approach. Clin Exp Dermatol. 2000;25(4):261–4.
29. Haeck IM, Rouwen TJ, Timmer-de Mik L, de Bruin-Weller MS, Bruijnzeel-Koomen CA. Topical corticosteroids in atopic dermatitis and the risk of glaucoma and cataracts. J Am Acad Dermatol. 2011;64(2):275–81.

30. Totri CR, Eichenfield LF, Logan K, Proudfoot L, Schmitt J, Lara-Corrales I, et al. Prescribing practices for systemic agents in the treatment of severe pediatric atopic dermatitis in the US and Canada: The PeDRA TREAT survey. J Am Acad Dermatol. 2017;76(2):281–5.
31. Prezzano JC, Beck LA. Long-term treatment of atopic dermatitis. Dermatol Clin. 2017;35(3):335–49.
32. Carr WW. Topical calcineurin inhibitors for atopic dermatitis: review and treatment recommendations. Paediatr Drugs. 2013;15(4):303–10.
33. Ohtsuki M, Morimoto H, Nakagawa H. Tacrolimus ointment for the treatment of adult and pediatric atopic dermatitis: review on safety and benefits. J Dermatol. 2018;45(8):936–42.
34. Paul C, Cork M, Rossi AB, Papp KA, Barbier N, de Prost Y. Safety and tolerability of 1% pimecrolimus cream among infants: experience with 1133 patients treated for up to 2 years. Pediatrics. 2006;117(1):e118–28.
35. Iskedjian M, Piwko C, Shear NH, Langley RG, Einarson TR. Topical calcineurin inhibitors in the treatment of atopic dermatitis: a meta-analysis of current evidence. Am J Clin Dermatol. 2004;5(4):267–79.
36. Paller A, Eichenfield LF, Leung DY, Stewart D, Appell M. A 12-week study of tacrolimus ointment for the treatment of atopic dermatitis in pediatric patients. J Am Acad Dermatol. 2001;44(1 Suppl):S47–57.
37. Hebert AA, Koo J, Fowler J, Berman B, Rosenberg C, Levitt J. Desoximetasone 0.25% and tacrolimus 0.1% ointments versus tacrolimus alone in the treatment of atopic dermatitis. Cutis. 2006;78(5):357–63.
38. Reitamo S, Rustin M, Harper J, Kalimo K, Rubins A, Cambazard F, et al. A 4-year follow-up study of atopic dermatitis therapy with 0.1% tacrolimus ointment in children and adult patients. Br J Dermatol. 2008;159(4):942–51.
39. Hanifin JM, Paller AS, Eichenfield L, Clark RA, Korman N, Weinstein G, et al. Efficacy and safety of tacrolimus ointment treatment for up to 4 years in patients with atopic dermatitis. J Am Acad Dermatol. 2005;53(2 Suppl 2):S186–94.
40. Oranje AP, Verbeek R, Verzaal P, Haspels I, Prens E, Nagelkerken L. Wet-wrap treatment using dilutions of tacrolimus ointment and fluticasone propionate cream in human APOC1 (+/+) mice with atopic dermatitis. Br J Dermatol. 2009;160(1):54–61.
41. Luger T, De Raeve L, Gelmetti C, Kakourou T, Katsarou A, Lambert J, et al. Recommendations for pimecrolimus 1% cream in the treatment of mild-to-moderate atopic dermatitis: from medical needs to a new treatment algorithm. Eur J Dermatol. 2013;23(6):758–66.
42. Van Leent EJ, Graber M, Thurston M, Wagenaar A, Spuls PI, Bos JD. Effectiveness of the ascomycin macrolactam SDZ ASM 981 in the topical treatment of atopic dermatitis. Arch Dermatol. 1998;134(7):805–9.
43. Meurer M, Folster-Holst R, Wozel G, Weidinger G, Junger M, Brautigam M, et al. Pimecrolimus cream in the long-term management of atopic dermatitis in adults: a six-month study. Dermatology. 2002;205(3):271–7.
44. Eichenfield LF, Thaci D, de Prost Y, Puig L, Paul C. Clinical management of atopic eczema with pimecrolimus cream 1% (Elidel) in paediatric patients. Dermatology. 2007;215(Suppl 1):3–17.
45. Sigurgeirsson B, Boznanski A, Todd G, Vertruyen A, Schuttelaar ML, Zhu X, et al. Safety and efficacy of pimecrolimus in atopic dermatitis: a 5-year randomized trial. Pediatrics. 2015;135(4):597–606.
46. Reitamo S, Rustin M, Ruzicka T, Cambazard F, Kalimo K, Friedmann PS, et al. Efficacy and safety of tacrolimus ointment compared with that of hydrocortisone butyrate ointment in adult patients with atopic dermatitis. J Allergy Clin Immunol. 2002;109(3):547–55.
47. Doss N, Reitamo S, Dubertret L, Fekete GL, Kamoun MR, Lahfa M, et al. Superiority of tacrolimus 0.1% ointment compared with fluticasone 0.005% in adults with moderate to severe atopic dermatitis of the face: results from a randomized, double-blind trial. Br J Dermatol. 2009;161(2):427–34.
48. Frankel HC, Qureshi AA. Comparative effectiveness of topical calcineurin inhibitors in adult patients with atopic dermatitis. Am J Clin Dermatol. 2012;13(2):113–23.
49. Reitamo S, Ortonne JP, Sand C, Cambazard F, Bieber T, Folster-Holst R, et al. A multicentre, randomized, double-blind, controlled study of long-term treatment with 0.1% tacrolimus ointment in adults with moderate to severe atopic dermatitis. Br J Dermatol. 2005;152(6):1282–9.
50. Reitamo S, Van Leent EJ, Ho V, Harper J, Ruzicka T, Kalimo K, et al. Efficacy and safety of tacrolimus ointment compared with that of hydrocortisone acetate ointment in children with atopic dermatitis. J Allergy Clin Immunol. 2002;109(3):539–46.
51. Paller AS, Lebwohl M, Fleischer AB Jr, Antaya R, Langley RG, Kirsner RS, et al. Tacrolimus ointment is more effective than pimecrolimus cream with a similar safety profile in the treatment of atopic dermatitis: results from 3 randomized, comparative studies. J Am Acad Dermatol. 2005;52(5):810–22.
52. Kempers S, Boguniewicz M, Carter E, Jarratt M, Pariser D, Stewart D, et al. A randomized investigator-blinded study comparing pimecrolimus cream 1% with tacrolimus ointment 0.03% in the treatment of pediatric patients with moderate atopic dermatitis. J Am Acad Dermatol. 2004;51(4):515–25.
53. Cury Martins J, Martins C, Aoki V, Gois AF, Ishii HA, da Silva EM. Topical tacrolimus for atopic dermatitis. Cochrane Database Syst Rev. 2015;7:CD009864.
54. Mandelin JM, Remitz A, Virtanen HM, Malmberg LP, Haahtela T, Reitamo S. A 10-year open follow-up of eczema and respiratory symptoms in patients with atopic dermatitis treated with topical tacrolimus for the first 4 years. J Dermatol Treat. 2010;21(3):167–70.
55. Wollenberg A, Reitamo S, Atzori F, Lahfa M, Ruzicka T, Healy E, et al. Proactive treatment of atopic dermatitis in adults with 0.1% tacrolimus ointment. Allergy. 2008;63(6):742–50.

56. Thaci D, Reitamo S, Gonzalez Ensenat MA, Moss C, Boccaletti V, Cainelli T, et al. Proactive disease management with 0.03% tacrolimus ointment for children with atopic dermatitis: results of a randomized, multicentre, comparative study. Br J Dermatol. 2008;159(6):1348–56.
57. Undre NA, Moloney FJ, Ahmadi S, Stevenson P, Murphy GM. Skin and systemic pharmacokinetics of tacrolimus following topical application of tacrolimus ointment in adults with moderate to severe atopic dermatitis. Br J Dermatol. 2009;160(3):665–9.
58. Harper J, Smith C, Rubins A, Green A, Jackson K, Zigure S, et al. A multicenter study of the pharmacokinetics of tacrolimus ointment after first and repeated application to children with atopic dermatitis. J Investig Dermatol. 2005;124(4):695–9.
59. Krueger GG, Eichenfield L, Goodman JJ, Krafchik BR, Carlin CS, Pang ML, et al. Pharmacokinetics of tacrolimus following topical application of tacrolimus ointment in adult and pediatric patients with moderate to severe atopic dermatitis. J Drugs Dermatol. 2007;6(2):185–93.
60. Katoh N, Ohya Y, Ikeda M, Ebihara T, Katayama I, Saeki H, et al. Clinical practice guidelines for the management of atopic dermatitis 2018. J Dermatol. 2019;46(12):1053–101.
61. Ling M, Gottlieb A, Pariser D, Caro I, Stewart D, Scott G, et al. A randomized study of the safety, absorption and efficacy of pimecrolimus cream 1% applied twice or four times daily in patients with atopic dermatitis. J Dermatol Treat. 2005;16(3):142–8.
62. Staab D, Pariser D, Gottlieb AB, Kaufmann R, Eichenfield LF, Langley RG, et al. Low systemic absorption and good tolerability of pimecrolimus, administered as 1% cream (Elidel) in infants with atopic dermatitis—a multicenter, 3-week, open-label study. Pediatr Dermatol. 2005;22(5):465–71.
63. Wahn U, Bos JD, Goodfield M, Caputo R, Papp K, Manjra A, et al. Efficacy and safety of pimecrolimus cream in the long-term management of atopic dermatitis in children. Pediatrics. 2002;110(1) Pt 1:e2.
64. Lubbe J. Secondary infections in patients with atopic dermatitis. Am J Clin Dermatol. 2003;4(9):641–54.
65. Rustin MH. The safety of tacrolimus ointment for the treatment of atopic dermatitis: a review. Br J Dermatol. 2007;157(5):861–73.
66. https://www.fda.gov/drugs/postmarket-drug-safety-information-patients-and-providers/tacrolimus-marketed-protopic-ointment-information
67. Woo TE, Kuzel P. Crisaborole 2% ointment (Eucrisa) for atopic dermatitis. Skin Therapy Lett. 2019;24(2):4–6.
68. Eichenfield LF, Call RS, Forsha DW, Fowler J Jr, Hebert AA, Spellman M, et al. Long-term safety of crisaborole ointment 2% in children and adults with mild to moderate atopic dermatitis. J Am Acad Dermatol. 2017;77(4):641–9 e5.
69. Zane LT, Kircik L, Call R, Tschen E, Draelos ZD, Chanda S, et al. Crisaborole topical ointment, 2% in patients ages 2 to 17 years with atopic dermatitis: a phase 1b, open-label, maximal-use systemic exposure study. Pediatr Dermatol. 2016;33(4):380–7.
70. Yosipovitch G, Gold LF, Lebwohl MG, Silverberg JI, Tallman AM, Zane LT. Early relief of pruritus in atopic dermatitis with crisaborole ointment, a non-steroidal, phosphodiesterase 4 inhibitor. Acta Derm Venereol. 2018;98(5):484–9.
71. Paller AS, Tom WL, Lebwohl MG, Blumenthal RL, Boguniewicz M, Call RS, et al. Efficacy and safety of crisaborole ointment, a novel, nonsteroidal phosphodiesterase 4 (PDE4) inhibitor for the topical treatment of atopic dermatitis (AD) in children and adults. J Am Acad Dermatol. 2016;75(3):494–503 e6.
72. Hanifin JM, Ellis CN, Frieden IJ, Folster-Holst R, Stein Gold LF, Secci A, et al. OPA-15406, a novel, topical, nonsteroidal, selective phosphodiesterase-4 (PDE4) inhibitor, in the treatment of adult and adolescent patients with mild to moderate atopic dermatitis (AD): a phase-II randomized, double-blind, placebo-controlled study. J Am Acad Dermatol. 2016;75(2):297–305.
73. Saeki H, Baba N, Oshiden K, Abe Y, Tsubouchi H. Phase 2, randomized, double-blind, placebo-controlled, 4-week study to evaluate the safety and efficacy of OPA- 15406 (difamilast), a new topical selective phosphodiesterase type-4 inhibitor, in Japanese pediatric patients aged 2–14 years with atopic dermatitis. J Dermatol. 2020;47(1):17–24.
74. Bissonnette R, Papp KA, Poulin Y, Gooderham M, Raman M, Mallbris L, et al. Topical tofacitinib for atopic dermatitis: a phase IIa randomized trial. Br J Dermatol. 2016;175(5):902–11.
75. Nakagawa H, Nemoto O, Igarashi A, Nagata T. Efficacy and safety of topical JTE-052, a Janus kinase inhibitor, in Japanese adult patients with moderate-to-severe atopic dermatitis: a phase II, multicentre, randomized, vehicle-controlled clinical study. Br J Dermatol. 2018;178(2):424–32.
76. Peppers J, Paller AS, Maeda-Chubachi T, Wu S, Robbins K, Gallagher K, et al. A phase 2, randomized dose-finding study of tapinarof (GSK2894512 cream) for the treatment of atopic dermatitis. J Am Acad Dermatol. 2019;80(1):89–98.e3.
77. Suga H, Sato S. Novel topical and systemic therapies in atopic dermatitis. Immunol Med. 2019;42(2):84–93.
78. Lee YW, Won CH, Jung K, Nam HJ, Choi G, Park YH, et al. Efficacy and safety of PAC-14028 cream—a novel, topical, nonsteroidal, selective TRPV1 antagonist in patients with mild-to-moderate atopic dermatitis: a phase IIb randomized trial. Br J Dermatol. 2019;180(5):1030–8.
79. Man MQ, Feingold KR, Elias PM. Exogenous lipids influence permeability barrier recovery in acetone-treated murine skin. Arch Dermatol. 1993;129(6):728–38.
80. Chamlin SL, Kao J, Frieden IJ, Sheu MY, Fowler AJ, Fluhr JW, et al. Ceramide-dominant barrier repair lipids alleviate childhood atopic dermatitis: changes in barrier function provide a sensitive indicator of disease activity. J Am Acad Dermatol. 2002;47(2):198–208.

81. Sugarman JL, Parish LC. Efficacy of a lipid-based barrier repair formulation in moderate-to-severe pediatric atopic dermatitis. J Drugs Dermatol. 2009;8(12):1106–11.
82. Kao JS, Fluhr JW, Man MQ, Fowler AJ, Hachem JP, Crumrine D, et al. Short-term glucocorticoid treatment compromises both permeability barrier homeostasis and stratum corneum integrity: inhibition of epidermal lipid synthesis accounts for functional abnormalities. J Investig Dermatol. 2003;120(3):456–64.
83. Boguniewicz M, Zeichner JA, Eichenfield LF, Hebert AA, Jarratt M, Lucky AW, et al. MAS063DP is effective monotherapy for mild to moderate atopic dermatitis in infants and children: a multicenter, randomized, vehicle-controlled study. J Pediatr. 2008;152(6):854–9.
84. Hon KL, Ching GK, Leung TF, Choi CY, Lee KK, Ng PC. Estimating emollient usage in patients with eczema. Clin Exp Dermatol. 2010;35(1):22–6.
85. Elias PM, Wakefield JS. Therapeutic implications of a barrier-based pathogenesis of atopic dermatitis. Clin Rev Allergy Immunol. 2011;41(3):282–95.
86. Miller DW, Koch SB, Yentzer BA, Clark AR, O'Neill JR, Fountain J, et al. An over-the-counter moisturizer is as clinically effective as, and more cost-effective than, prescription barrier creams in the treatment of children with mild-to-moderate atopic dermatitis: a randomized, controlled trial. J Drugs Dermatol. 2011;10(5):531–7.
87. Kulthanan K, Maneeprasopchoke P, Varothai S, Nuchkull P. The pH of antiseptic cleansers. Asia Pacific Allergy. 2014;4(1):32–6.
88. Broberg A, Faergemann J. Topical antimycotic treatment of atopic dermatitis in the head/neck area. A double-blind randomised study. Acta Derm Venereol. 1995;75(1):46–9.
89. Ryan C, Shaw RE, Cockerell CJ, Hand S, Ghali FE. Novel sodium hypochlorite cleanser shows clinical response and excellent acceptability in the treatment of atopic dermatitis. Pediatr Dermatol. 2013;30(3):308–15.
90. Huang JT, Rademaker A, Paller AS. Dilute bleach baths for *Staphylococcus aureus* colonization in atopic dermatitis to decrease disease severity. Arch Dermatol. 2011;147(2):246–7.
91. Hon KL, Tsang YC, Lee VW, Pong NH, Ha G, Lee ST, et al. Efficacy of sodium hypochlorite (bleach) baths to reduce Staphylococcus aureus colonization in childhood onset moderate-to-severe eczema: a randomized, placebo-controlled cross-over trial. J Dermatol Treat. 2016;27(2):156–62.
92. Ludwig G. [On the topical effect of sea water tub-baths with and without addition of an oil emulsion]. Z Haut Geschlechtskr. 1968;43(16):683–8.
93. Hon KL, Tsang YC, Pong NH, Lee VW, Luk NM, Chow CM, et al. Patient acceptability, efficacy, and skin biophysiology of a cream and cleanser containing lipid complex with shea butter extract versus a ceramide product for eczema. Hong Kong Med J = Xianggang Yi Xue Za Zhi/Hong Kong Acad Med. 2015;21(5):417–25.
94. Lynde CW, Andriessen A. A cohort study on a ceramide-containing cleanser and moisturizer used for atopic dermatitis. Cutis. 2014;93(4):207–13.

Systemic Treatment

Chang Ook Park

Systemic Steroids

Action Mechanisms

Structure and Metabolism of Steroids

All steroids, including glucocorticoids, have four basic ring structures of cholesterols (three hexanes and one pentane). Figure 1 shows the chemical structure of hydrocortisone (cortisol). Glucocorticoids undergo numerous variations in their four-ring structures. Depending on such structural variations, glucocorticoids differ in glucocorticoidal and mineralcorticoidal intensities, action duration, and metabolism.

Absorption and Distribution of Systemic Steroids

Glucocorticoids are naturally occurring cortisones (hydrocortisone) synthesized from cholesterols in the adrenal cortex. They are absorbed in the jejunum and reach the maximum plasma concentration after 30–90 min of administration. If taken with food, it delays the absorption of glucocorticoids but the amount of absorption remains the same. Only less than 5% of the normally circulating cortisol stays unattached. This free cortisol becomes active. The rest of cortisol attaches to CBG (cortisol-binding globulin, transcortin) or albumin and becomes inactive. Cortisol is produced about 10–20 mg every day and peaks at 8 a.m. [1]. The half-life of cortisol in plasma is 90 min. Cortisol is initially metabolized in the liver and shows its hormonal effects in almost every tissue of the whole body. Its metabolites are secreted by the kidney and liver.

The Hypothalamic–Pituitary–Adrenal (HPA) Axis

In order to understand the physiology of glucocorticoids, it is necessary to learn about the normal functions of the HPA axis. Hypothalamus generates corticotropin-releasing hormone (CRH) and anterior pituitary gland reacts with CRH to create adrenocorticotropic hormone (ACTH). ACTH stimulates adrenocortical cells of the adrenal cortex to produce and secrete cortisol. The maximum level of cortisol is released early in the morning before wake up in humans with a normal circadian rhythm. However, its secretion increases up to ten times in a highly stressed condition. ACTH partially involves in the generation of adrenal androgens, but it does not significantly in that of aldosterone, which is a major mineralocorticoid.

There are three main mechanisms related to the internal secretion of cortisol. The first one is negative feedback by plasma cortisol. This mechanism suppresses the hypothalamus and pituitary

C. O. Park (✉)
Department of Dermatology, Cutaneous Biology Research Institute, Yonsei University College of Medicine, Seoul, Korea (Republic of)
e-mail: copark@yuhs.ac

K. H. Lee et al. (eds.), *Practical Insights into Atopic Dermatitis*,
https://doi.org/10.1007/978-981-15-8159-5_15

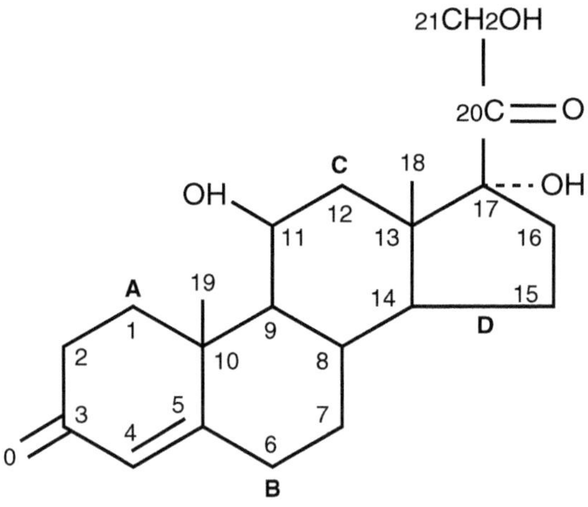

Fig. 1 A chemical structure of hydrocortisone (cortisol)

gland from releasing CRH and ACTH, respectively. Secondly, it is a pulsatile secretion that follows the circadian of ACTH. Cortisol level increases within a few hours after asleep and reaches a peak right before wake up. Finally, the third mechanism reacts to a variety of mental and physical stresses and can produce cortisol at the HPA axis internally as a neural effect. Such neural stimulants are catecholamine in the brainstem and CRH and Vasopressin in the rest of the regions except for the pituitary gland.

Molecular Genetic Action Mechanisms of Systemic Steroids

There are three major action mechanisms of glucocorticoids (Fig. 2).

Firstly, glucocorticoids not bound to cortisol-binding globulin (CBG) are diffused via cell membrane and combine with glucocorticoid receptor protein complex [2]. Glucocorticoid receptor is a protein complex that includes 90 kDa of Heat Shock protein 90 and FK506 binding protein 51 (FKBP51). After binding of glucocorticoids, this receptor replaces FKBP51 with FK506 binding protein 52 (FKBP52). It helps the glucocorticoids move to a nucleus and the receptor is then detached from the protein complex to move to a nucleus. Glucocorticoid receptors in a nucleus bind to specific DNA sequences, the glucocorticoid response elements (GREs) to form a duplex. This is a mechanism of the receptors binding to GREs so that they influence directly on the expression of the genes that induce proteins like annexin I or MAPK phosphatase I. Annexin reduces activities of phospholipase A2 and thus phospholipids of cell membrane release less arachidonic acids. Consequently, annexin diminishes the amount of prostaglandins and leukotrienes [3]. There are approximately 10–100 genes that glucocorticoids directly regulate in the above way.

Secondly, glucocorticoid receptors and other transcription factors interact with each other so that indirectly affect gene expression. One of the most important mechanisms is the suppression of transcription factors, activator protein 1 (AP-1), and nuclear factor-κB (NF-κB). The other one is an increase in IkB, an NF-kB inhibitor [4]. These two reactions indirectly decrease the synthesis of pro-inflammatory molecules such as cytokines, interleukins, adherents, and proteases so that they influence gene expression.

Finally, the third one is a mediating effect of glucocorticoid receptors for the second messenger cascade through the PI3K-Akt-eNOS pathway [5, 6].

mRNAs of human glucocorticoid receptors are splice variants, which have a glucocorticoid receptor (GR)-α and β. The difference in a relative amount of these two variations affects glucocorticoidal susceptibility and a high level of GR-β is associated with glucocorticoid resistance [6, 7].

Normally, there is a delay before pharmacological reactions of glucocorticoids after reaching the maximum plasma concentration. Even if some mechanisms occur regardless of the transcription process, the delay may be caused due to the time taken for transforming gene transcriptions [5]. In a non-genetic way, glucocorticoids show physiochemical interactions with receptors on the membrane or cell membrane. This action is much quicker than some actions of glucocorticoids to be mediated by genetic activities of glucocorticoids [8].

Glucocorticoids have a significant impact on the replication and movement of cells. They reduce blood monocyte, eosinophil, and lymphocyte count with a greater influence on T cells rather

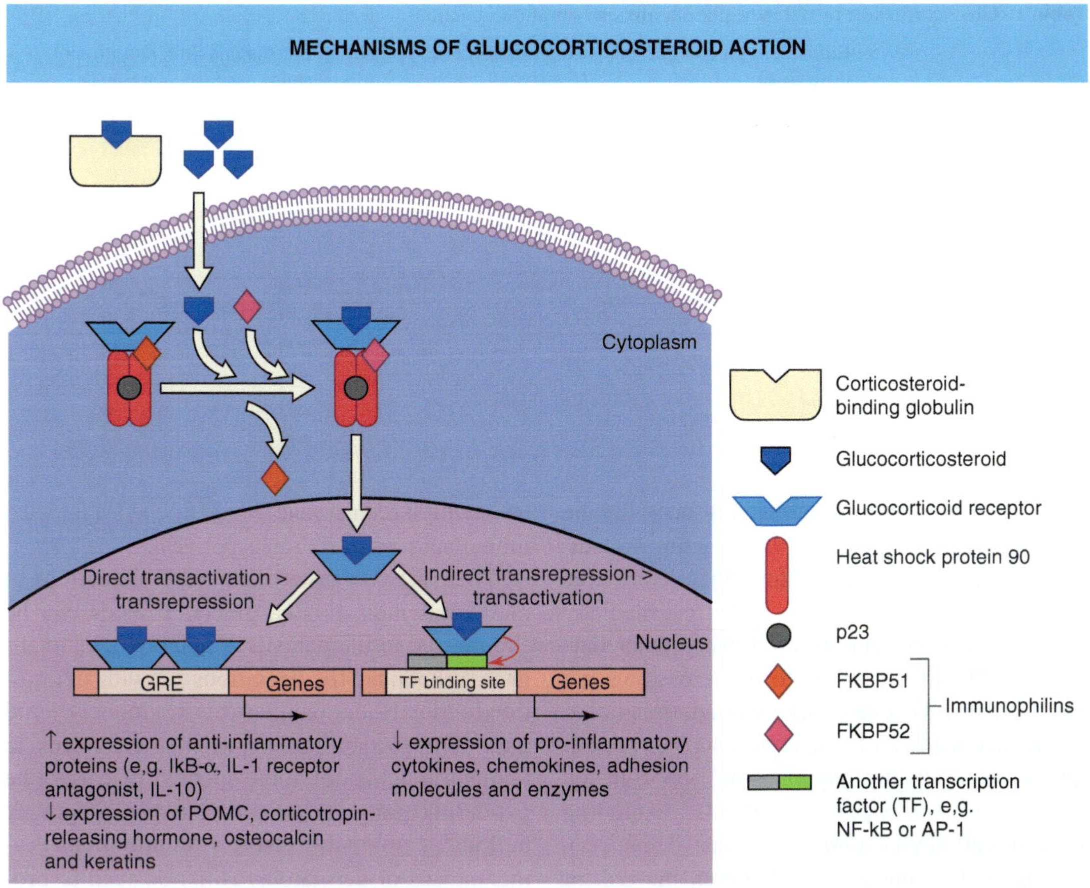

Fig. 2 Action mechanisms of systemic steroids

than B cells [9]. In contrast, neutrophils increase. Glucocorticoids also affect the activation, proliferation, and differentiation of cells. They regulate the levels of IL-1, IL-2, IL-6, and tumor necrosis factor, the mediators of inflammatory and immune responses, and they diminish functions of macrophages [10–13]. Glucocorticoids inhibit the activities of monocytes and lymphocytes more rather than those of neutrophils [14]. In the case of infectious granuloma diseases like tuberculosis, since the symptoms are likely to get better and worse back and forth during chronic glucocorticoid treatment, it is clinically critical. Mast cells display diminished levels of cell maturation, cytokine production, FcεRI (high-affinity IgE receptor) expression, and mediator releases. B cells that generate antibodies or keratinocytes are relatively resistant to glucocorticoid inhibition. A very high dosage of glucocorticoids is required for suspending antibody formation [15].

Types of Steroids (by Potency, for Injection, for Oral)

Table 1 presents the major pharmacological characteristics of glucocorticoids. Half-lives of glucocorticoids vary from 1 to 5 h. On the other hand, plasma half-life is not a good indicator during the biological activation periods of each drug. The biological efficacy duration of a specific glucocorticoids is the most well described as a period when the frontal lobe of the pituitary gland inhibits ACTH release.

As referred in Table 1, since the duration of action of intermediate-acting drugs ranges from

Table 1 Glucocorticoids: by potency, plasma life, and duration of action

	Equivalent glucocorticoid dose (mg)	Mineralocorticoid potency (relative)	Plasma half-life (min)	Duration of action (h)
Short-acting				
Hydrocortisone (Cortisol)	20	0.8	90	8–12
Cortisone	25	1	30	8–12
Intermediate-acting				
Prednisone	5	0.25	60	16–36
Prednisolone	5	0.25	200	12–36
Methylprednisolone	4	0	180	12–36
Triamcinolone	4	0	300	12–36
Long-acting				
Dexamethasone	0.75	0	200	36–54
Betamethasone	0.6	0	200	36–54

24 to 36 h, use intermediate-acting ones for the every-other-day-treatment. Long-acting medicines should be avoided because there is no time for the HPA axis to recover. If the intermediate-acting agents are administered every other day, there is 12 h of recovery for the HPA axis on a rest day. Furthermore, every-other-day-administration can reduce the risk of side effects such as growth inhibition, myopathy, hypertension, opportunistic infections, neuropsychiatric effects (excluding intermittent aggravation of bipolar behaviors), and electrolyte imbalance. However, the risk of osteoporosis and cataract still remains the same.

Glucocorticoids can be administered systemically by injections into the affected lesion (intralesional), IM (intramuscular) or IV (intravascular) injections or oral methods.

Injections into the affected areas can be used for a small number of lesions or those that are resistant to treatments. For intralesional injection, triamcinolone is usually selected for this type of injections and diluted to a target concentration. A small quantity of triamcinolone is injected normally with 30 gauge of a needle. Cautions should be taken for the overdose of triamcinolone, because it may cause atrophy of the dermis or subcutaneous fat.

IM injections present irregular patterns of absorption, and cannot control the dosage every day. The duration of action is within 1 week for IM injection of betamethasone or dexamethasone, whereas it is about 3 weeks for that of triamcinolone or methylprednisolone. Thus, triamcinolone and methylprednisolone should not be IM injected more than four to six times per year.

There are two cases that need IV injections of glucocorticoids. Firstly, glucocorticoids can be IV injected to the patients at acute phases of illness, scheduled for operations or with deteriorated adrenal functions due to daily glucocorticoid uses. The second case is when there needs to regulate quickly for some specific diseases like pyoderma gangrenosum, severe pemphigus or bullous pemphigoid, severe systemic lupus erythematosus or dermatomyositis, or need to provide less frequent oral treatments of high-dosage steroids for a long term. IV injection of methylprednisolone is recommended for such an event because of the high potency and low efficacy of mineralocorticoids, and the dosage ranges from 500 mg to 1 g for daily treatment. The serious adverse reactions related to IV injections are anaphylaxis, seizure, arrhythmia, and sudden death. Other adverse events are hypotension, hypertension, hyperglycemia, electrolyte imbalance, and acute mental diseases, etc. It is advised to slowly administer the drug for 2–3 h in order to minimize the risk of serious adverse reactions. The administration is not necessarily monitored for the patients without underlying kidneys or heart diseases if their vital signs are measured frequently [16]. It is especially important for patients who are co-administering diuretic agents to observe their electrolyte levels before and after a high dosage of systemic steroid treatments.

Prednisone is the most common oral glucocorticoid medicine. Oral glucocorticoids are usually administered once a day or once every other day. In order to control the progress after treatment, the initial dosage of oral glucocorticoids ranges from 2.5 mg to a few hundred milligrams for every day administration. If the oral ones are to be administered less than 3–4 weeks, the patient can suspend the intake without decreasing gradually. It minimizes the risk of side effects to taking the lowest dosage of the short-acting drugs every other day. Since a cortisol level is the highest at 8 a.m., administering drugs before noon effect reduction of HPA axis the least. Thus, intermediate-acting agents are normally administered once every morning to suppress the HPA axis. Before starting to use glucocorticoids, there should be more benefits expected than potential adverse reactions. If considering a long-term treatment, not only alternatives or supplements but also accompanying diseases like diabetes, hypertension, and osteoporosis must be evaluated.

There are a number of cautions to be taken when selecting glucocorticoids. Firstly, one must choose the drug that usually has the lowest mineralocorticoid effects. Next, use oral prednisolone or a similar one that has about a middle level of the half-life and weak bonding with steroid receptors especially if long-term uses are considered. Third, if cortisone or prednisone does not work on the patients, consider replacing cortisone or prednisone into biologically active forms, such as cortisol or prednisolone. Lastly, one must use methylprednisolone for the treatment with high dosage drugs due to their high potency and low mineralocorticoid effects.

Indications and Efficacy of Systemic Steroids for the Treatment of Atopic Dermatitis

In the recent guidelines from Korea, America, Europe, and Japan, there are similar opinions about indications and efficacy of systemic steroids for atopic dermatitis. However, there have not been any double-blinded randomized clinical trials to investigate the effects of systemic steroids for atopic dermatitis [17]. First of all, the following context is from the guideline of The Korean Atopic Dermatitis Association.

According to the guideline, systemic steroids can significantly improve clinical symptoms of atopic dermatitis, but patients should normally avoid using them due to their adverse reactions and rebound phenomenon. There is a frequent rebound phenomenon observed after an immediate withdrawal of systemic steroids. Thus, it is very critical to gradually reduce the dosage over time after the clinical symptoms improve. In the clinical study, it has been reported that skin glucocorticoid concentrations displayed similarities between patients who administered the strong topical steroids (clobetasol propionate 0.05%, hydrocortisone 2.3%, or triamcinolone 0.1%) and patients who administered oral prednisone. However, if the skin gets severe damage, the distribution of topical steroids becomes irregular. Therefore, oral administration is safer. It is not recommended for atopic dermatitis to the use of consecutive or chronic and intermittent steroids. Nonetheless, they can be considered as a transitional treatment for the cases that are progressing quickly or severe before starting non-steroidal systemic immune modulators or phototherapy. Dosage is determined depending on the body weights and administered at 0.5~1.0 mg/kg of dosage for an acute exacerbation phase. In conclusion, even though steroids are not recommended in terms of their risk and benefit ratio, they can be an option for treating acutely aggravating cases (The level of evidence is equivalent to that of an expert; level of evidence 5, strength of recommendation D) [18].

Similarly, in the guidelines of America, Europe, and Japan, it is not recommended to use systemic steroids for atopic dermatitis but rather it is advising to use them temporarily only for the acute exacerbation cases or for certain patients who just started using other types of systemic drugs or phototherapy and there has not been any efficacy shown yet. Furthermore, it also describes that there is a correlation between using systemic steroids for the short term without reducing the dosage gradually and a high recurrence rate or aggravation of the symptoms [17, 19, 20].

Adverse Events of Systemic Steroids

It is greatly normal to use glucocorticoids for acute skin disease for a short term. The common adverse events of administering glucocorticoids for a short term are mood changes, gastrointestinal disturbance (nausea, vomiting), high blood sugar, electrolyte imbalance, increased appetite, weight gain, acneiform eruption, increased infection, amenorrhea, muscle atrophy, and impact on wound healing. Table 2 gives a summary of adverse events when used glucocorticoids for a long term. Most of the adverse reactions are dependent on dosage.

Osteoporosis

Being one of the most common complications found in patients who are administering systemic glucocorticoids, osteoporosis occurs at a rate of about 40%. It especially affects children, adolescents, and females after menopause. Even if the patients receive therapy every other day, it is impossible to avoid osteoporosis [21]. Fracture of the spine is found in one-third of the patients who administered glucocorticoids for 5–10 years [22, 23]. Bone loss proceeds quickly within the first 6 months of glucocorticoid administration; however, the symptom continues at a slower pace after the initial period and 3~10% of additional bone loss happens every year [21, 24]. According to recent studies, it has been reported that a low dosage of prednisone (2.5 mg of every day) may affect the bone and cause spine and pelvic fracture [25]. Young patients may recover from bone loss after suspension of glucocorticoid intake [26].

Table 2 Adverse reactions when using glucocorticoids for a long term

Musculoskeletal system
Osteoporosis, avascular necrosis, growth retardation, muscle atrophy, myopathy
Ophthalmic system
Cataract, glaucoma, infection, bleeding, ocular proptosis
Gastrointestinal system
Nausea, vomiting, gastroesophageal reflux, gastric/duodenal ulcers, perforation, pancreatitis, (reflux or candida) esophagitis
Metabolic system
Hyperglycemia, hyperlipidemia, obesity, hypocalcemia, hypokalemic alkalosis
Cardiovascular system
Hypertension, peripheral edema, atherosclerosis
Gynecological system
Amenorrhea, fetal effect
Hematologic, Cellular system
Leukocytosis, neutrophilia, lymphocytopenia, eosinopenia, immunosuppression, impaired fibroplasia, reduced in mitosis rate, infection
Nervous system
Change in mood or personality, psychosis, seizures, pseudotumor cerebri, peripheral neuropathy
Skin
Skin atrophy, striae distensae, telangiectasia, vascular fragility, purpura, acne, acneiform eruption, hirsutism, infection
HPA Axis
HPA axis suppression, withdrawal syndrome, adrenal crisis

Glucocorticoids inhibit osteoblasts, increase excretion of calcium from the kidneys, reduce calcium absorption in gastrointestinal tracts, and elevate bone resorption of osteoclasts. Furthermore, glucocorticoids decrease the level of estrogens and testosterone, which are critical factors of osteoporosis. Administering prednisone of the daily dosage of 7.5 mg or more induces severe damage on bones and increase fracture rates [27]. With the release of the new drugs that can alleviate such bone loss, it is becoming more important to prevent osteoporosis. The primary treatments are supplements of calcium and Vitamin D, injecting sex hormones, weight-bearing exercise programs, and sodium restriction. Supplying calcium and Vitamin D simultaneously, bone mass can be maintained normally in the patients who are administering steroids for a long term. On the other hand, calcium monotherapy does not have such an effect. Patients who are administering glucocorticoids must take 1500 mg of calcium and 400 units of vitamin D2 twice every day. They should also get serum and 24 h of urine tests every 3 months.

Avascular Necrosis

Avascular necrosis refers to intraosseous hypertension, which causes bone ischemia and necrosis; it thus results in pain, and movement limit of one or more joints. Intraosseous fat cell hypertrophy is thought to induce intraosseous hypertension in the patients administering glucocorticoids [28]. Moreover, glucocorticoids promote cell death of osteoblasts and contribute to avascular necrosis. Glucocorticoids also increase the possibility of steroid-induced-avascular-necrosis in those who have systemic lupus erythematosus or other underlying diseases [29]. A number of studies have suggested that patients with avascular necrosis have excessive platelets or thrombotic blockade of vein excretion in the bones due to low fibrinogen, and consequently, arterial blood flow decreases to cause necrosis [30]. In order to prevent avascular necrosis from advancing to degenerative joint diseases that require replacement of joints, initial diagnosis and treatments are significant. In 20% of the avascular necrosis patients, their X-ray results seem to be normal. So, it is recommended to have more sensitive examinations such as bone scan and magnetic resonance imaging (MRI). Ask regularly about pain and joint movement impairment, and if there is any, perform an X-ray, bone scan, and MRI immediately. If the MRI result turned out to be avascular necrosis, the patient should get decompression therapy from orthopedists to inhibit any further progression of the disease. Joint replacement surgery may be required for the case of which avascular necrosis has progressed to destructive joint disease [31]. There may remain some risks to other joints in avascular necrosis patients, general care is necessary.

Myopathy

Myopathy, a rare complication of glucocorticoids, displays painless and symmetric proximal muscular atrophy mainly in legs. It usually occurs within a few weeks or months after administering an overdose of a systemic steroid, prednisolone 40 mg. It is not a common adverse event that happened when administering drugs like dexamethasone, betamethasone, and triamcinolone; however, it can occur by any type of medicine. It is difficult to diagnose myopathy because a level of serum muscle enzymes and electromyogram present normal results, and the majority of muscle biopsy tests seem to be non-specific. However, an elevation of urine creatinine excretion can prove the diagnosis.

Cataract

Posterior subcapsular cataract is likely to occur in the patients administering systemic glucocorticoids depending on their accumulated dosage and medication periods. This adverse event is also observed in the patients who have taken 10 mg of prednisone every day for a year, and administering every other day does not decrease the risk of cataract. Cataract, which develops in the course of atopic dermatitis, normally starts in the anterior portion of the papillary region, but also in the posterior position, making it difficult to distinguish cataracts from glucocorticoid-related cataracts.

Gastrointestinal Adverse Reactions

It is controversial whether the incidence of peptic ulcer diseases increases when taking glucocorticoids, but it has been reported to increase peptic ulcers by ninefold when co-administering glucocorticoids and non-steroidal anti-inflammatory drugs. If a patient has two or more risk factors (combining non-steroidal anti-inflammatory drugs, previous peptic ulcer history, progressive malignant diseases, total glucocorticoid doses greater than 1000 mg), take antacids, H2 receptor blockers, proton pump inhibitors, or others as a preventive medicine.

Metabolic Effects

Systemic treatment with glucocorticoids elevates the risk of hyperglycemia and hyperlipidemia. Glucocorticoids affect glucose metabolism and cause hyperglycemia. Thus, blood glucose testing should be conducted periodically at a high dose or for the long-term steroid use. Hyperlipidemia is also a common adverse reaction, and an elevation of triglycerides is common and there may be an increase in high-density or low-density lipoproteins in some patients. A low saturated fat and calorie diet are advised for long-term glucocorticoid treatment. In addition, glucocorticoids may cause weight gain, redistribution of fat to the central trunk, hypokalemic alkalosis, and rarely hypocalcemia. Depending on the cases, there may be a need for potassium supply and proper calorie intake is essential.

Atherosclerosis

Glucocorticoids increase atherosclerosis-related risk factors such as arterial hypertension, insulin resistance, glucose intolerance, hyperlipidemia, and central obesity. Therefore, it is not surprising that the risk of atherosclerosis increases in patients taking glucocorticoids. Patients with untreated Cushing's syndrome are known to have a fourfold increase in mortality from cardiovascular complications. In patients with Cushing's syndrome, the risk of atherosclerosis persists at least for 5 years after a level of serum cortisol returns to be normal, even in those who are chronically treated with glucocorticoids. Blood pressure, serum lipids, and glucose levels should be measured periodically. If there are any abnormalities, treat with food control or medications depending on the symptoms. Smokers should quit smoking.

Gynecological Effects

Glucocorticoids penetrate the placenta but do not cause malformation. There was controversy about the safety of glucocorticoids in the first trimester of pregnancy because of a cleft lip observed in the rat exposed to a very high dose of glucocorticoids at the early stage of pregnancy. However, clinical experiences and several clinical trials have presented that there is little effect in the fetus of pregnant women treated with glucocorticoids. Since placental enzymes, such as 11-hydroxysteroid dehydrogenase type 2, inactivate most of the prednisolone that go to the fetal circulatory system, only a small quantity of active form of prednisone is delivered to the fetus of pregnant patients. On the other hand, the enzymes are less in their ability to metabolize betamethasone and dexamethasone, which reach the fetus more in amount. There is a slightly elevated risk of hypertension and glucose intolerance in pregnant women undergoing glucocorticoid treatments. Administrating a high dosage of glucocorticoids near the time of pregnancy can result in fetal HPA axis depression. Cautions need to be taken about adrenal and growth limitations for the fetus exposed to glucocorticoids and the infants breastfed from mothers taking glucocorticoids. Although glucocorticoids can be excreted through breast milk, the American Academy of Pediatrics suggested that prednisone therapy is available in lactating mothers. In non-pregnant women, amenorrhea may occur when glucocorticoids are injected intramuscularly. To prevent unnecessary concerns, this possibility of adverse events should be explained to premenopausal women who are treated with glucocorticoids.

Nervous System Effects

Adverse reactions such as mood changes, anxiety, and insomnia are dose-dependent of glucocorticoids. Depression and fatigue are common symptoms during glucocorticoid tapering, and psychosis is a rare side effect that is common in people with major psychiatric disorders previously. Pseudotumor Cerebri is a possible complication of high-dose long-term glucocorticoid treatment and are manifested as headaches, nausea, vomiting, abnormal vision, and papillary edema. These symptoms can occur when you taper or stop glucocorticoids quickly. Seizure is a rare but possible complication of high-dose glucocorticoid treatment.

Skin

Skin adverse reactions similar to those of Cushing's syndrome may occur, such as purpura, telangiectasia, skin atrophy, stretch marks, and acneiform eruption. Topical or intralesional glucocorticoid injections can cause skin atrophy and hypopigmentation. Acne or folliculitis caused by systemic steroids occurs mainly in the trunk and appears as monomorphous pustules or papules. In addition, acne itself can usually worsen after continuous glucocorticoid treatment. Other skin side effects may include acanthosis nigricans, telogen effluvium, and hirsutism. Systemic steroids inhibit wound healing by inhibiting fibroblast function and collagen production. Besides, systemic steroids inhibit angiogenesis, production of extracellular matrix, and wound re-epithelialization.

Adrenal Suppression

Gradual tapering of glucocorticoid therapy may help prevent disease exacerbations, but gradual tapering is usually not necessary with respect to adrenal function recovery if it is used for a short-term period of about less than 3 weeks. However, gradual tapering is important for adrenal recovery in the case of more than 3 weeks of treatment. Symptoms of glucocorticoid withdrawal syndrome include joint pain, muscle pain, emotional changes, fatigue, headache, and gastrointestinal symptoms (nausea, vomiting, and anorexia). Patients with steroid withdrawal syndrome experience symptoms of adrenal insufficiency despite normal cortisol response to ACTH. Common symptoms of adrenal insufficiency include drowsiness, weakness, anorexia, fever, orthostatic hypotension, hypoglycemia, and weight loss. If this syndrome occurs, it is recommended to return to the previous glucocorticoid dose and reduce it more slowly. The best reduction is to change from daily dose to every other day and then gradually reduce the amount of medicine. After prednisolone is reduced to 5 mg every other day, it should be evaluated whether maintenance therapy is necessary. Reduce to 5 mg dose and measure plasma cortisol levels at 8 am after 4 weeks. If plasma cortisol levels are less than 10 μg/dL, the every-other-day dose should be reduced by 1 mg every 1–2 weeks until the maintenance dose reaches 2 mg/day [32]. Later on, plasma cortisol levels at 8 am should be measured every 2 months until they become higher than 10 μg/dL. Recovery of the HPA axis can take more than 9 months. At steroid tapering, acute adrenal insufficiency may result from inappropriate stresses due to trauma, surgery, diarrhea, high fever, and the like. Adrenal insufficiency usually recovers within 1 year of glucocorticoid discontinuation. ACTH (cosyntropin) stimulation tests may be performed to assess adrenal function following glucocorticoid discontinuation.

Mental Effects

Mood and cognitive changes are dose-dependent and may appear immediately after glucocorticoid initiation. Hypomania and mania are the most common symptoms early on, but continued use of glucocorticoids is more often associated with depression. Although there are no clinical trials, antipsychotics, anticonvulsants, and antidepressants can improve mood swings.

Drug Interaction

Glucocorticoids interact with many drugs. Drugs that induce liver microsomal enzymes, such as barbiturate, phenytoin, and rifampin, can promote glucocorticoid metabolism. Drugs such as cholestyramine, colestipol, and antacid reduce glucocorticoid absorption. Glucocorticoids reduce serum salicylate levels and one should increase the warfarin dose to maintain the anticoagulant effect of warfarin upon co-administration.

Immunological Adverse Events

Patients treated with glucocorticoids are highly susceptible to bacterial, viral, fungal, and parasitic infections. Staphylococcal and superficial fungal infections of the skin are very common. During glucocorticoid treatment, the expression of fever and signs of inflammation are hidden, making it difficult to detect early infections. Every other day administration and less than 10 mg of prednisone decrease the risk of opportunistic infections. Glucocorticoids interfere with lymphocytes and monocytes, reducing delayed hypersensitivity. Although reactivation of tuberculosis has been a concern in patients chronically treated with glucocorticoids, it is reported to be less harmful than previously thought. A tuberculosis examination is required, and a tuberculin skin test or interferon-gamma secretion test should also be conducted if necessary. Chest X-rays are taken in those who show positive results for tuberculin skin test and interferon-gamma secretion tests, and a history of tuberculosis among patients administering prednisolone greater than 15 mg. Patients receiving chronic glucocorticoid treatment may develop an inappropriate antibody response to the vaccine. Patients taking more than 20 mg of prednisone (no less than 2 mg/kg/day for children weighing below 10 kg) should not get injections of live vaccines within 1 month after glucocorticoid discontinuation.

Special Consideration When Used in Pediatric Patients

In children, glucocorticoids can cause developmental impairment and early osteoporosis. Growth delays are caused by direct effects on cell metabolism, calcium and phosphorous metabolism, growth hormone decrease, and inhibition of bone matrix formation, and cannot be prevented even by administering glucocorticoids every other day.

Other Systemic Immunomodulatory Therapies

The most basic treatment for atopic dermatitis is the use of topical steroids and topical calcineurin inhibitors. In most patients with atopic dermatitis, topical steroids or topical calcineurin inhibitors improve symptoms, but in some cases, topical treatments are not effective and topical steroids are difficult to use due to "steroid phobia." Short-term use of systemic steroids can be highly effective for acute exacerbation of severe atopic dermatitis. However, if systemic steroids have been administered for a long-term period, they are known to cause various serious adverse reactions such as diabetes, hypertension, osteoporosis, and the like, including the ones related to the endocrine system. Therefore, it is advised to administer systemic steroids restrictively for acute exacerbation of severe cases. As a result, systemic immunomodulators are used when severe atopic dermatitis patients who do not respond to topical agents continue to relapse and get worse. Here we introduce systemic immunomodulators that have been widely used so far (Table 3) [33].

Table 3 Overview of systemic therapies in severe atopic dermatitis

Ingredient	Approved/not approved for AD therapy	Mechanism of action	Significant adverse reactions
Azathioprine	Not approved	Inhibition of Purine synthesis → inhibit proliferation of lymphocytes	Change in a blood count, gastrointestinal diseases, hepatotoxicity, pancreatitis, fetal toxicity
Systemic corticosteroids	Approved	Anti-inflammation, anti-proliferation, vasoconstriction	Increase in a risk of infection, delay in wound healing, muscle weakness, osteoporosis, glaucoma, occurrence or exacerbation of diabetes, increase in risk of thrombosis, stomach ulcer, moon-face, obesity, hirsutism, steroid rebound reactions, delayed growth in children
Cyclosporine A	Approved in adult patients with severe intolerant AD	Inhibitor of calcineurin Inhibit IL-2 → reduced T cell proliferation	Renal toxicity, increased bilirubin and liver enzyme levels, elevated blood lipids, hypertension, gum hypertrophy, central nervous system disturbances, gastrointestinal disorders, susceptible to infections, tumorigenesis, change in a blood count, fetal toxicity
Tacrolimus	Systemic agents are not approved Only topical ones are approved	Inhibitor of calcineurin Inhibit IL-2 → reduced T cell proliferation	Renal toxicity, neurotoxicity, central nervous system disturbance, metabolic syndrome, gastrointestinal diseases, susceptible to infections, tumor incidence, changes in blood count, fetal toxicity
Mycophenolate mofetil	Not approved	Inhibitor of lymphocyte proliferation Prevent de novo synthesis of Purine → decreased cell proliferation	Gastrointestinal disorders, leukopenia, susceptible to infections, sepsis, fetal toxicity, neurotoxicity, nephrotoxicity, hypertension, hyperglycemia
Methotrexate	Not approved	Antifolate Inhibit Purine and thymidine (DNA synthesis) → decreased cell proliferation	Hepatotoxicity, nephrotoxicity, change in a blood cell count, infections, lymphadenopathy, malformations

Cyclosporine

Cyclosporine is a polypeptide isolated from *Tolypocladium inflatum gams* and *Cyclindrocarpon lucidum* fungi and is known as a potent inhibitor of T cell-dependent immune reactions, usually for the treatment and management of organ transplant patients. Recently, it is used as a treatment for numerous immune-mediated skin diseases such as psoriasis, pemphigus, Behçet's disease, and atopic dermatitis. Cyclosporine selectively acts on CD4+ helper T cells without inhibiting bone marrow to inhibit the production of IL-1 and IL-2, proliferation of helper T cells, ultimately preventing activation of helper T cells and maturation of cytotoxic T cells. By blocking T cell-dependent immune reactions, it can thus be applied to patients with severe atopic dermatitis who do not respond with the conventional treatments. As a treatment method, it is common to administer 3–5 mg/kg daily for 6–8 weeks as an initial dosage, and the symptoms appear to enhance very quickly within 2 weeks of the start of treatment. If the treatment is stopped, the disease usually recurs within 8 weeks, but the symptoms are more alleviated than before treatment and no rebound phenomenon occurs. Maintenance therapies include a method of reducing 1 mg/kg every 2 weeks, increasing the medication interval every 2 weeks, 4 mg/kg daily for the first 4–8 weeks, and then 0.5–0.7 mg daily for 13–34 months, and other methods. Side effects of cyclosporine include hypertension, nephrotoxicity, hyperlipidemia, vomiting, diarrhea, elevated liver enzymes, hirsutism, gum hypertrophy, anemia, encephalitis, and drug interactions (Table 4). Especially cyclosporine may cause severe adverse reactions, such as hypertension and renal toxicity, thus measuring blood pressure, blood cyclosporine concentrations, and performing renal function tests are recommended while administering cyclosporine (Table 5). Cautions need to be taken because cyclosporine may interact with drugs like azoles, macrolide antibiotics, hormonal contraceptives, calcium channel blockers, anti-epileptics, and sulfones. It is contraindicated in patients with active skin infection of *Staphylococcus aureus* or *Herpes simplex*, immunosuppressed patients, patients with severe chronic diseases, patients with renal dysfunction, patients with hypertension and malignancy, and those who do not follow the instructions of the physicians (Table 6). It has been reported to cause less adverse reactions if the drug is administered initially at 5 mg/kg and then decrease the dose gradually to 1–2 mg/kg and

Table 4 Adverse reactions of cyclosporine

Organ	Symptoms
Kidney	Elevation in BUN/creatinine and uric acid, decrease in glomerular filtration rate (GFR)
Cardiovascular system	Hypertension, hyperlipidemia
Gastrointestinal system	Vomiting, diarrhea, elevation in SGOT, and alkaline phosphatase
Mucocutaneous system	Hirsutism, gum hypertrophy
Hematological system	Anemia
Nervous system	Encephalitis, tremor
Others	Hands and feet burning sensation, drug interactions (Azoles, macrolide antibiotics, hormonal contraceptives, calcium channel blockers, anticonvulsants, sulfones)

Table 5 Monitoring of renal function and blood pressure during cyclosporine treatment

Main monitoring issues
Renal function
(i) Measure serum creatinine at 2-weekly intervals for first 3 months, then measure monthly thereafter (ii) For patients on long-term therapy (>12 months continuous treatment), assess annual renal function using creatinine clearance to estimate glomerular filtration rate
Blood pressure
Measure blood pressure at +2 weeks, +4 weeks, and +8 weeks, then measure monthly thereafter

Table 6 Cyclosporine contraindications

• Patients administering erythromycin and azole antifungal agents, which inhibit the metabolism of cyclosporine
• Patients with active skin infection of *Staphylococcus aureus* or *Herpes simplex*
• Patients with immunosuppression, severe chronic diseases, renal dysfunction, hypertension, or malignant tumors
• Patients who do not follow the instructions of the physicians

maintain it when the patients show clinical improvement. Cyclosporine has been reported to be effective in children, but cautions should be taken to adverse reactions [34–38].

Azathioprine

Azathioprine is a systemic immunomodulator secondarily used when primary treatment with cyclosporine is ineffective or has side effects in Korea. Azathioprine is an imidazole derivative of 6-mercaptopurine (MP), which is known to inhibit the proliferation of B and T cells by blocking DNA and RNA synthesis. In atopic dermatitis patients, after azathioprine therapy, more than 80% of patients showed significant improvement. When the patients administered azathioprine per 2.5 mg/kg daily, their clinical symptoms significantly improved than those of a placebo group in a double-blind clinical study [39]. Therefore, azathioprine may be appropriately used in patients with severe atopic dermatitis who do not respond to conventional treatments. When azathioprine was used in Korean atopic dermatitis patients who did not respond to previous treatments, the skin symptoms and pruritus of atopic dermatitis improved, thus it was confirmed that azathioprine could be used as a secondary drug for intractable atopic dermatitis [40]. Azathioprine is rarely associated with gastrointestinal disturbance, liver dysfunction, and pancytopenia. However, pancytopenia caused by bone marrow suppression is particularly a fatal case and it occurs when thiopurine methyltransferase (TPMT) activity decreases. Thus, before administering azathioprine, it is better to begin the therapy after taking a genetic test that evaluates TPMT activity and confirming the TPMT function is normal.

There have been reports about various uses of azathioprine in atopic dermatitis, and most of the cases used 1–3 mg/kg a day. No optimal dose is recommended yet, but the most common method is to initiate with a lower dose and gradually increase the dose to minimize any adverse events. Some patients require administering azathioprine for at least 12 weeks because this drug shows its efficacy slowly. When symptoms of atopic dermatitis improve, it is advised to reduce the amount of the drug and maintain the therapy with topical and moisturizing supplements. Concomitant use of azathioprine and phototherapy is not recommended due to elevated DNA damage and a risk of carcinogenicity. Although there are no suggested optimal usage and duration of treatment for atopic dermatitis in children because there are not many studies on the use of azathioprine for pediatric atopic dermatitis groups, they usually administer at 2.5 mg/kg/day and it has been also reported to use maximum at 4 mg/kg/day.

Methotrexate (MTX)

Methotrexate (MTX) is a folic acid antagonist that inhibits DNA and RNA synthesis by blocking the synthesis of purine and pyrimidine. By preventing the proliferation of lymphocytes, MTX shows its pharmacological actions. It also hinders lymphocyte migration and cytokine secretion and ultimately induces lymphocyte apoptosis. MTX is known to be effective in patients with moderate and severe atopic dermatitis and can be in patients with severe atopic dermatitis in children who do not respond to conventional therapies. Before using MTX, it is necessary to perform a liver function test to confirm that liver function is normal in advance. Continuous accumulation of MTX may lead to hepatotoxicity, which requires periodic monitoring. Oral administration of folic acid is sometimes recommended to prevent adverse reactions.

MTX is usually administered once per week as done for psoriasis. Doses have been reported to be 7.5–25 mg/week, and the regimen is sometimes three times a week at a 12-h interval. The average time to show its maximum efficacy is reported to be 10 weeks and consider increasing the dose if it does not work even after 12–16 weeks of administration. However, it is advised to discontinue the therapy if administering more than 15 mg/week turns out to be ineffective. If the symptoms of atopic dermatitis improve with MTX treatment, consider decreasing the dose. Moisturizers and topical treatments may be used as maintenance therapy, and phototherapy may be considered [41, 42].

Mycophenolate Mofetil (MMF)

Mycophenolate mofetil (MMF) is a 2-morpholinoethyl ester precursor of mycophenolic acid and isolated from Penicillium species. To date, it has been used in patients with acute kidney graft rejection or as an immunosuppressant for patients who had heart transplantation. Since the 1970s, MMF also has been administered to patients with psoriasis and bullous disease. By inhibiting inosine monophosphate (IMP) dehydrogenase, MMF prevents de novo synthesis of purine. IMP dehydrogenase converts IMP into xanthosine monophosphate (XMP), which promotes the production of GTP required for RNA, DNA, and protein synthesis. Thus, MMF acts as an inhibitor of guanosine nucleotide synthesis. Lymphocytes depend more on the de novo pathway than on the salvage pathway during the process of purine biosynthesis, by which MMF hinders the proliferation of T and B cells. MMF also inhibits glycoproteins, which play a role in leukocyte adhesion to vascular endothelial cells. MMF treatment improved symptoms of severe or moderate atopic dermatitis patients who did not respond to any of the systemic steroids, phototherapy, or cyclosporine treatments. The usual dosage of MMF is 0.5–1 g twice a day, and the overdose may cause nausea, abdominal pain, gastritis, neurotoxicity, nephrotoxicity, hypertension, hyperglycemia, and infections, but MMF has relatively fewer adverse events than azathioprine or cyclosporine does [43–45].

Other Alternative Therapies

Antihistamines

Mechanisms and Types of Antihistamine Agents

Antihistamines were first synthesized in the 1930s and have been used in clinical practices since the 1940s, and as antiallergic drugs since the 1950s. In the 1980s, so-called second-generation antihistamines, which have a low frequency of adverse drug reactions, were developed and have been used worldwide. Depending on their chemical structures, antihistamines are classified into six groups: alkylamine, piperazine, piperidine, ethanolamine, ethylendiamine, and phenothiazine. Each antihistamine acts through four different receptors (H1, H2, H3, H4). Table 7 describes expression sites of each receptor, types of representative antihistamines, clinical use [46].

Mainly symptoms like vasodilation, urticaria, and itching are associated with H1 receptors. By blocking H1 receptors, antihistamines relieve the itching caused by histamine in the treatment of atopic dermatitis [47]. However, other various mediators can cause itching in atopic dermatitis other than histamines. Thus, some patients do not respond to antihistamine therapies. Although it is controversial how effective antihistamines can be in treating the pruritus of atopic dermatitis, many physicians prefer oral administration of antihistamines in real clinical practice. Table 8 includes representative therapeutic targets of H1 antihistamines (Table 8).

There are two types of H1 antihistamines: (1) the first-generation H1 antihistamines that pass through the blood–brain barrier and (2) the second-generation H1 antihistamines that cannot pass through the blood–brain barrier. Typical first-generation H1 antihistamines include hydroxyzine, chlorpheniramine, tripelennamine, cyproheptadine, diphenhydramine. The major efficacy of these drugs is reducing erythema, size, and number of acute urticaria and relieving itchiness. Adverse reactions of the first-generation H1 antihistamines are lack of concentration, difficulty in learning and multitasking, shortening of restful rapid eye movement (REM) sleep periods, and increasing latency of the onset of REM sleep. Alcohols enhance the sedative effects of these drugs, and there are other adverse reactions such as arrhythmia, tachycardia, anxiety, hypotension, difficulty passing urine, etc. These adverse reactions occur more especially in children, the elderly, and those with liver or kidney diseases. Diphenhydramine can induce QT interval prolongation and torsades de pointes. Representative second-generation H1 antihistamines are fexofenadine, loratadine, cetirizine, ebastine, levo-

Table 7 The types of histamine receptors

Receptor	GPCR signaling	Expression	Representative antihistamine	Clinical use/potential use
H1	Gq/G11 family to phospholipase C stimulation	CNS neurons, smooth muscle cells (vascular, respiratory, and GI), CVS, neutrophils, eosinophils, monocytes, macrophages, DCs, T and B cells, endothelial cells, epithelial cells	Chlorpheniramine, diphenhydramine, hydroxyzine, cetirizine, desloratadine, fexofenadine, levocetirizine, loratadine, and 40 others	Allergic rhinitis, allergic conjunctivitis, urticaria; used in many other allergic diseases and nonallergic diseases, including CNS diseases
H2	Gs family to adenylate cyclase stimulation and cyclic AMP	Gastric parietal cells, smooth muscle, CNS, CVS, neutrophils, eosinophils, monocytes, macrophages, DCs, T and B cells, endothelial cells, epithelial cells	Cimetidine, ranitidine, famotidine, nizatidine	Peptic ulcer disease and gastroesophageal reflux disease
H3	Gi/o family to adenylate cyclase inhibition and Y cyclic AMP	CNS and peripheral neurons, CVS, lungs, monocytes, eosinophils, endothelial cells	No agents approved for use to date; those in clinical trials include JNJ 39220675 and PF-03654746 for allergic rhinitis	Potentially useful in allergic rhinitis and neurologic disorders, including Alzheimer disease, attention-deficit hyperactivity disorder, schizophrenia, epilepsy, narcolepsy, and neuropathic pain; also in obesity
H4	Gi/o family to adenylate cyclase inhibition and Y cyclic AMP	Neutrophils, eosinophils, monocytes, DCs, Langerhans cells, T cells, basophils, mast cells, fibroblasts, bone marrow, endocrine cells, and CNS	No agents approved for use to date; those in clinical trials have included JNJ 7777120 for allergic rhinitis and pruritus, UR 65380 and UR 63825 for pruritus	Potentially useful in allergic rhinitis, atopic dermatitis/eczema, and asthma and in other chronic inflammatory disorders and autoimmune disorders

cetirizine, etc. These agents have less sedative effects because they have lower lipophilicity thus cannot penetrate the blood–brain barrier. In the past, terfenadine and astemizole were used for the treatment; however, they are no longer in use due to their serious adverse reactions like QT interval prolongation and torsades de pointes. Fexofenadine is known to be the least sedative drug. Cetirizine acts on H1 receptors of the CNS in proportion to its dose. Ebastine is metabolized by cytochrome P450 enzymes of the liver, whereas fexofenadine, desloratadine, and cetirizine are less metabolized in the liver and therefore interact with other drugs less. Ebastine should not be co-administered with antifungals, macrolide antibiotics, and doxepin. As an active metabolite of terfenadine, fexofenadine causes fewer adverse reactions and is effective in treating chronic idiopathic urticaria and allergic rhinitis. Patients with kidney disease, including the elderly, need to adjust the dose, but fexofenadine is not well metabolized in the liver so it is safe to use for liver disease. Loratadine has less sedative actions and can be administered to patients with cardiac arrhythmias. However, it is relatively less effective because it cannot inhibit histamine release well enough. Cetirizine is a metabolite of hydroxyzine and has a sedative action slightly. However, it is not well metabolized in the liver, so it is safe to co-administer with antifungals, macrolide antibiotics, and doxepin, inducing less sedative or anticholinergic effects. Since it has efficacy for treating diseases with high eosinophil infiltration by restricting chemotaxis, it also works well for treating physical urticaria. In children, second-generation antihistamines are safe

Table 8 Clinical uses of H1 antihistamines

Strong evidence base for second-generation H1-antihistamine use	Weak evidence base for H1-antihistamine use	Weak evidence base for first-generation H1-antihistamine use in CNS and vestibular disorders
Allergic rhinitis Allergic conjunctivitis Urticaria	Atopic dermatitis Asthma Anaphylaxis Nonallergic angioedema Upper respiratory tract infection Otitis media Sinusitis Nasal polyps Non-specific cough Nonallergic, non-specific itching	Insomnia Conscious sedation Perioperative sedation Analgesia Anxiety Serotonin syndrome Akathisia Migraine Motion sickness Vertigo

due to their low sedative actions, while the first-generation antihistamines can cause irritability and insomnia upon overdose. H2 antihistamines in children are safe at moderate doses, but they may induce necrotizing enterocolitis according to some reports. It is not safe to administer antihistamines during the first trimester of pregnancy, but chlorpheniramine, loratadine, and levocetirizine are the least dangerous types of antihistamine to administer during pregnancy because there is no evidence of teratogenicity. Table 9 summarizes the dose adjustments of H1 antihistamines [46].

Table 9 The dose adjustments of H1 antihistamines

Drug	Dosage	Conditions requiring dosage adjustment
Fist-generation H1 antihistamines		
Chlorpheniramine	4 mg three or four times daily 12 mg (sustained release formulation) twice daily	
Diphenhydramine	25–50 mg three or four times daily or at bedtime	Hepatic impairment
Doxepin	25–50 mg three times daily or at bedtime	Hepatic impairment
Hydroxyzine	25–50 mg three times daily or at bedtime	Hepatic impairment
Second-generation H1 antihistamines		
Acrivastine	8 mg three times daily	
Cetirizine	5–10 mg daily	Renal and hepatic impairment
Desloratadine	5 mg daily	Renal and hepatic impairment
Ebastine	10–20 mg daily	Renal and hepatic impairment
Fexofenadine	60 mg twice daily or 120 or 180 mg daily	Renal impairment
Levocetirizine	5 mg daily	Renal and hepatic impairment
Loratadine	10 mg daily	Hepatic impairment

Atopic Dermatitis and Antihistamines

Oral antihistamines do not improve pruritus as much as expected because the symptom is not caused only by histamine; however, they are still traditionally used as a basic drug. There are advantages of first-generation antihistamines, which induce drowsiness as an adverse reaction, and of the second-generation antihistamines that do not cause such event, respectively. Some clinicians prefer first-generation antihistamines such as diphenhydramine and chlorpheniramine for atopic dermatitis because drowsiness reduces symptoms of pruritus, and others prefer second-generation antihistamines such as loratadine and cetirizine due to their antiallergic effects [46]. Nevertheless, these antihistamines cannot be prescribed uniformly because their efficacy and a degree of adverse reactions are different depending on each individual. Thus, it is better to change the type of antihistamines or adjust the dose while administering. Even if the effects of H2 antihistamines are not obvious, a combination of drugs such as cimetidine and famotidine may work in some cases of dermatitis that does not respond to conventional H1 antihistamines. Doxepin, an antidepressant, has the advantages of H1–H2-antagonistic effects and long action time, but it is not common to use in children [46].

It is controversial about how much effective antihistamines are in treating pruritus of atopic dermatitis; however, antihistamines are given orally in most cases. Sedative H1 antihistamines such as hydroxyzine and diphenhydramine are effective, and they can effectively control pruritus severe enough to cause sleep disturbance. It is known that antihistamines that have no sedative effects have little effect on the regulation of pruritus in atopic dermatitis patients, but recently developed second-generation antihistamines have an antiallergic effect that inhibits activities of leukotrienes or platelet-activating factors. Although a majority of antihistamines are safe without concerns about significant side effects, cautions need to be taken when administering terfenadine and astemizole because concomitant administration with hypotensive drugs or erythromycin has been reported to have severe cardiovascular toxicity [48]. Antihistamines are known to cause sedation or drowsiness often due to their central nervous system suppression activities. However, infants may experience excitation and the prolonged therapies with antihistamines may induce tachyphylaxis. If night pruritus is critical, it may be possible to add antidepressants or sedatives such as tricyclic antidepressants (doxepin) for a short term [49].

Control of Skin Infections

Atopic dermatitis may frequently accompany infections by bacteria, virus, and fungi, and gets worse by these skin infections in many cases. Consequently, it is highly significant to identify the types of skin infections that aggravate atopic dermatitis and to understand the relevant treatments.

Staphylococcus aureus

Staphylococcus aureus produces a toxin, which acts as a superantigen and exacerbates atopic dermatitis. If atopic dermatitis suddenly worsens, systemic administration of antibiotics may work, and antibiotic ointments may help treating local lesions. Semisynthetic penicillin or erythromycin is a common oral medication. First- or second-generation cephalosporin antibiotics are generally used. In atopic dermatitis, the application of mupirocin ointment topically for 7–10 days could reduce Staphylococcal colonies. Detergents that include antimicrobial agents are effective but usually irritating.

Eczema Herpeticum

Eczema herpeticum is a skin disease mainly caused by *herpes simplex* virus type 1 infection in patients with preexisting dermatitis, such as atopic dermatitis. It occurs at an acute phase of multiple blisters within a few days after exposure to the virus or in the preexisting lesions of atopic dermatitis. Distributed in clusters, eczema herpeticum develops into pustules and crusts, and may accompany systemic symptoms such as high fever and lymphadenitis. The adverse reactions can happen in all age groups but do most frequently in pediatrics and around facial areas. Besides, there are whole body involved in some severe cases. The formation of chickenpox-like blisters over the whole skin is called as Kaposi's varicelliform eruption. If this severe eruption occurs in infants and pediatrics, it is a medical emergency and requires immediate initial treatment with antiviral agents. Most *herpes simplex* virus infections do not need treatment and can be cured naturally by simply maintaining the lesion clean and dry. Treatment is required only when the lesion is long-lasting and accompanied by symptoms and complications. There are various types of antivirals that can be used for eczema herpeticum. First, acyclovir is a very potent and selective inhibitor of *herpes simplex* virus type 1 and type 2. In order for the drug to work, it first needs to be phosphorylated and converted into monophosphate acyclovir. This phosphorylation process rarely occurs in uninfected cells, resulting in the selective accumulation of acyclovir inside infected cells. Monophosphate acyclovir is transformed again into triphosphate acyclovir to inhibit viral DNA polymerase, thereby preventing virus growth and replication in early stages. Acyclovir can be administered intravenously, orally, and topically. Patients with immunosuppression are recommended to receive intravenous injection of acyclovir, reducing recovery time, duration of pain, and the spread of viruses. According to recent studies, famciclovir and valacyclovir, which are for oral administration, have an advantage that their bioavailability is about three to five times higher and they are easier to take when compared to acyclovir [50].

Molluscum Contagiosum

Molluscum contagiosum is caused by molluscipoxvirus, one of the poxvirus types, and is a relatively common viral disease that primarily affects the skin and mucous membranes of young children. In particular, patients with atopic dermatitis are usually susceptible to molluscum contagiosum because they have damaged skin barriers and poor cellular immune function, resulting in increased susceptibility to infections. In atopic dermatitis patients, there are widely distributed, many in number for a long term. In most cases, there is no need for treatment because the lesions are naturally healed if there are no secondary bacterial infections. On the other hand, atopic dermatitis patients tend to scratch their skin lesions, causing the lesions to spread widely. Therefore, they may need more aggressive treatments. To treat molluscum contagiosum, it usually involves topical anesthesia on the lesion followed by a curettage method that scrapes the lesion using a curette or small tweezers. Although it is possible to freeze the larger lesions, it is not common due to scars and pain. Topical chemotherapy with cytotoxic agents such as podophyllin and trichloroacetic acid (TCA) can also be applicable, but atopic dermatitis patients are better to avoid this therapy because it can irritate their weakened skin barriers. Nowadays, there have been a number of clinical cases and researches that use imiquimod, an immune modulator, as a treatment for molluscum contagiosum in children and it has been proved to cure molluscum contagiosum relatively more effectively without pain than the physical method of curettage [51]. According to the reports of Choi et al. in Korea, it has shown a high morbidity rate of molluscum contagiosum in pediatric atopic dermatitis patients. Nevertheless, there have been some adverse reactions of applying imiquimod in the molluscum contagiosum lesions, such as erythema, itching, tenderness, nodule, erosion, scales, etc. Thus, it takes a caution to use only a small amount of imiquimod on the molluscum contagiosum lesion for atopic dermatitis patients.

Fungal Infection

Malassezia infection has recently emerged as a cause of worsening atopic dermatitis, and *Malassezia furfur* which belongs to the genus Malassezia is known to be representative. Especially in patients with atopic dermatitis, it is known to be involved mainly around head and neck areas and to aggravate atopic dermatitis chronically. According to numerous reports, there has been a higher detection rate of fungi in skin lesions of atopic dermatitis patients than that of normal patients. Furthermore, atopic dermatitis patients with head and neck are likely to have high levels of Malassezia-specific IgE antibodies [52]. For this reason, topical antifungal agents like ketoconazole have been reported to decrease Malassezia species and improve atopic dermatitis including head and neck areas among atopic dermatitis patients with severe head and neck dermatitis. One recent study also reported that itraconazole, an antifungal agent, maintained the improved symptoms of 17 subjects with atopic dermatitis out of 24 in total when they administered this drug for an average of 8 months [53]. The result indicates that oral azole antifungal agents can be considered as a method of treatment for adult patients with head and neck atopic dermatitis that do not respond to conventional treatments. Antifungal drugs inhibit the growth of fungi by preventing the synthesis of ergosterol, an essential component of fungal cell membranes. In dermatologic fields, antifungal agents commonly used include terbinafine, itraconazole, and fluconazole. One of the main triazole-group agents, itraconazole hinders 14-α-demethylase, an enzyme required to convert lanosterol into ergosterol. Itraconazole has a broad range of antifungal activity and thus can be widely used for almost every fungal strain. It binds easily to skin tissues and works well against ringworm, candidiasis, and Malassezia infections. Its typical dose is 100 mg a day, but it may be administered at a high dose of 200–400 mg for a short-term period, and in the case of ringworm, it has been used at a dose of 400 mg/day for 7 days recently [54]. However, cautions need to be taken regarding drug interactions. Contraindicated drugs include the following: (1) simvastatin, lovastatin, which are HMG CoA reductases that are metabolized by CYP3A4, (2) tranquilizers like triazolam, midazolam, and (3) quinidine that can prolong QT intervals. The elderly patients should be prescribed with proper types of antifungal drugs not related with drug interactions because many of them are taking medications related to systemic diseases such as hypertension, cardiovascular disease, and diabetes. It is effective to administer itraconazole right after a meal since it is well absorbed in the presence of high stomach acids. Fluconazole, another triazole-group antifungal agent, displays its antifungal effects by inhibiting 14-α-demethylase, like itraconazole does. It is usually excreted through the kidneys and at a slower rate due to its long half-life. Therefore, fluconazole can maintain the duration of antifungal efficacy long enough even with fewer number of administrations. In the case of ringworm, 150 mg once a week shows its effects in 2–3 weeks. Contraindicated drugs include cisapride. Fluconazole rarely causes nausea and indigestion. Unlike itraconazole, it is not affected by meals or antacids when absorbed into the body. Since it is usually excreted through the kidneys, its dose should be adjusted in patients with kidney disease.

Terbinafine, an allylamine-group antifungal agent similar to naphthylamine, displays its antifungal effects by inhibiting squalene epoxidase, which is required for synthesis of ergosterol in fungal cell membranes, thereby hindering cell membrane formation. In particular, terbinafine is known to have a selective therapeutic effect on dermatophytes, and its administration dose is 250 mg once per day for 2–6 weeks in treating tinea pedis and the same dose for 4 weeks to treat tinea corporis. In the case of onychomycosis, it has been reported that continuous therapy with terbinafine is relatively superior to pulse therapy with itraconazole. However, it is comparatively ineffective against cutaneous candidiasis and Malassezia infections that frequently occur in patients with atopic dermatitis [52]. There are no specific contraindicated drugs interacted with terbinafine. Even though adverse reactions rarely happen, it causes very rarely some like indigestion, anorexia, skin rashes, and liver dysfunction. The recurrence rate of Malassezia infection is high, being 60% after 1 year and 80% after 2 years of the treatment because Malassezia species are normal flora of the skin so it is difficult to remove them completely even after the above-mentioned therapies. Thus, the recurrence of Malassezia infection may be one of the reasons to be considered in the case of exacerbation in the head and neck areas in patients with atopic dermatitis [55].

References

1. Esteban NV, Loughlin T, Yergey AL, Zawadzki JK, Booth JD, Winterer JC, et al. Daily cortisol production rate in man determined by stable isotope dilution/mass spectrometry. J Clin Endocrinol Metab. 1991;72(1):39–45.
2. Bloom E, Matulich DT, Lan NC, Higgins SJ, Simons SS, Baxter JD. Nuclear binding of glucocorticoid receptors: relations between cytosol binding, activation and the biological response. J Steroid Biochem. 1980;12:175–84.
3. Flower RJ, Rothwell NJ. Lipocortin-1: cellular mechanisms and clinical relevance. Trends Pharmacol Sci. 1994;15(3):71–6.
4. Adcock IM, Ito K. Molecular mechanisms of corticosteroid actions. Monaldi Arch Chest Dis. 2000;55(3):256–66.
5. Rhen T, Cidlowski JA. Antiinflammatory action of glucocorticoids—new mechanisms for old drugs. N Engl J Med. 2005;353(16):1711–23.
6. Buttgereit F, Saag KG, Cutolo M, da Silva JA, Bijlsma JW. The molecular basis for the effectiveness, toxicity, and resistance to glucocorticoids: focus on the treatment of rheumatoid arthritis. Scand J Rheumatol. 2005;34(1):14–21.
7. Lu NZ, Cidlowski JA. The origin and functions of multiple human glucocorticoid receptor isoforms. Ann N Y Acad Sci. 2004;1024:102–23.
8. Buttgereit F, Wehling M, Burmester GR. A new hypothesis of modular glucocorticoid actions: steroid treatment of rheumatic diseases revisited. Arthritis Rheum. 1998;41(5):761–7.

9. Cupps TR, Fauci AS. Corticosteroid-mediated immunoregulation in man. Immunol Rev. 1982;65:133–55.
10. Amano Y, Lee SW, Allison AC. Inhibition by glucocorticoids of the formation of interleukin-1 alpha, interleukin-1 beta, and interleukin-6: mediation by decreased mRNA stability. Mol Pharmacol. 1993;43(2):176–82.
11. Kitajima T, Ariizumi K, Bergstresser PR, Takashima A. A novel mechanism of glucocorticoid-induced immune suppression: the inhibiton of T cell-mediated terminal maturation of a murine dendritic cell line. J Clin Invest. 1996;98(1):142–7.
12. Balow JE, Rosenthal AS. Glucocorticoid suppression of macrophage migration inhibitory factor. J Exp Med. 1973;137(4):1031–41.
13. Hogan MM, Vogel SN. Inhibition of macrophage tumoricidal activity by glucocorticoids. J Immunol. 1988;140(2):513–9.
14. Parrillo JE, Fauci AS. Mechanisms of glucocorticoid action on immune processes. Annu Rev Pharmacol Toxicol. 1979;19:179–201.
15. Butler WT, Rossen RD. Effects of corticosteroids on immunity in man. I. Decreased serum IgG concentration caused by 3 or 5 days of high doses of methylprednisolone. J Clin Invest. 1973;52(10):2629–40.
16. Levis S, Altman R. Bone densitometry: clinical considerations. Arthritis Rheum. 1998;41(4):577–87.
17. Saeki H, Nakahara T, Tanaka A, Kabashima K, Sugaya M, Murota H, et al. Clinical practice guidelines for the management of atopic dermatitis 2016. J Dermatol. 2016;43(10):1117–45.
18. Kim JE, Kim HJ, Lew BL, Lee KH, Hong SP, Jang YH, et al. Consensus guidelines for the treatment of atopic dermatitis in Korea (part II): systemic treatment. Ann Dermatol. 2015;27(5):578–92.
19. Sidbury R, Davis DM, Cohen DE, Cordoro KM, Berger TG, Bergman JN, et al. Guidelines of care for the management of atopic dermatitis: section 3. Management and treatment with phototherapy and systemic agents. J Am Acad Dermatol. 2014;71(2):327–49.
20. Wollenberg A, Oranje A, Deleuran M, Simon D, Szalai Z, Kunz B, et al. ETFAD/EADV Eczema task force 2015 position paper on diagnosis and treatment of atopic dermatitis in adult and paediatric patients. J Eur Acad Dermatol Venereol. 2016;30(5):729–47.
21. Lukert BP, Raisz LG. Glucocorticoid-induced osteoporosis: pathogenesis and management. Ann Intern Med. 1990;112(5):352–64.
22. Adachi JD, Bensen WG, Brown J, Hanley D, Hodsman A, Josse R, et al. Intermittent etidronate therapy to prevent corticosteroid-induced osteoporosis. N Engl J Med. 1997;337(6):382–7.
23. Luengo M, Picado C, Del Rio L, Guanabens N, Montserrat JM, Setoain J. Vertebral fractures in steroid dependent asthma and involutional osteoporosis: a comparative study. Thorax. 1991;46(11):803–6.
24. Reid IR, Heap SW. Determinants of vertebral mineral density in patients receiving long-term glucocorticoid therapy. Arch Intern Med. 1990;150(12):2545–8.
25. Ton FN, Gunawardene SC, Lee H, Neer RM. Effects of low-dose prednisone on bone metabolism. J Bone Miner Res. 2005;20(3):464–70.
26. Rizzato G, Montemurro L. Reversibility of exogenous corticosteroid-induced bone loss. Eur Respir J. 1993;6(1):116–9.
27. Buckley LM, Leib ES, Cartularo KS, Vacek PM, Cooper SM. Effects of low dose methotrexate on the bone mineral density of patients with rheumatoid arthritis. J Rheumatol. 1997;24(8):1489–94.
28. Solomon L. Idiopathic necrosis of the femoral head: pathogenesis and treatment. Can J Surg. 1981;24(6):573–8.
29. Zizic TM, Marcoux C, Hungerford DS, Dansereau JV, Stevens MB. Corticosteroid therapy associated with ischemic necrosis of bone in systemic lupus erythematosus. Am J Med. 1985;79(5):596–604.
30. Glueck CJ, Freiberg R, Tracy T, Stroop D, Wang P. Thrombophilia and hypofibrinolysis: pathophysiologies of osteonecrosis. Clin Orthop Relat Res. 1997;334:43–56.
31. Mont MA, Fairbank AC, Petri M, Hungerford DS. Core decompression for osteonecrosis of the femoral head in systemic lupus erythematosus. Clin Orthop Relat Res. 1997;334:91–7.
32. Dixon RB, Christy NP. On the various forms of corticosteroid withdrawal syndrome. Am J Med. 1980;68(2):224–30.
33. Bußmann C, Bieber T, Novak N. Systemic therapeutic options for severe atopic dermatitis. J Dtsch Dermatol Ges. 2009;7(3):205–19.
34. Berth-Jones J, Graham-Brown RA, Marks R, Camp RD, English JS, Freeman K, et al. Long term efficacy and safety of cyclosporin in severe atopic dermatitis. Br J Dermatol. 1997;136(1):76–81.
35. Denby KS, Beck LA. Update on systemic therapies for atopic dermatitis. Curr Opin Allergy Clin Immunol. 2012;12(4):421–6.
36. Harper JI, Berth-Jones J, Camp RD, Dillon MJ, Finlay AY, Holden CA, et al. Cyclosporin for atopic dermatitis in children. Dermatology. 2001;203(1):3–6.
37. Haw S, Shin MK, Haw CR. The efficacy and safety of long-term oral cyclosporine treatment for patients with atopic dermatitis. Ann Dermatol. 2010;22(1):9–15.
38. Kim SW, Park YW, Kwon IH, Kim KH. Cyclosporin treatment of atopic dermatitis: is it really associated with infectious diseases? Ann Dermatol. 2010;22(2):170–2.
39. Berth-Jones J, Takwale A, Tan E, Barclay G, Agarwal S, Ahmed I, et al. Azathioprine in severe adult atopic dermatitis: a double-blind, placebo-controlled, crossover trial. Br J Dermatol. 2002;147(2):324–30.
40. Lee H, Shin JU, Lee KH. The clinical efficacy of azathioprine in Korean patients with atopic dermatitis. Ann Dermatol. 2015;27(6):774–5.
41. Park YW, Yeom KB, Kim KH. Refractory atopic dermatitis in childhood: improvement with methotrexate? Ann Dermatol. 2013;25(1):114–6.
42. Weatherhead SC, Wahie S, Reynolds NJ, Meggitt SJ. An open-label, dose-ranging study of methotrex-

ate for moderate-to-severe adult atopic eczema. Br J Dermatol. 2007;156(2):346–51.
43. Lee SW, Park YM, Kim HO, Kim CW. Therapeutic efficacy of mycophenolate mofetil in atopic dermatitis. Korean J Dermatol. 2002;40(8):908–13.
44. Assmann T, Ruzicka T. New immunosuppressive drugs in dermatology (Mycophenolate mofetil, Tacrolimus): unapproved uses, dosages, or indications. Clin Dermatol. 2002;20(5):505–14.
45. Grundmann-Kollmann M, Podda M, Ochsendorf F, Boehncke WH, Kaufmann R, Zollner TM. Mycophenolate mofetil is effective in the treatment of atopic dermatitis. Arch Dermatol. 2001;137(7):870–3.
46. Simons FE, Simons KJ. Histamine and H1-antihistamines: celebrating a century of progress. J Allergy Clin Immunol. 2011;128(6):1139–50.
47. Simons FE. Advances in H1-antihistamines. N Engl J Med. 2004;351(21):2203–17.
48. Zechnich AD, Hedges JR, Eiselt-Proteau D, Haxby D. Possible interactions with terfenadine or astemizole. West J Med. 1994;160(4):321–5.
49. Kim HS, Cho SH. Treatment for atopic dermatitis. J Korean Med Assoc. 2014;57(3):226–33.
50. Micali G, Lacarrubba F. Eczema herpeticum. N Engl J Med. 2017;377(7):e9.
51. Choi WS, Kim JW, Park HS, Jang SJ, Choi JC. Treatment of molluscum contagiosum in children by topical imiquimod cream therapy. Korean J Dermatol. 2007;45(6):541–4.
52. Bayrou O, Pecquet C, Flahault A, Artigou C, Abuaf N, Leynadier F. Head and neck atopic dermatitis and malassezia-furfur-specific IgE antibodies. Dermatology. 2005;211(2):107–13.
53. Kaffenberger BH, Mathis J, Zirwas MJ. A retrospective descriptive study of oral azole antifungal agents in patients with patch test-negative head and neck predominant atopic dermatitis. J Am Acad Dermatol. 2014;71(3):480–3.
54. Svejgaard E, Larsen PO, Deleuran M, Ternowitz T, Roed-Petersen J, Nilsson J. Treatment of head and neck dermatitis comparing itraconazole 200 mg and 400 mg daily for 1 week with placebo. J Eur Acad Dermatol Venereol. 2004;18(4):445–9.
55. Darabi K, Hostetler SG, Bechtel MA, Zirwas M. The role of Malassezia in atopic dermatitis affecting the head and neck of adults. J Am Acad Dermatol. 2009;60(1):125–36.

Emerging Treatment of AD: Biologics and Small Molecules

Jiyoung Ahn

Biologics

Dupilumab, the first biologic drug approved for AD, has filled this large void for a safe and effective therapy for long-term use. Since the advent of dupilumab, several biologics are now being developed and investigated to provide alternatives to dupilumab (Table 1). Several antibodies targeting cytokines have been developed as therapeutic agents against AD (Fig. 1).

Th2 Cell Inhibition

IL-4, 13 Inhibition

IL-4 is the most critical cytokine among Th2 cytokines and plays an essential role in the differentiation of Th2 cells and the production of IgE. IL-4 acts on Th0 cells to promote differentiation and growth into Th2 cells, and the newly dispersed and grown Th2 cells produce IL-4 again; it makes to amplify and sustain Th2 reactions. IL-4 receptors are expressed in T cells, B cells, and macrophages, and when IL-4 is attached to these receptors, low-affinity IgE receptors are displayed on the surface of B cells, monocyte, and macrophages.

In B cells, Janus Kinase-1and 3 are activated when IL-4 stimulates IL-4 receptors, which induces activation of STAT6 and increases IgE production. Moreover, IL-4 and IL-13 suppress the production of f antimicrobial peptide in the epidermis to facilitate microbial intrusion, and suppress the lipid production of the stratum corneum, causing epidermal barrier damage.

Also, IL-4 and IL-13 induce the expression of thymic stromal lymphopoietin (TSLP), which contributes to linking barrier abnormality and Th2 activation responses, and activates the dendritic cells and induce OXO-40L to appear on the surface of the activated dendritic cells; it results in increasing Th2 cells.

Dupilumab

Dupilumab is a human monoclonal antibody (mAb) against IL-4 receptor α (Fig. 2). IL-4 receptor α is shared with IL-4 and IL-13 receptors. The randomized, placebo-controlled, phase III trials (SOLO 1 and SOLO 2) confirmed the efficacy and safety of dupilumab in moderate-to-severe atopic dermatitis (AD) [1]. In this study, the primary outcome was 0 or 1 of the Investigator's Global Assessment (IGA) score and a reduction of 2 points or more from baseline at week 16. The primary outcome reached

J. Ahn (✉)
Department of Dermatology, National Medical Center, Seoul, Korea (Republic of)
e-mail: jiyoung.ahn@nmc.or.kr

K. H. Lee et al. (eds.), *Practical Insights into Atopic Dermatitis*,
https://doi.org/10.1007/978-981-15-8159-5_16

Table 1 Novel systemic biologics; targeted therapies of AD

Category	Target	Name	Development status
Th2 inhibitors	IL-4Rα	Dupilumab	Approved by EMA/FDA/MFDS
	IL-13	Tralokinumab	Ph III On-going
		Lebrikizumab	Ph II Completed
	IL-33	Etokimab	Ph II On-going
		REGN3500	Ph II On-going
		PF-067817024	Ph I On-going
	IL-31	Nemolizumab	Ph III On-going
		BMS-981164	Ph I Completed
	TSLP	Tezepelumab	Ph II On-going
	OX40	KHK4083	Ph II On-going
		GBR830	Ph II On-going
	IL-5	Mepolizumab	Ph II Completed
Th1/17/22 inhibitors	IL12/23	Ustekinumab	Ph II Completed
	IL-17	Secukinumab	Ph II On-going
		MOR106	Ph II On-going
	IL-22	Fezakinumab	Ph II Completed

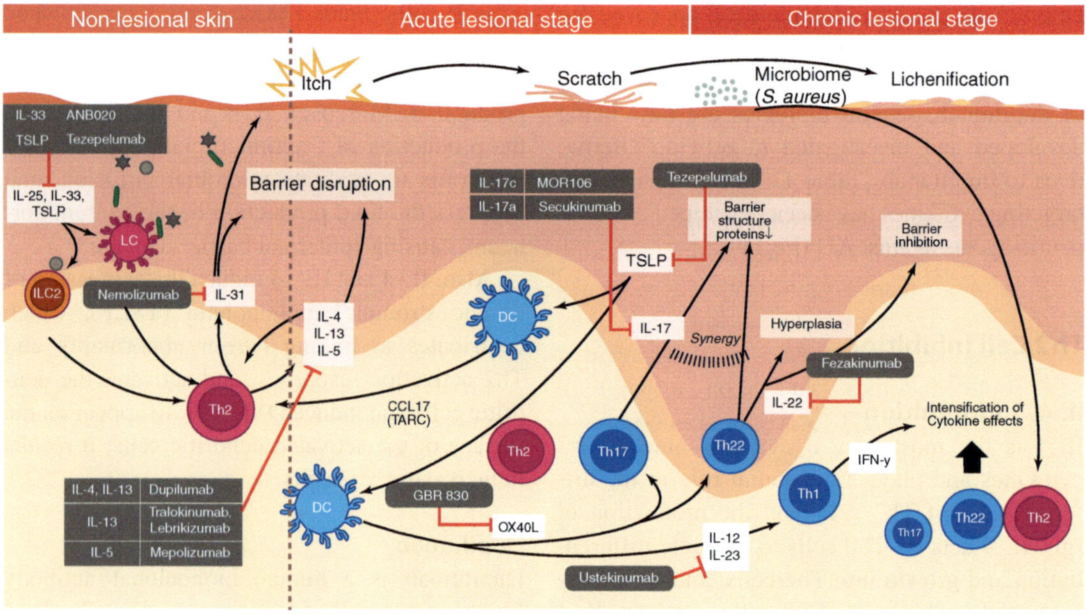

Fig. 1 Biologics targeted the immunologic aspect of AD

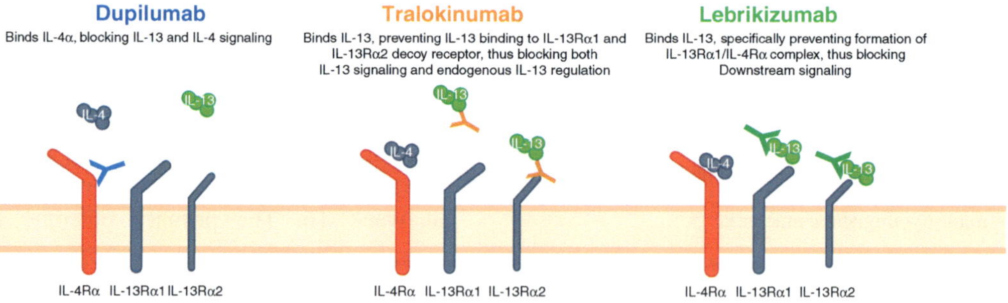

Fig. 2 Mechanism of dupilumab, tralokinumab, and lebrikizumab

36–38% of all patients who received dupilumab compared with 8–10% in patients who received a placebo. These studies found that there was no significant difference between every 2 weeks in IGA scores, Eczema Area and Severity Index (EASI), Numerical Rating Scale (NRS), Patient-Oriented Eczema Measure (POEM), and Dermatology Life Quality Index (DLQI) compared with a week [1]. In a more recently published 1-year, randomized, double-blinded, placebo-controlled, phase III study (CHRONOS), 740 adults with moderate-to-severe AD, and inadequate response to topical corticosteroids (TCS) were enrolled. This study allows that all patients were given concomitant topical corticosteroids with or without topical calcineurin inhibitors (TCI). The results after 16 weeks were similar to those in the SOLO studies and proved to be stable over the extension period of 52 weeks [2]. No significant dupilumab-induced laboratory abnormalities were noted. Injection-site reactions and conjunctivitis were more common in patients treated with dupilumab than in patients treated with placebo. This study reported that Dupilumab added to standard TCS treatment for 1 year improved atopic dermatitis signs and symptoms, with acceptable safety.

And to evaluate efficacy and safety of dupilumab with TCS in adults with atopic dermatitis with inadequate response to/intolerance of Cyclosporin A (CsA), or for whom CsA treatment was medically inadvisable. In this 16-week, double-blind, randomized, placebo-controlled, phase 3 trial (café), patients were randomized 1: 1: 1 to subcutaneous dupilumab 300 mg qw or q2w or placebo. This study expands upon the previous studies in two principal ways. Firstly, unlike previous studies, the patients in this study were candidates for having experienced intolerance to CsA, or for whom the use of CsA treatment was medically inadvisable. Secondly, this study evaluated dupilumab on a background of treatment with TCS, and patients could not discontinue TCS, unless for safety reasons, unlike in previous studies of dupilumab with concomitant TCS use, in which TCS could be stopped [3]. In total, 390 patients were screened, 325 were randomized, and 318 completed the trial. Treatment groups had similar baseline characteristics. Significantly more patients in the dupilumab qw + TCS and q2w + TCS groups achieved ≥75% improvement from baseline in the EASI at Week 16 vs. the placebo + TCS group (primary end point) (59.1% and 62.6% vs. 29.6%, respectively; $P < 0.001$ vs. placebo + TCS, both doses). Conjunctivitis was more frequent with dupilumab + TCS; skin infections were more frequent with placebo + TCS. We can know through this study, Dupilumab + TCS significantly improved signs and symptoms of atopic dermatitis and QoL in adults with a history of inadequate response to/intolerance of CsA, or for whom CsA treatment was medically inadvisable. No new safety signals were identified [3].

The most common adverse events in clinical trials were the deterioration of atopic dermatitis, which was more prevalent in placebo populations [1–3]. Reported adverse back effects in the dupilumab patient group include nasopharyngitis, conjunctivitis, headache, herpes simplex infection, and injection site reaction. In particular, conjunctivitis was more frequent and has been reported after the market.

Currently, patients are prescribed to patients in South Korea and other countries, and real-world data is being reported in many countries. In the French multicenter adult cohort, they demonstrated a similar result as that seen in clinical trials, but it also revealed a higher frequency of conjunctivitis and eosinophilia [4]. Conjunctivitis with dupilumab treatment was significantly associated with a history of atopic conjunctivitis in their study. However, they could not explain pathophysiology of dupilumab induced eye disorders, but several therapeutics were prescribed from artificial tears to cyclosporine eye drops for relieving eye symptoms [4]. Furthermore, they have hypothesized hypereosinophilia of dupilumab treatment that dupilumab blocks the migration of eosinophils into the tissue by inhibiting the IL-4 and IL-13 mediated production of eotaxins and vascular cell adhesion molecule but not in bone marrow [4].

In Korea (National Medical Center, South Korea), we conducted a study on the real-world use of dupilumab in patients with moderate-to-severe AD in Korea. A total of 101 patients were

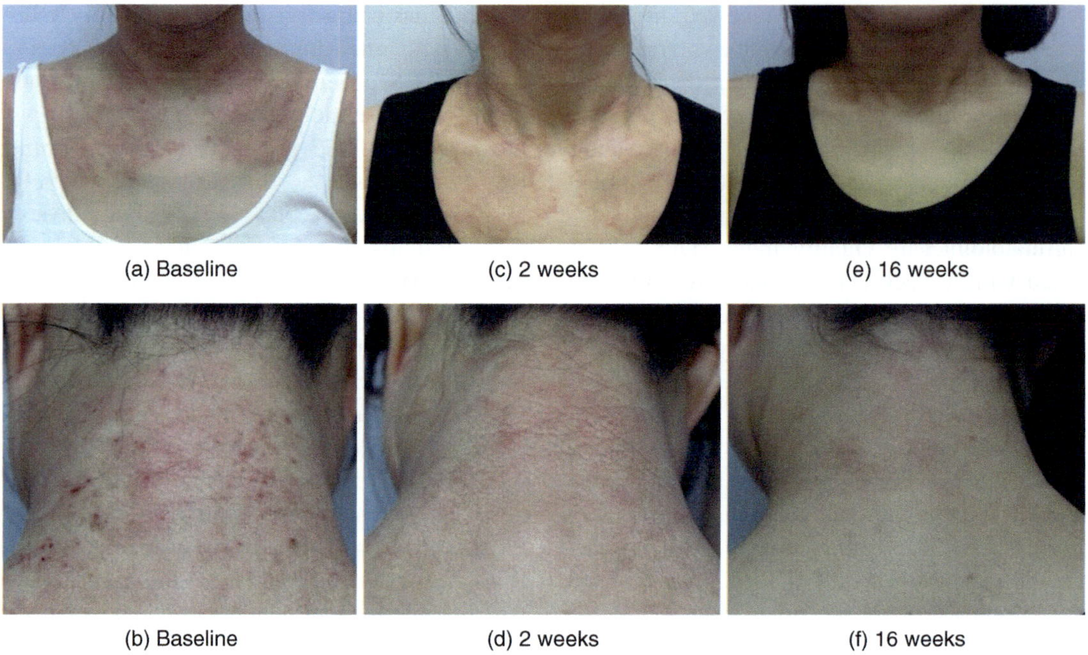

Fig. 3 Case showing a good treatment response

included. All showed a significant decrease after 16 weeks; EASI 74.6% (Fig. 3 showed the best responder in EASI), NRS 62.4%, POEM 58.0%, and DLQI 60.4%. In the laboratory test, only LDH showed a significant decrease after 16 weeks. In the demographics, the proportion of allergic conjunctivitis and asthma was less than allergic rhinitis. In this study, EASI was characterized by a marked improvement of nearly 50% in just 2 weeks, which is more significant than in previous clinical trials. Factors affecting the therapeutic effect of dupilumab have not been revealed in previous clinical trials and other studies. In this study, the only significant difference was gender, with an odds ratio for women achieving EASI 75 equaling 5.4 ($P = 0.04$), this result is consistent with other previous real-world data [4–6]. Furthermore, persistent elevation of LDH after 16 weeks was related to inadequate treatment response about subjective efficacy tools. Although not related to EASI, it is consistent with a recent real-world study of dupilumab in that it is associated with therapeutic response [6]. About the adverse event, facial erythema is another major issue associated with dupilumab treatment in other countries [7, 8]. The mechanism and cause of this are not well understood, but we thought that facial erythema might be related to the worsening of existing AD lesions, withdrawal of systemic treatment, concomitant allergic contact dermatitis, or adverse effects of dupilumab.

Further research and attention to facial erythema will be needed. For conjunctivitis, the cause is not well understood, but it seems to be aggravated in people who have previously had allergic conjunctivitis [4]. An accurate diagnosis will be important not to misdiagnose, such as itching of the eyelids and eyes or exacerbation of a periorbital facial-skin problem [9].

In Japan, real-world data revealed that some patients showed poor improvement on the head and neck while obtaining an excellent response to dupilumab on the trunk and the limbs and that conjunctivitis as an adverse event was more common in the real-world setting than in the clinical trials, although this was controllable in most patients. They explain that the issues raised by their study could be race-specific [10].

Dupilumab also is approved for use in adolescents aged ≥ 12 years with inadequately controlled moderate-to-severe atopic dermatitis (AD). Dupilumab significantly improved AD signs/symptoms in a 16-week, randomized, placebo-controlled phase III trial in adolescents. The phase IIa study and phase III OLE were the earliest studies of dupilumab in adolescents to characterize its PK and long-term safety and efficacy profile. The results from these studies support the use of dupilumab for the long-term management of moderate-to-severe AD in adolescents [11].

IL-13 Inhibition

IL-13, also significant type 2 cytokine secreted from T lymphocytes, is elevated in atopic dermatitis patients [12]. Additionally, IL-13 is considered to be an essential cytokine of type 2 inflammation with a number of effects on a variety of cells [13]. Two antibodies against IL-13 have been studied.

Tralokinumab

Tralokinumab, an IgG4λ anti-IL-13 monoclonal antibody derived from a human phage display library, prevents IL-13 from binding to both IL-13Rα1 and IL-13Rα2 [14] (Fig. 2). IL-13Rα2 has a short cytoplasmic tail and no known signaling motifs, decoy function via internalization of excess IL-13 [15, 16]. Tralokinumab prevents both IL-13-mediated signalings downstream of IL-4Rα/IL-13Rα1 hetero-dimerization (type 2 receptor), but it may also interfere with endogenous regulation of IL-13 that is mediated by IL-13Rα2. Loss of function of the IL-13 decoy receptor was shown to be deleterious in a mouse model of cutaneous inflammation [17].

Tralokinumab was studied in different doses in adults with moderate-to-severe AD in a phase IIb study with concomitant topical steroid [18]. Coprimary endpoints were the change of EASI and the percentage of participants with an IGA response with 0 or 1 score and reduction of two grades or more from baseline at week 12. The highest applied dose of tralokinumab (300 mg) showed significant improvement. Moreover, more excellent responses were higher concentrations of IL-13 activity [18]. IL-13 upregulate DDP-4 and periostin, which are considered a biomarker of IL-13 signaling, in high DDP-4, and periostin groups showed a good response. The safety profile was similar to asthma study, upper respiratory tract infections, and headache were reported.

Lebrikizumab

Lebrikizumab is a humanized, IgG4κ monoclonal antibody that also binds soluble IL-13, but at a different epitope compared with tralokinumab [19] (Fig. 3). Lebrikizumab-bound IL-13 can still bind to its cell surface receptors, but the biologic prevents IL-4Rα/IL-13Rα1 hetero-dimerization (type 2 receptor) and downstream signaling. The two antibodies interfere with IL-13-mediated signaling by different mechanisms. Tralokinumab prevents access of the prebound IL-13/IL-13Rα1 complex to the receptor signaling subunit IL-4Rα, while lebrikizumab interferes with IL-13 binding to IL-13Rα1. Trolokinumab blocks binding of IL-13 to IL-13Rα2, and lebrikizumab does not. Lebrikizumab was studied in different doses in a randomized, placebo-controlled, double-blind, phase II study of adults with moderate-to-severe AD in combination with topical corticosteroids twice daily. Achieving EASI-50 at week 12 was significantly higher with lebrikizumab than with placebo (82.4% in the treatment group vs. 62.3% in the placebo group) [20].

IL-33 Inhibjition

IL-33 is an IL-1 family cytokine produced by innate immune cells, produced by stimuli by allergen or microbes. IL-33 acted on Th2 cells in the in vitro experiment to produce IL-5 and IL-13 and in vivo experiment increased the number of eosinophils and immunoglobulin in the peripheral blood. IL-33 also stimulates the mast cell to create cytokines and chemokines such as IL-5, IL-6, IL-10, IL-13, CXCL8, and CCL1 [21].

Etokimab

There is a phase 2 study; this study is designed to evaluate the efficacy, safety, and pharmacokinetic (PK) profiles of multiple doses of Etokimab in subjects with atopic dermatitis (AD) [21].

IL-31 Inhibition

IL-31, as a knownTh2 cytokine, acts as an itch-causing role in atopic dermatitis and reduces the expression of filaggrin and loricrin to interfere with the final differentiation of the epidermis. IL-31 works in combination with receptors composed of IL-31RA and oncostatin M receptor beta complex and IL-31RA is found in keratinocyte, macrophage, eosinophil, and nerve fiber in AD patients and dorsal root ganglion in healthy people [22].

Nemolizumab

Nemolizumb is a humanized mAb that targets the IL-31 receptor alpha subunit; it binds to the IL-31 receptor on a spectrum of cells and neurons, which is relieving pruritus. There are two published clinical trial results. In phase 2 clinical study, nemolizumab improved EASI, IGA, and NRS with 30 mg dose being most effective, it (30 mg) reduced EASI scores vs. placebo at 24 weeks (−68.8 vs. −52.1%, $P < 0.016$) NRS scores were improved at 16 weeks (−68.6 vs. −34.31%, $P < 0.0001$). Moreover, it was safe and tolerated; the most common adverse events were nasopharyngitis and upper respiratory tract infection [22].

In randomized, phase 2, long-term extension study, they showed that the long-term efficacy and safety of nemolizumab injected every 4 weeks or every 8 weeks in 52 weeks. They concluded nemolizumab for up to 64 weeks was effective and well-tolerated in moderate and severe AD patients [23].

BMS-981164

BMS-981164 ended phase I clinical trials, but no results were reported [24].

TSLP Inhibition

Thymic stromal lymphopoietin (TSLP), an epithelial cell-derived cytokine, is produced in response to pro-inflammatory stimuli. TSLP-activated dendritic cells induce the production of Th2 cytokines (Fig. 4), IL-4, -5, and -13, and tumor necrosis factor-α [25]. TSLP supports a role for Th2 inflammation in AD pathogenesis [26].

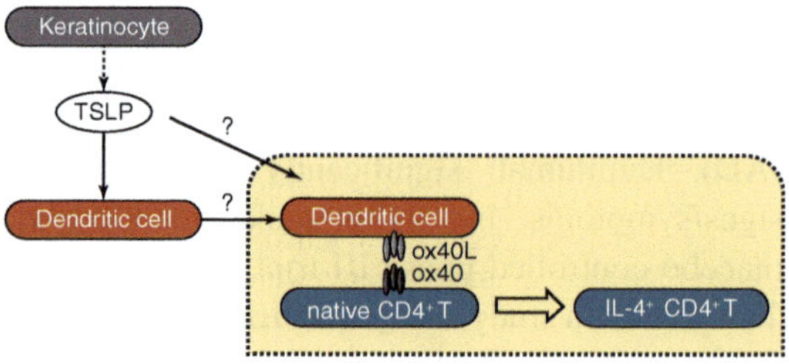

Fig. 4 TSLP-OX40 axis. Keratinocyte-derived TSLP activates dendritic cells to induce the production of Th2 immunity cytokines, IL-33 appears to amplify TSLP's effect of inducing expression of OX40 ligand on dendritic cells

Tezepelumab

Tezepelumab, a first monoclonal antibody, targets TSLP. In the phase 2a study, 113 patients were randomized 1:1 to subcutaneous tezepelumab 280 mg or placebo every 2 weeks, plus class 3 TCS. A higher percentage of tezepelumab plus TCS treated patients achieved EASI 50 (64.7%) vs. placebo plus TCS for 12 weeks (48.2%; $P = 0.091$) [26].

OX40 Inhibition

OX40 (CD134), a costimulatory molecule of TNF receptor, is expressed predominantly on T cells, including effector cells and forkhead box P3 $(Foxp^3)^+$ regulatory T (Treg) cells. OX40 ligand (OX40L; CD252) is expressed on activated antigen-presenting cells. OX40-OX40L engagement is critical to potentiate T-cell response (Fig. 4). In AD patients, numbers of $OX40L^+$ DCs are highly increased [27].

GBR830

GBR830 is a humanized mAb against OX40. In the phase 2a study, two doses of GBR830 administered 4 weeks apart were well tolerated and induced significant progressive tissue and clinical changes until day 71 (42 days after the last dose) [28].

IL-5 Inhibition

Mepolizumab

Mepolizumab is a humanized immunoglobulin G (IgG) monoclonal antibody (IgG1, kappa) with human heavy and light chain frameworks. It binds to IL-5, which is responsible for the growth, differentiation, recruitment, activation, and survival of eosinophils. In the phase 2 study, there is no meaningful difference with control to placebo group [29].

Th1/Th17/Th22 Cell Inhibition

IL12/23 Inhibition

Ustekinumab

Ustekinumab is an IL-12/IL-23p40 antagonist that suppresses Th1, Th17, and Th22 activation, commonly used for psoriasis patients. The ustekinumab group achieved higher SCORAD50 responses at 12, 16 (the primary endpoint), and 20 weeks compared to the placebo, but the difference between groups was not significant. Ustekinumab had clear clinical and molecular effects, but a profound "placebo" effect might have obscured clinical outcomes, most likely due to background topical glucocorticosteroids and possibly insufficient dosing for AD [30].

IL-17 Inhibition

Secukinumab

Secukinumab is a humanized anti-IL-17A monoclonal antibody. Since Secukinumab is well established in the therapy of psoriasis with a highly favorable benefit to risk ration and IL-17 has been described in atopic dermatitis. In the phase 2 study, randomized, placebo-controlled, multicenter, double-blinded study to evaluate the efficacy and safety of subcutaneous Secukinumab compared to placebo in 45 adults with atopic dermatitis. However, no results were reported [31].

MOR106

17-C is a keratinocyte-produced cytokine that is overexpressed in atopic dermatitis and psoriasis; it stimulates the synthesis of many inflammatory products also induced by IL-17A/F. This may help leat ultimately to the induction of S100As and other molecules that accompany epidermal hyperplasia. MOR106 is IL-17C neutralizing Ab, which is able to inhibit both T helper type2 cells and T helper type 17/22-skewed inflammatory loops that drive different features of AD and psoriasis. The therapeutic potential of IL-17C antagonism in AD is supported by a small phase 1 clinical trial [32].

IL-22 Inhibition

Key pathogenic features of AD include a disturbed skin barrier with epidermal hyperplasia and abnormal keratinocyte differentiation well as robust activation of the Th2 and Th22 T-cell pathways. In vivo research and animal studies suggest that IL-22, the Th22 cytokine, promotes hyperplasia and inhibits keratinocyte differentiation and skin barrier formation, two hallmarks of AD [33].

Fezakinumab

FezakinumB is the IL-22 antagonist; in phase 2a study, at 12 weeks, the mean declines are SCORD for the entire study population were 13.8 ± 2.7 in the fazekinumab arm ad 8.03 ± 0.1 in the placebo arm ($P = 0.134$). All scores showed progressive improvements after the last dosing (10 weeks) until the end of the study (20 weeks). Frequent adverse events were upper respiratory tract infections [33].

Small Molecules

Beyond biologics, several small molecule inhibitors are in various stages of clinical development (Table 2).

JAK Inhibitor

The Janus kinase (JAK)–signal transducer and activator of transcription (STAT) and spleen tyrosine kinase (SYK) pathways are involved in signaling of several cytokines, mediating

Table 2 Small molecules; targeted therapies of AD

Category	Target(s)	Name	Formulation	Development status
JAK inhibitors	JAK1	Upadacitinib	Oral	Ph III On-going
		Abrocitinib	Oral	Ph III Completed
	JAK1/2	Baricitinib	Oral	Ph III On-going
		Ruxolitinib	Topical	Ph III On-going
	JAK1/3	Tofacitinib	Oral/Topical	Ph II Completed (Topical)
	Pan JAK	ASN002	Oral	Ph II On-going
		Delgocitinib	Topical	Ph II On-going
PDE4 inhibitors	PDE4	Apremilast	Oral	Ph II Completed
		Roflumilast	Topical	Ph II Completed
		Crisaborole	Topical	Approved by FDA
		Opa-15406	Topical	Ph III On-going
		DRM-02	Topical	Ph II Completed
		LEO29102	Topical	Ph II Completed

downstream inflammation, and related other inflammatory diseases (Table 3, Figs. 5 and 6). Spleen tyrosine kinases (SYK) is involved in the release of cytokines during the pro-inflammatory process, including IL-1b, IL-10, and IL-17,14 and regulates dendritic cells, B lymphocytes, and keratinocyte differentiation, suggesting that SYK inhibitors could improve inflammatory skin diseases with aberrant differentiation, such as AD. The JAK kinases family (JAK1, JAK2, JAK3, and TYK2) is also involved in signaling pathways of several cytokines involved in AD, such as IL-4, IL-13, IL-31, and IL33. Besides, JAK inhibitors, targeting mostly JAK1, have been shown to be useful for the treatment of AD.

JAK1 Inhibition

Upadacitinib

Upadacitinib is developed for the treatment of rheumatoid arthritis, the first generation of JAK inhibitors, tofacitinib, and ruxolitinib, lacked subtype selectivity, affecting JAK1/JAK3 and JAK1/JAK2, respectively. This has led to dose-limiting side effects. Upadacitinib is a second-generation Janus kinase inhibitor that is selective for the JAK1 subtype of this enzyme over the JAK2 (74-fold), JAK3 (58-fold), and tyrosine kinase 2 subtypes [34]. A Phase 3 study has continued [35], including younger patients with moderate-to-severe AD are also currently underway.

Abracitinib

Abrocitinib is an oral JAK1 selective inhibitor under investigation for the treatment of atopic dermatitis. In this randomized, double-blinded, phase 2b clinical trial, including 267 participants, the proportion of patients achieving substantial improvement from baseline was significantly more significant for those receiving 200 mg and 100 mg of abrocitinib compared with placebo. Dose-related decreases in platelet count were observed for all doses higher than 10 mg, but platelet values trended upward toward baseline after the maximum decrease at week 4, and despite ongoing treatment with abrocitinib; most adverse events were mild and considered unrelated to treatment. Now the phase 3 clinical trial has been processing.

JAK 1/2 Inhibition

Baricitinib

Baricitinib is a selective JAK1 and JAK2 inhibitor that is currently approved for the treatment of RA. The phase 2 trial included a standardization period with the use of TCS to identify individuals whose AD was inadequately controlled by TCS. Significantly more patients who received baricitinib, 4 mg, achieved EASI 50 than the placebo group (61 vs. 37%, $P = 0.027$) at 16weeks. The increase in CPK level observed with barici-

Table 3 Signaling JAKs for cytokines in immune homeostasis and immune-mediated disease

Type I cytokines	Signaling JAKs	Immune function and potential role in Immune-mediated disease
Common γc		
IL-2	JAK1, JAK3	Enhances effector and regulatory responses
IL-4	JAK1, JAK3	Allergies and asthma—Th2-mediated diseases
IL-7	JAK1, JAK3	T cell development and homeostasis
IL-9	JAK1, JAK3	Atopic disease, IBD
IL-13	JAK1, JAK3, JAK2, TYK2	Airway hyperresponsiveness, goblet cell metaplasia and mucus hypersecretion, fibrosis
IL-15	JAK1, JAK3	Memory T cells, NK cells, induction of cell proliferation
IL-21	JAK1, JAK3	Tfh cells
Common βχ		
GM-CSF	JAK2	Macrophages, T cells, mast cells, NK cells, endothelial cells, and fibroblasts, stem cell stimulation and differentiation
IL-3	JAK2	Differentiation of multipotent hematopoietic stem cells, the proliferation of all cells in the myeloid lineage
IL-5	JAK2	Allergies, asthma, eosinophilic disease
gp130		
IL-6	JAK1, JAK2, TYK2	Prototypic proinflammatory cytokine broadly relevant for many autoimmune diseases
IL-11	JAK1, JAK2, TYK2	Hematopoiesis, bone remodeling
IL-27	JAK1, JAK2, TYK2	Regulation of the activity of B- and T-lymphocytes
Dimeric		
IL-12	JAK2, TYK2	Th1-associated disease
IL-23	JAK2, TYK2	Th17-mediated disease
IL-27	JAK1, JAK2	Enhance Th1 and inhibit Th17 responses
IL-35	JAK1, JAK2	Anti-inflammatory responses
IFN family		
IFNα/β	JAK1, TYK2	Enhance immunity against infections and drive autoimmunity
IFNγ	JAK1, JAK2	Enhance immunity against infections and drive autoimmunity
IL-28	JAK1, TYK2	Enhance immunity against infections
IL-29	JAK1, TYK2	Enhance immunity against infections
IL-10 family		
IL-10	JAK1, JAK2, TYK2	Anti-inflammatory actions
IL-19	JAK1, JAK2, TYK2	B cell activation, antibody production
IL-20	JAK1, JAK2, TYK2	Synoviocyte migration, osteoclast formation
IL-22	JAK1, JAK2, TYK2	Promote barrier immunity, augment IL-17 function

tinib group likely related to an as-yet-unknown pharmacological effect of JAK inhibition. It was not associated with muscle-related side events, as previously reported with other JAK inhibitions and in other studies [36]. Now the phase 3 clinical trial has been processing.

Ruxolitinib

Ruxolitinib, a selective inhibitor of JAK-1 and JAK-2, in the phase 2 study, 307 adult patients with AD, an IGA score of 2 or 3 (mild or moderate), and 3–20% affected body surface area were equally randomized for 8 weeks of double-blind treatment to Ruxolitinib (1.5% twice daily [BID], 1.5% once daily [QD], 0.5% QD, 0.15% QD), vehicle, or triamcinolone cream (0.1% BID for 4

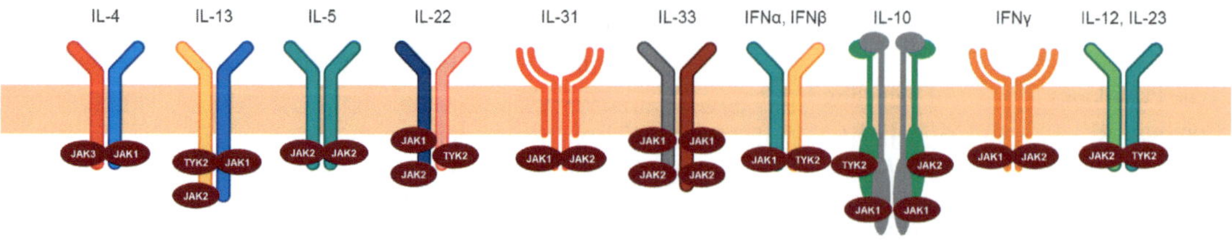

Fig. 5 Signaling JAKs for cytokines in immune homeostasis and immune-mediated disease

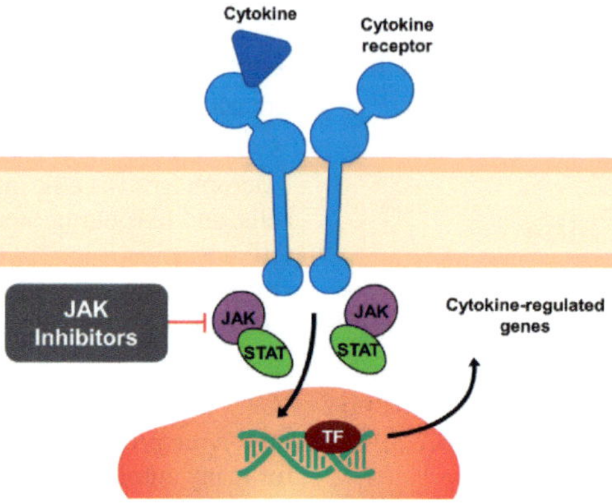

Fig. 6 JAK-STAT pathway. A cytokine binds to its cell surface receptor. A Janus kinase (JAK) family of receptor-associated kinases phosphorylate intracellular receptors and increase the production of a group of signal transducer and activator of transcription (STAT). Phosphorylated STATs dimerize and translocate to the nucleus, leading to the activation of targeted gene expression

weeks then vehicle for 4 weeks). All Ruxolitinib regimens demonstrated therapeutic benefit at Week 4; 1.5% BID provided the most considerable improvement in EASI (71.6 vs. 15.5%; $P < 0.0001$) and IGA responses (38.0 vs. 7.7%; $P < 0.001$) vs. vehicle. No serious side effects were observed in patients treated with Ruxolitinib cream and well tolerated [37]. Now the phase 3 clinical trial has been processing.

JAK 1/3 Inhibition

Tofacitinib

Tofacitinib is an inhibitor of the enzyme JAK 1 and JAK 3, in a mouse model of established arthritis, tofacitinib rapidly improved disease by inhibiting the production of inflammatory mediators and suppressing STAT1-dependent genes in joint tissue. Common side effects include diarrhea, headache, and high blood pressure. Serious side effects may include infections, cancer, and pulmonary embolism. In 2019, the safety committee of the European Medicines Agency (EMA) began a review of tofacitinib and recommended that doctors temporarily not prescribe the 10 mg twice-daily dose to people at high risk for pulmonary embolism. In 2015, there was a study about six AD patients treated with oral tofacitinib citrate, but a small sample size, lack of placebo control group, and the possibility of bias were limitations [38]. In 4-week, phase 2a, randomized, double-blind, vehicle-controlled study, 69 adults with mild-to-moderate AD were randomized 1:1 to 2% tofacitinib or vehicle ointment twice daily. The mean percentage change at week 4 in the EASI score was significantly more enormous ($P < 0.001$) for tofacitinib (−81.7%) vs. vehicle (−29.9%). Patients treated with tofacitinib showed significant ($P < 0.001$) improvements vs. vehicle across all prespecified efficacy endpoints and for pruritus at week 4 [39]. However, there is no ongoing research.

Pan JAK Inhibition

ASN002

ASN002 is a potent, dual inhibitor of JAK and SYK kinases, a total of 36 patients with moderate-to-severe AD were randomized (3:1) to ASN002 or placebo in the phas1b study. Three dosage cohorts were studied over 28 days (20 mg, 40 mg, and 80 mg once daily). ASN002 was superior to placebo for the proportion of patients achieving EASI 50 (20 mg 20%, $P = 0.093$; 40 mg 100%, $P = 0.0003$; 80 mg 83%, $P = 0.003$; placebo 22%), EASI 75 (20 mg 0%, $P = 0.027$; 40 mg 71%, $P = 0.006$; 80 mg 33%, $P = 0.065$; placebo 22%). Adverse events were generally mild and similar across all groups. ASN002 showed dose-dependent plasma exposure with low interpatient variability, significantly downregulated several serum biomarkers involved in Th1, Th2, and Th17/Th22 immunity, and decreased the atherosclerosis-associated biomarker E selectin/SELE [40]. There is a phase 2, extension study to evaluate the long-term safety, tolerability, and efficacy of ASN002 in subjects with moderate-to-severe atopic dermatitis until 2021 [41].

Delgocitinib

Delgocitinib is another pan JAK inhibitor, which has inhibitory effects on all types of JAK family kinase (JAK1, 2, 3, and tyrosine kinase 2). In non-clinical studies, the topical application of delgotinib suppressed skin inflammation in animal dermatitis model; improved skin barrier dysfunction by promotion production of terminal differentiation proteins, including filaggrin; and suppressed pruritus.

In the phase 2 study modified EASI in both delgocitinib groups was significantly reduced compared with that in the vehicle group. This study showed that the 4-week treatment with delgocitinib ointment was well tolerated in pediatric patient with AD [42].

Phosphodiesterase Enzyme 4 Inhibition

Phosphodiesterase Enzyme 4 (PDE4) hydrolyzes cyclic adenosine monophosphate (cAMP) to inactive adenosine monophosphate (AMP). Inhibition of PDE4 blocks hydrolysis of cAMP, thereby increasing levels of cAMP within cells. The resulting increase in cAMP levels downregulates the expression of several pro-inflammatory factors like TNFα, IL-17, IL-23, and many others, and upregulates the anti-inflammatory IL-10 [43].

Apremilast

Apremilast, an orally available PDE4 inhibitor that is approved for the treatment of adults with moderate-to-severe psoriasis and active psoriatic arthritis, regulates several proinflammatory signals involved in AD, including IL-17, 22, 13, 31, 33, 5, and S100A7/A8. Patients were randomly assigned to receive a placebo, apremilast 30 mg twice daily (APR30), or apremilast 40 mg twice daily (APR40) for 12 weeks. APR40, but not APR30, led to statistically significant improvement (vs. placebo, $n = 64$) in EASI (−31.6 vs. −11.0%; $P < 0.04$) mRNA expression of Th17/22 related markers (IL17, 22, and S100A7/A8; $P < 0.05$) showed the highest reduction with APR40 [43].

Roflumilast

Roflumilast is a topical PDE4 inhibitor; there was a phase 2 clinical trial, but no benefit in AD [44].

Crisaborole

Crisaborole is mainly acting on phosphodiesterase 4B (PDE4B), which causes inflammation. Inhibition of PDE4B appears to suppress the release of TNFα, IL-12, IL-23, and other cytokines, proteins believed to be involved in the immune response and inflammation. In some phase 3 studies, cisaborole ointment improved disease severity and pruritus with a favorable safety profile in mild-to-moderate AD [45]. The mechanism through which PDE4 regulates pruritus is not well understood but is believed to be partially an indirect result of reducing inflammation similar to the antipruritic effects observed with treatment [45].

OPA15406

OPA15406 is a highly selective inhibitory activity against PDE4 subtype, also subtype B. In the phase 2 study, IGA of Disease Severity Score of 1 or 1 with greater than or equal to 2-grade reduction, was met at 4 weeks in the OPA15406 1% group (*P* = 0.016 vs. vehicle). Incidence of adverse events mild in intensity [46]. Now the phase 3 study is under process [47].

DRM-02, LEO29102

They are also topical PDE4 inhibitor; phase 2 clinical trials are currently underway [48, 49].

Conclusion

Many novel biologic and small molecule agents that are clinically effective in AD treatment have emerged, even though effective management of AD is complicated due to its multifaceted pathophysiology, variable clinical manifestations, and chronic course of the disease. In the future, more data regarding ongoing development programs can be published for other biologics and small molecule inhibitors. Of all the treatments, the ability to change the disease progress, drug safety, and cost-effectiveness should be essential factors. Further studies are required in the real world before the promise of a therapeutic revolution.

References

1. Simpson EL, Bieber T, Guttman-Yassky E, Beck LA, Blauvelt A, Cork MJ, et al. Two phase 3 trials of dupilumab versus placebo in atopic dermatitis. N Engl J Med. 2016;375:2335–48.
2. Blauvelt A, de Bruin-Weller M, Gooderham M, Cather JC, Weisman J, Pariser D, et al. Long-term management of moderate-to-severe atopic dermatitis with dupilumab and concomitant topical corticosteroids (LIBERTY AD CHRONOS): a 1-year, randomised, double-blinded, placebo-controlled, phase 3 trial. Lancet. 2017;389:2287–303. https://doi.org/10.1016/S0140-6736(17)31191-1.
3. de Bruin-Weller M, Thaçi D, Smith CH, Reich K, Cork MJ, Radin A, et al. Dupilumab with concomitant topical corticosteroid treatment in adults with atopic dermatitis with an inadequate response or intolerance to ciclosporin A or when this treatment is medically inadvisable: a placebo-controlled, randomized phase III clinical trial (LIBERTY AD CAFÉ). Br J Dermatol. 2018;178:1083–101. https://doi.org/10.1111/bjd.16156.
4. Faiz S, Giovannelli J, Podevin C, Jachiet M, Bouaziz JD, Reguiai Z, et al. Effectiveness and safety of dupilumab for the treatment of atopic dermatitis in a real-life French multicenter adult cohort. J Am Acad Dermatol. 2019;81:143–51. https://doi.org/10.1016/j.jaad.2019.02.053.
5. Wang C, Kraus CN, Patel KG, Ganesan AK, Grando SA. Real-world experience of dupilumab treatment for atopic dermatitis in adults: a retrospective analysis of patients' records. Int J Dermatol. 2019;59(2):253–6. https://doi.org/10.1111/ijd.14573.
6. Ruiz-Villaverde R, Dominguez-Cruz J, Armario-Hita JC, Martinez-Pilar L, Alcantara-Luna S, Pereyra-Rodriguez JJ. Fifty-two week follow-up safety and effectiveness results of dupilumab treatment of moderate-to-severe atopic dermatitis from a retrospective, multicentric series. Dermatol Ther. 2019;32:e12931. https://doi.org/10.1111/dth.12931.
7. Allergy Asthma Clinical Immunology, Facial erythema after the treatment of dupilumab in SLE patient. Dong Hyek Jang, Jae In Lee, Joo Yoon Bae, Hye Jung Jung, Mi Yeon Park, Jiyoung Ahn. 2020;16:60
8. Sakhar A, Abdulmajeed A, Rakan A, et al. Dupilumab side effect in a patient with atopic dermatitis: a case report study. Biologics. 2019;13:79–82.
9. Jang DH, Ahn JY, et al. Treatment of moderate to severe atopic dermatitis with dupilumab: real world practice in Korea: free communication therapy presented at the 71st Korean Dermatological Association Annual Meeting, October 19–20, 2019, Seoul. Program book. p. 321. Abstract.
10. Uchida H, Kamata M, Mizukawa I, Watanabe A, Agematsu A, Nagata M, et al. Real-world effectiveness and safety of dupilumab for the treatment of atopic dermatitis in Japanese patients: a single-centre retrospective study. Br J Dermatol. 2019;181(5):1083–5. https://doi.org/10.1111/bjd.18163.
11. Cork MJ, Thaçi D, Eichenfield LF, Arkwright PD, Hultsch T, Davis JD, et al. Dupilumab in adolescents with uncontrolled moderate-to-severe atopic dermatitis: results from a phase IIa open-label trial and subsequent phase III open-label extension. Br J Dermatol. 2019;182(1):85–96. https://doi.org/10.1111/bjd.18476.
12. Werfel T, Allam JP, Biedermann T, et al. Cellular and molecular immunologic mechanisms in patients with atopic dermatitis. J Allergy Clin Immunol. 2016;138:336–49.
13. Karo-Atar D, Bitton A, Benhar I, et al. Therapeutic targeting of the interleukin-4/interleukin-13 signaling pathway: in allergy and beyond. BioDrugs. 2018;32:201–20.
14. Popovic B, Breed J, Rees DG, Gardener MJ, Vinall LM, Kemp B, Spooner J, Keen J, Minter R, Uddin F, Colice G, Wilkinson T, Vaughan T, May

RD. Structural characterisation reveals mechanism of IL-13-neutralising monoclonal antibody tralokinumab as inhibition of binding to IL-13Rα1 and IL-13Rα2. J Mol Biol. 2017;429(2):208.
15. Chandriani S, DePianto DJ, N'Diaye EN, Abbas AR, Jackman J, Bevers J 3rd, Ramirez-Carrozzi V, Pappu R, Kauder SE, Toy K, Ha C, Modrusan Z, Wu LC, Collard HR, Wolters PJ, Egen JG, Arron JR. Endogenously expressed IL-13Rα2 attenuates IL-13-mediated responses but does not activate signaling in human lung fibroblasts. J Immunol. 2014;193(1):111.
16. Kasaian MT, Raible D, Marquette K, Cook TA, Zhou S, Tan XY, Tchistiakova L. IL-13 antibodies influence IL-13 clearance in humans by modulating scavenger activity of IL-13Rα2. J Immunol. 2011;187(1):561.
17. Braddock M, Hanania NA, Sharafkhaneh A, Colice G, Carlsson M. Potential risks related to modulating interleukin-13 and interleukin-4 signalling: a systematic review. Drug Saf. 2018;41(5):489.
18. Wollenberg A, Howell MD, Guttman-Yassky E, Silverberg JI, Kell C, Ranade K, et al. Treatment of atopic dermatitis with tralokinumab, an anti-IL-13 mAb. J Allergy Clin Immunol. 2019;143:135–41. https://doi.org/10.1016/j.jaci.2018.05.029.
19. Ultsch M, Bevers J, Nakamura G, Vandlen R, Kelley RF, Wu LC, Eigenbrot C. Structural basis of signaling blockade by anti-IL-13 antibody Lebrikizumab. J Mol Biol. 2013;425(8):1330.
20. Simpson EL, Flohr C, Eichenfield LF, Bieber T, Sofen H, Taïeb A, et al. Efficacy and safety of lebrikizumab (an anti-IL-13 monoclonal antibody) in adults with moderate-to-severe atopic dermatitis inadequately controlled by topical corticosteroids: a randomized, placebo-controlled phase II trial (TREBLE). J Am Acad Dermatol. 2018;78:863–71.e11. https://doi.org/10.1016/j.jaad.2018.01.017.
21. Clinicaltrial.gov. (2019). https://clinicaltrials.gov/ct2/show/NCT03533751. Accessed 23 Oct 2019 (online database).
22. Silverberg JI, Pinter A, Pulka G, Poulin Y, Bouaziz JD, Wollenberg A, et al. Phase 2B randomized study of nemolizumab in adults with moderate-to-severe atopic dermatitis and severe pruritus. J Allergy Clin Immunol. 2019;145(1):173–82. https://doi.org/10.1016/j.jaci.2019.08.013.
23. Kabashima K, Furue M, Hanifin JM, Pulka G, Wollenberg A, Galus R, et al. Nemolizumab in patients with moderate-to-severe atopic dermatitis: randomized, phase II, long-term extension study. J Allergy Clin Immunol. 2018;142:1121–30.e7. https://doi.org/10.1016/j.jaci.2018.03.018.
24. Clinicaltrials.gov. (2019). https://clinicaltrials.gov/ct2/show/NCT01614756. Accessed 23 Oct 2019 (online database).
25. Soumelis V, Reche PA, Kanzlwe H, et al. Human epithelial cells trigger dendritic cell mediated allergic inflammation by producing TSLP. Nat Immunol. 2002;3:673–80.
26. Simpson EL, Parnes JR, She D, Crouch S, Rees W, Mo M, et al. Tezepelumab, an anti-thymic stromal lymphopoietin monoclonal antibody, in the treatment of moderate to severe atopic dermatitis: a randomized phase 2a clinical trial. J Am Acad Dermatol. 2019;80:1013–21. https://doi.org/10.1016/j.jaad.2018.11.059.
27. Kroemer A, Xiao X, Vu MD, et al. OX40 controls functionally different T cell subsets and their resistance to depletion therapy. J Immunol. 2007;179:5584–91.
28. Guttman-Yassky E, Pavel AB, Zhou L, Estrada YD, Zhang N, Xu H, et al. GBR 830, an anti-OX40, improves skin gene signatures and clinical scores in patients with atopic dermatitis. J Allergy Clin Immunol. 2019;144:482–93.e7. https://doi.org/10.1016/j.jaci.2018.11.053.
29. Kang EG, Narayana PK, Pouliquen IJ, Lopez MC, Ferreira-Cornwell MC, Getsy JA. Efficacy and safety of mepolizumab administered subcutaneously for moderate to severe atopic dermatitis. Allergy. 2019;75(4):950–3. https://doi.org/10.1111/all.14050.
30. Khattri S, Brunner PM, Garcet S, Finney R, Cohen SR, Oliva M, et al. Efficacy and safety of ustekinumab treatment in adults with moderate-to-severe atopic dermatitis. Exp Dermatol. 2017;26:28–35. https://doi.org/10.1111/exd.13112.
31. Clinicaltrials.gov. (2019). https://clinicaltrials.gov/ct2/show/NCT03568136. Accessed 23 Oct 2019 (online database).
32. Guttman-Yassky E, Krueger JG. IL-17C: a unique epithelial cytokine with potential for targeting across the spectrum of atopic dermatitis and psoriasis. J Invest Dermatol. 2018;138:1467–9. https://doi.org/10.1016/j.jid.2018.02.037.
33. Guttman-Yassky E, Brunner PM, Neumann AU, Khattri S, Pavel AB, Malik K, et al. Efficacy and safety of fezakinumab (an IL-22 monoclonal antibody) in adults with moderate-to-severe atopic dermatitis inadequately controlled by conventional treatments: a randomized, double-blind, phase 2a trial. J Am Acad Dermatol. 2018;78:872–881.e6. https://doi.org/10.1016/j.jaad.
34. Riese RJ, Krishnaswami S, Kremer J. Inhibition of JAK kinases in patients with rheumatoid arthritis: scientific rationale and clinical outcomes. Best Pract Res Clin Rheumatol. 2010;24(4):513–26.
35. Clinicaltrials.gov. (2019). https://clinicaltrials.gov/ct2/show/NCT03607422. Accessed 5 Nov 2019 (online database).
36. Guttman-Yassky E, Silverberg JI, Nemoto O, Forman SB, Wilke A, Prescilla R, et al. Baricitinib in adult patients with moderate-to-severe atopic dermatitis: a phase 2 parallel, double-blinded, randomized placebo-controlled multiple-dose study. J Am Acad Dermatol. 2019;80:913–921.e9. https://doi.org/10.1016/j.jaad.2018.01.018.
37. Kim BS, Howell MD, Sun K, Papp K, Nasir A, Kuligowski ME, et al. Treatment of atopic dermatitis with ruxolitinib cream (JAK1/JAK2 inhibitor) or triamcinolone cream. J

Allergy Clin Immunol. 2019;145(2):572–82. https://doi.org/10.1016/j.jaci.2019.08.042.
38. Levy LL, Urban J, King BA. Treatment of recalcitrant atopic dermatitis with the oral Janus kinase inhibitor tofacitinib citrate. J Am Acad Dermatol. 2015;73:395–9. https://doi.org/10.1016/j.jaad.2015.06.045.
39. Bissonnette R, Papp KA, Poulin Y, Gooderham M, Raman M, Mallbris L, et al. Topical tofacitinib for atopic dermatitis: a phase IIa randomized trial. Br J Dermatol. 2016;175:902–11. https://doi.org/10.1111/bjd.14871.
40. Bissonnette R, Maari C, Forman S, Bhatia N, Lee M, Fowler J, et al. The oral Janus kinase/spleen tyrosine kinase inhibitor ASN002 demonstrates efficacy and improves associated systemic inflammation in patients with moderate-to-severe atopic dermatitis: results from a randomized double-blind placebo-controlled study. Br J Dermatol. 2019;181(4):733–42. https://doi.org/10.1111/bjd.17932.
41. Clinicaltrails.gov. (2019). https://clinicaltrials.gov/ct2/show/NCT03654755. Accessed 5 Nov 2019 (online database).
42. Nakagawa H, Nemoto O, Igarashi A, Saeki H, Oda M, Kabashima K, et al. Phase 2 clinical study of delgocitinib ointment in pediatric patients with atopic dermatitis. J Allergy Clin Immunol. 2019;144(6):1575–83. https://doi.org/10.1016/j.jaci.2019.08.004.
43. Simpson EL, Imafuku S, Poulin Y, Ungar B, Zhou L, Malik K, et al. A phase 2 randomized trial of apremilast in patients with atopic dermatitis. J Invest Dermatol. 2019;139:1063–72. https://doi.org/10.1016/j.jid.2018.10.043.
44. Clinicaltrials.gov. (2019). https://clinicaltrials.gov/ct2/show/results/NCT01856764. Accessed 5 Nov 2019 (online database).
45. Paller AS, Tom WL, Lebwohl MG, Blumenthal RL, Boguniewicz M, Call RS, et al. Efficacy and safety of crisaborole ointment, a novel, nonsteroidal phosphodiesterase 4 (PDE4) inhibitor for the topical treatment of atopic dermatitis (AD) in children and adults. J Am Acad Dermatol. 2016;75:494–503.e6. https://doi.org/10.1016/j.jaad.2016.05.046.
46. Hanifin JM, Ellis CN, Frieden IJ, Fölster-Holst R, Stein Gold LF, Secci A, et al. OPA-15406, a novel, topical, nonsteroidal, selective phosphodiesterase-4 (PDE4) inhibitor, in the treatment of adult and adolescent patients with mild to moderate atopic dermatitis (AD): a phase-II randomized, double-blind, placebo-controlled study. J Am Acad Dermatol. 2016;75:297–305. https://doi.org/10.1016/j.jaad.2016.04.001.
47. Clinicaltrials.gov. (2019). https://clinicaltrials.gov/ct2/show/NCT03911401. Accessed 5 Nov 2019 (online database).
48. Clinicaltrials.gov. (2019). https://clinicaltrials.gov/ct2/show/NCT01993420. Accessed 5 Nov 2019 (online database).
49. Clinicaltrials.gov. (2019). https://clinicaltrials.gov/ct2/show/NCT01037881. Accessed 5 Nov 2019 (online database).

Phototherapy

Sang Ho Oh

Introduction

The management of atopic dermatitis (AD) includes regular use of emollient, avoidance of irritants and allergens, topical steroids or calcineurin inhibitors, and systemic immune modulators. Most patients with AD respond well to usual treatment, however, some may not get adequate disease control due to repeated relapses and aggravation.

This chapter addresses phototherapy, which can be considered as a second-line or adjuvant therapy for patients with AD who are not controlled with the use of emollient and topical steroids or calcineurin inhibitors. One questionnaire-based clinical study supported the hypothesis that phototherapy can be effectively used for the treatment of AD. The study showed that 74% of patients affected by mild-to-moderate AD had complete resolution during summer holidays and patients with seaside holidays produced a significantly greater improvement than those with mountain holidays [1]. Phototherapy is considered before the use of other systemic therapy [2] and recommended in patients with moderate-to-severe AD (SCORAD > 25), especially in adults and older children [3, 4]. European guideline for treatment of AD published in 2012 suggested that phototherapy in children younger than 12 years should not be applied [5]. However, according to recent European guideline [6], phototherapy is not contraindicated, although it is rarely used in prepubertal children. Therefore, phototherapy can be also efficacious in the pediatric population, considering the long-term risk of skin cancer, especially in fair-skinned individuals who might use systemic immunosuppressants later in life [2]. This chapter includes the mechanism of phototherapy in AD, various light sources for AD and practical consideration of phototherapy in AD and finally recommendation of phototherapy will be summarized based on evidence.

Biological Mechanism of Phototherapy in AD

Phototherapy is used for the treatment of skin disorders by various biologic effects in the skin through the energy transferred from natural or artificial light sources. As photochemical and photobiological characteristics in the skin vary according to the wavelengths of light sources, effective light sources can also be different depending on skin disorders. The main mechanism of phototherapy used for the treatment of AD is photo-immunologic effect, caused by a combination of immunosuppressive, immunomodulating, and anti-inflammatory effects. Second, phototherapy has an antimicrobial effect suppressing the colonization of

S. H. Oh (✉)
Department of Dermatology, Cutaneous Biology Research Institute, Severance Hospital, Yonsei University College of Medicine, Seoul, Korea (Republic of)
e-mail: oddung93@yuhs.ac

K. H. Lee et al. (eds.), *Practical Insights into Atopic Dermatitis*,
https://doi.org/10.1007/978-981-15-8159-5_17

Staphylococcus aureus in the skin, which is an aggravation factor in AD via upregulation of antimicrobial peptides and barrier recovery [7]. Third, phototherapy could improve symptoms of AD by attenuating penetration of allergens into the skin through increased epidermal thickness.

The evidence of the use of phototherapy for AD will be more detailedly addressed in the aspect of photoimmunology. Phototherapy induces apoptosis of T cells, which are the main culprit for the pathogenesis of AD. In particular, UVB decreases the activity of effector T cells infiltrated into the skin, while regulatory T cells are relatively unaffected, finally resulting in decrease in cellular immune responses. The mechanism of UVA phototherapy is associated with induction of singlet oxygen-induced T helper cell apoptosis [8]. In addition, UVA1 phototherapy suppresses gene expression of Th2-associated cytokines such as Il-5, IL-13, and IL-31 [9].

Regarding the role of regulatory T cells in the pathogenesis of AD [10, 11] and the change in blood and tissue regulatory T cells after phototherapy [12, 13], there are conflicting data depending on studies. There was a study in which other skin disorders including AD were enrolled, suggesting that induction of regulatory T cells is associated with increase in vitamin D following phototherapy [14]. However, a recent study reported that NBUVB phototherapy was associated with increased vitamin D concentrations, but not changes in circulating regulatory T cells in patients with AD [15]. Nevertheless, increased vitamin D following phototherapy could improve symptoms of AD through unknown vitamin D-mediated immune regulation.

UVB also affects dendritic cells in the skin directly or indirectly by IL-10 and prostaglandin E2, which show decreased function of antigen presentation to T cells [16]. Other mediators such as platelet-activating factor, melanocortin stimulating hormone, and calcitonin gene-related peptide also have immunosuppressive function [17]. In addition, phototherapy induces immunosuppression through depletion and loss of function of antigen-presenting cells in the epidermis and dermis. Decreased expression of ICAM-1 in the keratinocytes, which is enhanced via IL-10-induced reduction of IFN-Ɣ by phototherapy reduces migration and adhesion of T cells into the epidermis [18, 19].

As for mast cells, which play an important role in the pathogenesis of AD, it is known that high-dose UVA1, in particular, but not medium-dose UVA/UVB induces a minor decrease in dermal mast cells in addition to decreased number of dermal T cells and epidermal Langerhans cells [18, 20].

Various Light Sources and Practical Consideration of Phototherapy for the Treatment of AD

Light Sources in AD

Various types of phototherapy and light sources including broadband UVB (BB-UVB, 280–320 nm), narrowband UVB (NB-UVB, 311–313 nm), full-spectrum UVA (320–400 nm), ultraviolet A1 (UVA1, 340–400 nm), UVA+UVB (280–400 nm), photochemotherapy (psoralen plus UVA, PUVA), full-spectrum light (320–5000 nm, including UVA, visible light and infrared), and light-emitting diodes (LEDs) can be applied for patients with AD. In fact, a lot of studies have been performed to suggest the most effective phototherapy methods for the treatment of AD and NB-UVB and UVA1 are known as the mainstay for phototherapy in AD [2, 6, 21].

Generally, phototherapy is principally used for chronic lichenified lesions of AD except for UVA1, which is effective in acute flares of AD. Phototherapy is not recommended in patients with a history of photosensitivity.

From now, several studies addressing the effect and safety of phototherapy in AD will be stated depending on the devices of phototherapy with different wavelengths.

Heliotherapy

Heliotherapy, called climatotherapy, is one of phototherapy using natural sunlight under controlled conditions. The dose of sunlight is slowly raised by increasing sun exposure time.

Climatotherapy of AD at the Dead Sea was reported to highly effective in AD [22] and heliotherapy improved vitamin D balance along with marked healing of AD [23].

BB-UVB, Full-Spectrum UVA, UVA+UVB, Full-Spectrum Light, and Blue Light

A split-body study with BB-UVB on one half of the body and with visible light on the other showed that BB-UVB was more effective than visible light [24]. And a paired-comparison study between UVA+UVB and UVB in AD showed combined UVA and UVB was more effective than UVB only [25]. The same group performed two paired comparison study to compare the effect of UVA, low-dose UVB, and combined UVA and UVB. As a result, UVA+UVB showed a much higher effect on AD compared to UVA or low-dose UVB [26]. However, another group reported that cyclosporin was significantly better than UVA+UVB for the improvement of SCORAD [27]. As another light source for AD, there was one study that full-spectrum phototherapy significantly reduced SCORAD directly after treatment compared to control group with only emollients [28]. And it has been reported blue light irradiation (short-wave visible light, >380 nm) could have some effect in AD providing long-term control of disease [29]. However, based on the results of small uncontrolled studies of low quality, BB-UVB, full-spectrum UVA, UVA+UVB, full-spectrum light, and blue light are not recommended for the treatment of AD in recent times [21]. Interestingly, one study suggested BB-UVB needs to be revisited in AD even in the situation of NB-UVB fad because there are a significant proportion of AD patients who do not tolerate NB-UVB but show an excellent response to BB-UVB [30].

Photochemotherapy

In a randomized observer-blinded crossover study using oral psoralen and UVA (PUVA) photochemotherapy and medium dose UVA1 in 40 patients with severe AD, both phototherapies resulted in clinical improvement; however, PUVA showed a better response with long-term remission than medium-dose UVA1 [31]. In addition, in a randomized investigator-blinded half-side comparison study on 12 patients with severe chronic AD, both bath PUVA and NB-UVB phototherapy showed equally effective in equi-erythemogenic doses [32]. Normalization of abnormal semaphorin 3A and nerve growth factor by photochemotherapy was suggested as the mechanism of photochemotherapy for AD [33]. However, photochemotherapy is hardly accepted for the treatment modality of AD highly prevalent in young ages, because of the long-term risks of skin cancer and skin aging.

NB-UVB

George et al. [34] first reported NB-UVB is an effective, steroid-sparing treatment for chronic severe AD. In an open study of 21 severe AD patients, NB-UVB phototherapy three times weekly for 12 weeks achieved a 68% reduction in AD severity scores, with a concomitant 88% reduction in potent topical steroid. Since then, there have been many studies reporting that NB-UBV is effective for AD. In addition, one study reported that clinical improvement in AD patients with NB-UVB is accompanied with suppression of Th2/Th22-associated cytokines and chemokines and normalized expression of barrier proteins [35].

According to a randomized controlled study comparing the effect of NB-UVB, UVA, and visible fluorescent light in adult AD patients, two groups assigned to NB-UVB and UVA showed significantly more reductions in total disease activity compared to visible light [36]. As described earlier in photochemotherapy, both PUVA and NB-UVB are reported to be equally effective in AD [32]. There were several studies to compare the effect of medium dose UVA1 and NB-UVB phototherapy on AD. According to one initial, half-side comparison study in nine patients with chronic AD, NB-UVB had a greater therapeutic effect than medium dose UVA1 [37]. However, generally, medium dose UVA and NB-UVB phototherapy are known to have a comparable effect and similar tolerability for the treatment of AD [38, 39]. However, the total amount of irradiation required for effective phototherapy is lower for NB-UVB than for medium dose UVA1. NB-UVB is more comfortable than medium dose UVA1 because exposure time is much lower and less heat is produced in NB-UVB [39]. Consequently, NB-UVB is indicated for chronic AD, while UVA1 is more preferably prescribed in acute severe flares [6]. However, considering the low accessibility of UVA1 in the dermatology clinics compared to other devices, NB-UVB is regarded most effective, cost-effective, and evidence-based phototherapy in chronic AD [4]. And there was a first prospective randomized controlled study showing that synchronous bathing in 10% Dead Sea salt solution combined with NB-UVB (balneophototherapy) has a clear advantage over NB-UVB alone through measurement of SCORAD [40] (Fig. 1).

NB-UVB phototherapy also has advantage that it can be safely and effectively used in children with AD. Several retrospective reviews about the treatment outcomes of NB-UVB reported NB-UVB achieved significant improvement or clearance without serious adverse effects in children with AD [41–43]. Also in a recent retrospective study regarding phototherapy in children, 76% of 44 patients with AD aged 3–17 years who received NB-UVB showed clear to almost clear improvement [44]. The comparative

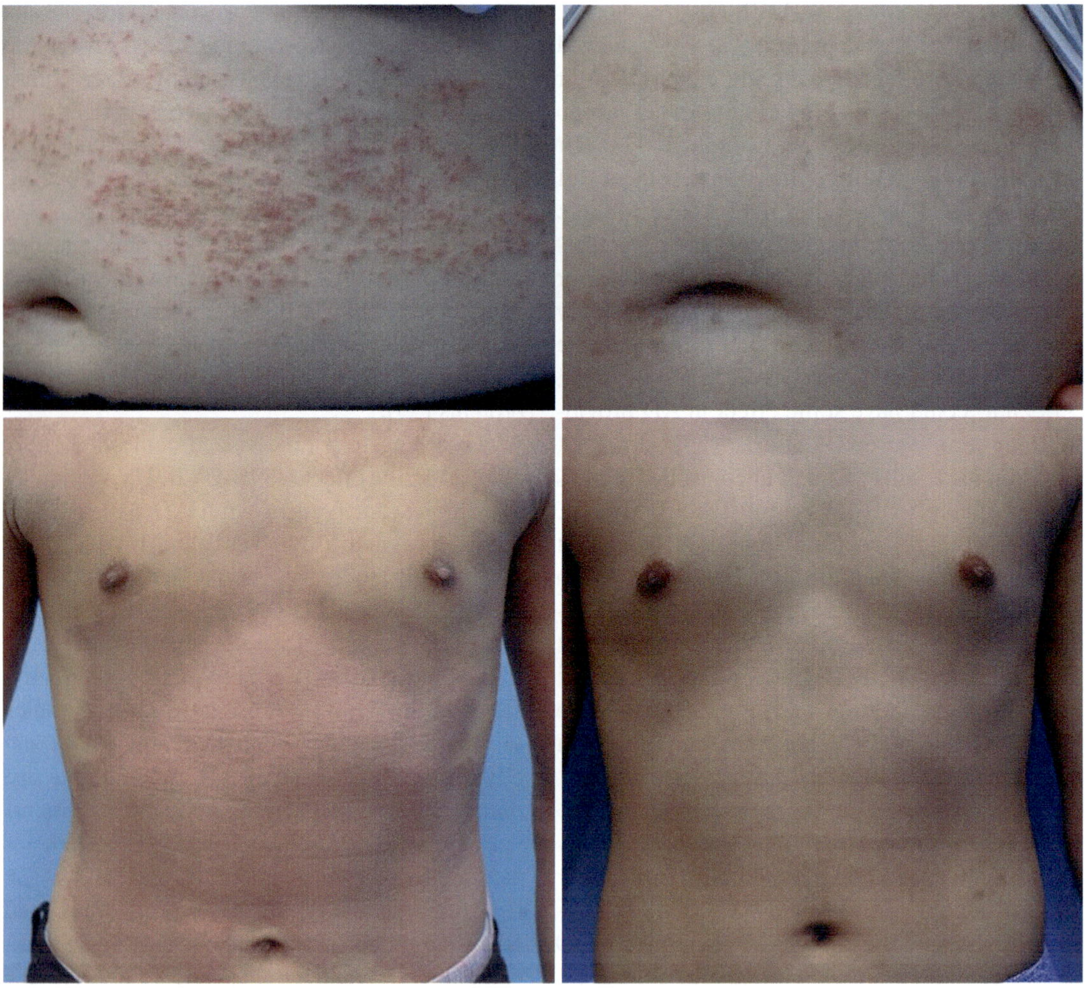

Fig. 1 Upper: Improvement of eczematous lesion on abdomen after total 24 times NBUVB during 3 months (Left: before NBUVB, Right: after NBUVB), Lower: Improvement of eczematous lesion on anterior trunk after total 40 times NBUVB during 5 months (Left: before NBUVB, Right: After NBUVB)

prospective cohort study was performed to evaluate the effect of NB-UVB in 29 children aged 3–16 years using Six Area Six Sign Atopic dermatitis (SASSAD) score. As a result, NBUVB is suggested to be effective and improve quality of life in children with moderate-to-severe AD, based on the findings that the NB-UVB cohort showed more significant reduction in mean SASSAD compared to the unexposed cohort [45]. In conclusion, NB-UVB is regarded as the first-line phototherapy because of several advantages such as its efficacy, steroid sparing, long remission, tolerability, easy administration, and low side effect [46].

UVA1

UVA1 is also reported to be very effective in AD and in particular, is indicated in acute flares of AD. UVA1 therapy has been introduced by Krutmann et al. for a novel treatment for AD and other inflammatory skin disorders [47]. In that comparison study between high dose UVA1 and UVA+UVB therapy, high dose UVA1 showed a favorable clinical improvement and significantly reduced serum levels of eosinophilic actionic protein in AD patients compared to UVA+UVB therapy. A randomized multicenter trial in the comparison of effectiveness among high dose UVA1, topical steroid therapy, and UVA-UVA therapy in AD confirmed that high dose UVA1 showed superior effect in clinical scores in addition to significantly decreased levels in serum eosinophil cation protein and eosinophil count [48]. However, high dose UVA1 can make patients intolerable to heat and sweating. Therefore, UVA1 cold light has been developed by filtering the infrared, making better improved remission than conventional UVA1 along with advantages of low heating and sweating [49]. And several studies were performed to compare their efficacies in AD among low, medium, and high dose UVA1. First, medium dose UVA1 was more effective for severe AD than low dose UVA1 [50]. A controlled within-subject comparison study of high dose and medium dose UVA1 demonstrated that medium dose UVA1 is known to be comparably as effective as high dose UVA1 [51]. In addition, a randomized, controlled prospective pilot study evaluated the efficacy of three kinds of UVA1 doses in patients with acute exacerbated AD. Even if low dose group did not show any clinical improvement, both high dose and medium dose groups showed a statistical reduction of the SCORAD, but medium dose was more tolerable in the aspect of patients' compliance [52]. Another recent randomized controlled, open trial showed both high and medium dose UVA1 resulted in a significant reduction of SCORAD in all AD patients. While high dose UVA1 was more effective than medium dose in AD patients with darker skin types, there were no significant differences between high and medium dose UVA1 in patients with fair skin types [53]. Despite highly therapeutic effect of medium dose UVA1 in acute exacerbated AD, there was one study to evaluate long-term efficacy of medium dose UVA1 in AD, suggesting the limitation of medium dose UVA1 such as short-term remission and recurrence after stopping treatment [54]. As mentioned in NB-UVB section, medium-dose UVA1 appears to have similar efficacy to NB-UVB phototherapy [38, 39]. To find out the mechanism of medium dose UVA1 in AD, the profiles of mRNA expression of hβ-defensin 1, IL-4, IL-10, and IL-31 were evaluated from the AD skins before and after phototherapy. Medium dose UVA1 improved SCORAD and pruritus but increased the expression of IL-4 without affecting other molecules, suggesting other unknown mediators might be involved in the mechanisms of UVA1 in AD [55].

308 nm Monochromatic Excimer Light or Laser

Targeted phototherapy using 308-nm monochromatic excimer light or laser could be a therapeutic option for localized and treatment-resistant AD despite no well-designed controlled study [56, 57]. In fact, the 308-nm excimer laser was reported to have a therapeutic effect on AD-like skin lesions in Nc/Nga mice [58] and one recent study suggested that excimer light treatment significantly change the composition of the bacterial microbiome in the lesional skins of AD patients along with clinical improvement [59]. However, excimer light or laser cannot be applied to generalized and widespread lesions of AD due to drawback of characteristics of the devices. Recently, as gain-switched 311-nm Ti-Sapphire laser as a new device was reported to improve AD-like skin lesions in Nc/Nga mouse model [60], it could be alternative option for localized AD lesions as like excimer laser.

Practical Consideration of Phototherapy for the Treatment of AD

Even if NB-UVB and medium-dose UVA1 are recommended for the treatment of AD, NB-UVB is more preferably used due to low availability of UVA1 device, which is more expensive to purchase and to maintain. And the exposure time is much longer and more heat is highly produced in UVA1 device compared to NB-UVB.

The disadvantage of phototherapy is that the patients have to visit a hospital to receive phototherapy for several weeks or more. Therefore, home-based phototherapy device is suggested as another option. However, there are still doubts about irradiances and wavelengths of light sources because the devices are not regulated thoroughly.

There is still no standardized protocol for optimal energy, duration, and frequency of phototherapy in AD. However, recommended treatment duration is 6–12 weeks or longer, twice or three times per week to induce sustained remission. If there is no response within 8–12 weeks, further phototherapy is not encouraged [2]. In general, phototherapy is not recommended for acute inflamed AD except UVA1, which is the best option for acute flares in AD and is rather appropriate to treat chronic, lichenified lesions of AD. The use of emollients and topical steroids is encouraged to control acute disease and prevent possible flare-up before the beginning of phototherapy [6]. If AD repeatedly flares during phototherapy, discontinuation of phototherapy is required. If AD shows rapid relapse despite improvement with phototherapy, other systemic treatment should be considered because long-term or frequent phototherapy can bring out safety issues. Phototherapy can decrease bacterial or fungal colonization and reduce the amount of topical drugs. The use of topical calcineurin inhibitor is not recommended in phototherapy. Concomitant use of systemic immunosuppressants such as cyclosporin, azathioprine, and mycophenolate mofetil should be avoided during phototherapy due to the risk of skin cancers but methotrexate is unrestricted in the combination with phototherapy compared to other systemic drugs [61].

Summary and Recommendation of Phototherapy in AD

Phototherapy is recommended as a second-line or adjunctive treatment option for moderate-to-severe AD, especially in adults and older children. Although phototherapy is rarely used for young children, it is not contraindicated. In particular, NB-UVB can be used safely in young children with AD but other modalities of phototherapy still have lack of evidence in safety. NB-UVB and medium dose UVA-1 phototherapy are the most effective phototherapy modalities with well-proven evidences in AD. NB-UVB has been shown to be most effective in managing chronic AD, whereas UVA-1 may be used for acute severe flares. NB-UVB is more preferably recommended for the treatment of AD than BB-UVB, which is more erythemogenic. Combined use of topical steroid and emollient is recommended at the beginning of phototherapy to prevent acute flare. All of phototherapy treatments have a long-term risk of skin aging and skin cancer. Therefore, long-term studies for safety issues of phototherapy are required. PUVA phototherapy is not recommended as a first-line phototherapy because of safety concerns. A 308-nm excimer laser or light could be a good option for localized refractory AD lesions. And new devices such as visible light including blue light may widen treatment options for AD but need to be assessed for their efficacy and safety. In the future, large-scale randomized controlled studies for phototherapy in AD regarding the most effective modality, optimal protocol, maintenance therapy, long-term effect or safety, and newly developed devices are required.

References

1. Patrizi A, Savoia F, Giacomini F, Tabanelli M, Gurioli C. The effect of summer holidays and sun exposure on atopic dermatitis. G Ital Dermatol Venereol. 2009;144(4):463–6.
2. Simpson EL, Bruin-Weller M, Flohr C, Ardern-Jones MR, Barbarot S, Deleuran M, et al. When does atopic dermatitis warrant systemic therapy? Recommendations from an expert panel of the International Eczema Council. J Am Acad Dermatol. 2017;77(4):623–33.
3. Sidbury R, Davis DM, Cohen DE, Cordoro KM, Berger TG, Bergman JN, et al. Guidelines of care for the management of atopic dermatitis: section 3. Management and treatment with phototherapy and systemic agents. J Am Acad Dermatol. 2014;71(2):327–49.
4. Kim JE, Kim HJ, Lew BL, Lee KH, Hong SP, Jang YH, et al. Consensus guidelines for the treatment of atopic dermatitis in Korea (part II): systemic treatment. Ann Dermatol. 2015;27(5):578–92.
5. Ring J, Alomar A, Bieber T, Deleuran M, Fink-Wagner A, Gelmetti C, et al. Guidelines for treatment of atopic eczema (atopic dermatitis) Part II. J Eur Acad Dermatol Venereol. 2012;26(9):1176–93.
6. Wollenberg A, Barbarot S, Bieber T, Christen-Zaech S, Deleuran M, Fink-Wagner A, et al. Consensus-based European guidelines for treatment of atopic eczema (atopic dermatitis) in adults and children: part I. J Eur Acad Dermatol Venereol. 2018;32(5):657–82.
7. Hong SP, Kim MJ, Jung MY, Jeon H, Goo J, Ahn SK, et al. Biopositive effects of low-dose UVB on epidermis: coordinate upregulation of antimicrobial peptides and permeability barrier reinforcement. J Invest Dermatol. 2008;128(12):2880–7.
8. Morita A, Werfel T, Stege H, Ahrens C, Karmann K, Grewe M, et al. Evidence that singlet oxygen-induced human T helper cell apoptosis is the basic mechanism of ultraviolet-A radiation phototherapy. J Exp Med. 1997;186(10):1763–8.
9. Gambichler T, Kreuter A, Tomi NS, Othlinghaus N, Altmeyer P, Skrygan M. Gene expression of cytokines in atopic eczema before and after ultraviolet A1 phototherapy. Br J Dermatol. 2008;158(5):1117–20.
10. Reefer AJ, Satinover SM, Solga MD, Lannigan JA, Nguyen JT, Wilson BB, et al. Analysis of CD25(hi) CD(4+) "regulatory" T-cell subtypes in atopic dermatitis reveals a novel T(H)2-like population. J Allergy Clin Immunol. 2008;121(2):415–22.
11. Roesner LM, Floess S, Witte T, Olek S, Huehn J, Werfel T. Foxp3(+) regulatory T cells are expanded in severe atopic dermatitis patients. Allergy. 2015;70(12):1656–60.
12. Schnopp C, Rad R, Weidinger A, Weidinger S, Ring J, Eberlein B, et al. Fox-P3-positive regulatory T cells are present in the skin of generalized atopic eczema patients and are not particularly affected by medium-dose UVA1 therapy. Photodermatol Photoimmunol Photomed. 2007;23(2–3):81–5.
13. El Samahy MH, Attia EAS, Saad AA, Mahmoud EY. Circulating CD4(+)CD25(high)FoxP3(+) T-regulatory cells in patients with atopic dermatitis after narrowband-ultraviolet B phototherapy. Int J Dermatol. 2015;54(10):E424–E9.
14. Milliken SV, Wassall H, Lewis BJ, Logie J, Barker RN, Macdonald H, et al. Effects of ultraviolet light on human serum 25-hydroxyvitamin D and systemic immune function. J Allergy Clin Immunol. 2012;129(6):1554–61.
15. Simonsen S, Bonefeld CM, Thyssen JP, Geisler C, Skov L. Increase in vitamin D but not regulatory T cells following ultraviolet B phototherapy of patients with atopic dermatitis. Acta Derm Venereol. 2019;99(2):139–45.
16. Pentland AP, Mahoney M, Jacobs SC, Holtzman MJ. Enhanced prostaglandin synthesis after ultraviolet injury is mediated by endogenous histamine stimulation—a mechanism for irradiation erythema. J Clin Invest. 1990;86(2):566–74.
17. Zhang QW, Yao YX, Konger RL, Sinn AL, Cai SB, Pollok KE, et al. UVB radiation-mediated inhibition of contact hypersensitivity reactions is dependent on the platelet-activating factor system. J Invest Dermatol. 2008;128(7):1780–7.
18. Grabbe J, Welker P, Humke S, Grewe M, Schopf E, Henz BM, et al. High-dose ultraviolet A1 (UVA1), but not UVA/UVB therapy, decreases IgE-binding cells in lesional skin of patients with atopic eczema. J Invest Dermatol. 1996;107(3):419–22.
19. Grewe M, Gyufko K, Krutmann J. Interleukin-10 production by cultured human keratinocytes—regulation by ultraviolet-B and ultraviolet A1 radiation. J Invest Dermatol. 1995;104(1):3–6.
20. Breuckmann F, von Kobyletzki G, Avermaete A, Kreuter A, Altmeyer P, Gambichler T. Mast cells in atopic dermatitis: resistance against medium-dose UVA1 phototherapy? Dermatology. 2003;207(3):334–6.
21. Garritsen FM, Brouwer MWD, Limpens J, Spuls PI. Photo(chemo) therapy in the management of atopic dermatitis: an updated systematic review with implications for practice and research. Br J Dermatol. 2014;170(3):501–13.
22. Harari M, Shani J, Seidl V, Hristakieva E. Climatotherapy of atopic dermatitis at the Dead Sea: demographic evaluation and cost-effectiveness. Int J Dermatol. 2000;39(1):59–69.
23. Vahavihu K, Ylianttila L, Salmelin R, Lamberg-Allardt C, Viljakainen H, Tuohimaa P, et al.

Heliotherapy improves vitamin D balance and atopic dermatitis. Br J Dermatol. 2008;158(6):1323–8.
24. Jekler J, Larko O. UVB phototherapy of atopic dermatitis. Br J Dermatol. 1988;119(6):697–705.
25. Jekler J, Larko O. Combined Uva-Uvb versus Uvb phototherapy for atopic-dermatitis—a paired-comparison study. J Am Acad Dermatol. 1990;22(1):49–53.
26. Jekler J, Larko O. Phototherapy for atopic-dermatitis with ultraviolet-a (Uva), low-dose Uvb and combined Uva and Uvb—2 paired-comparison studies. Photodermatol Photoimmunol Photomed. 1991;8(4):151–6.
27. Granlund H, Erkko P, Remitz A, Langeland T, Helsing P, Nuutinen M, et al. Comparison of cyclosporin and UVAB phototherapy for intermittent one-year treatment of atopic dermatitis. Acta Derm Venereol. 2001;81(1):22–7.
28. Byun HJ, Lee HI, Kim B, Kim MN, Hong H, Choi Y, et al. Full-spectrum light phototherapy for atopic dermatitis. Int J Dermatol. 2011;50(1):94–101.
29. Becker D, Langer E, Seemann M, Seemann G, Fell I, Saloga J, et al. Clinical efficacy of blue light full body irradiation as treatment option for severe atopic dermatitis. PLoS One. 2011;6(6):e20566.
30. Pugashetti R, Lim HW, Koo J. Broadband UVB revisited: is the narrowband UVB fad limiting our therapeutic options? J Dermatol Treat. 2010;21(6):326–30.
31. Tzaneva S, Kittler H, Holzer G, Reljic D, Weber M, Honigsmann H, et al. 5-Methoxypsoralen plus ultraviolet (UV) A is superior to medium-dose UVA1 in the treatment of severe atopic dermatitis: a randomized crossover trial. Br J Dermatol. 2010;162(3):655–60.
32. Der-Petrossian M, Seeber A, Honigsmann H, Tanew A. Half-side comparison study on the efficacy of 8-methoxypsoralen bath-PUVA versus narrowband ultraviolet B phototherapy in patients with severe chronic atopic dermatitis. Br J Dermatol. 2000;142(1):39–43.
33. Tominaga M, Tengara S, Kamo A, Ogawa H, Takamori K. Psoralen-ultraviolet A therapy alters epidermal Sema3A and NGF levels and modulates epidermal innervation in atopic dermatitis. J Dermatol Sci. 2009;55(1):40–6.
34. George SA, Bilsland DJ, Johnson BE, Ferguson J. Narrow-band (TL-01) UVB air-conditioned phototherapy for chronic severe adult atopic dermatitis. Br J Dermatol. 1993;128(1):49–56.
35. Tintle S, Shemer A, Suarez-Farinas M, Fujita H, Gilleaudeau P, Sullivan-Whalen M, et al. Reversal of atopic dermatitis with narrow-band UVB phototherapy and biomarkers for therapeutic response. J Allergy Clin Immunol. 2011;128(3):583–93 e1-4.
36. Reynolds NJ, Franklin V, Gray JC, Diffey BL, Farr PM. Narrow-band ultraviolet B and broadband ultraviolet A phototherapy in adult atopic eczema: a randomised controlled trial. Lancet. 2001;357(9273):2012–6.
37. Legat FJ, Hofer A, Brabek E, Quehenberger F, Kerl H, Wolf P. Narrowband UV-B vs medium-dose UV-A1 phototherapy in chronic atopic dermatitis. Arch Dermatol. 2003;139(2):223–4.
38. Majoie IM, Oldhoff JM, van Weelden H, Laaper-Ertmann M, Bousema MT, Sigurdsson V, et al. Narrowband ultraviolet B and medium-dose ultraviolet A1 are equally effective in the treatment of moderate to severe atopic dermatitis. J Am Acad Dermatol. 2009;60(1):77–84.
39. Gambichler T, Othlinghaus N, Tomi NS, Holland-Letz T, Boms S, Skrygan M, et al. Medium-dose ultraviolet (UV) A1 vs. narrowband UVB phototherapy in atopic eczema: a randomized crossover study. Br J Dermatol. 2009;160(3):652–8.
40. Heinlin J, Schiffner-Rohe J, Schiffner R, Einsele-Kramer B, Landthaler M, Klein A, et al. A first prospective randomized controlled trial on the efficacy and safety of synchronous balneophototherapy vs. narrow-band UVB monotherapy for atopic dermatitis. J Eur Acad Dermatol. 2011;25(7):765–73.
41. Collins P, Ferguson J. Narrowband (TL-01) UVB air-conditioned phototherapy for atopic eczema in children. Br J Dermatol. 1995;133(4):653–5.
42. Jury CS, McHenry P, Burden AD, Lever R, Bilsland D. Narrowband ultraviolet B (UVB) phototherapy in children. Clin Exp Dermatol. 2006;31(2):196–9.
43. Pavlovsky M, Baum S, Shpiro D, Pavlovsky L, Pavlotsky F. Narrow band UVB: is it effective and safe for paediatric psoriasis and atopic dermatitis? J Eur Acad Dermatol Venereol. 2011;25(6):727–9.
44. Eustace K, Dolman S, Alsharqi A, Sharpe G, Parslew R. Use of phototherapy in children. Pediatr Dermatol. 2017;34(2):150–5.
45. Darne S, Leech SN, Taylor AE. Narrowband ultraviolet B phototherapy in children with moderate-to-severe eczema: a comparative cohort study. Br J Dermatol. 2014;170(1):150–6.
46. Rodenbeck DL, Silverberg JI, Silverberg NB. Phototherapy for atopic dermatitis. Clin Dermatol. 2016;34(5):607–13.
47. Krutmann J, Czech W, Diepgen T, Niedner R, Kapp A, Schopf E. High-dose Uva1 therapy in the treatment of patients with atopic-dermatitis. J Am Acad Dermatol. 1992;26(2):225–30.
48. Krutmann J, Diepgen TL, Luger TA, Grabbe S, Meffert H, Sonnichsen N, et al. High-dose UVA1 therapy for atopic dermatitis: results of a multicenter trial. J Am Acad Dermatol. 1998;38(4):589–93.
49. von Kobyletzki G, Pieck C, Hoffmann K, Freitag M, Altmeyer P. Medium-dose UVA1 cold-light phototherapy in the treatment of severe atopic dermatitis. J Am Acad Dermatol. 1999;41(6):931–7.
50. Kowalzick L, Kleinheinz A, Neuber K, Weichenthal M, Kohler I, Ring J. Elevated serum levels of soluble adhesion molecules Icam-1 and Elam-1 in patients with severe atopic eczema and influence of Uva1 treatment. Dermatology. 1995;190(1):14–8.
51. Tzaneva S, Seeber A, Schwaiger M, Honigsmann H, Tanew A. High-dose versus medium-dose UVA1 phototherapy for patients with severe gen-

eralized atopic dermatitis. J Am Acad Dermatol. 2001;45(4):503–7.
52. Dittmar HC, Pflieger D, Schopf E, Simon JC. UVA1 phototherapy. Pilot study to determine dosage in acute exacerbated atopic dermatitis. Hautarzt. 2001;52(5):423–7.
53. Pacifico A, Iacovelli P, Damiani G, Ferraro C, Cazzaniga S, Conic RRZ, et al. 'High dose' vs. 'medium dose' UVA1 phototherapy in Italian patients with severe atopic dermatitis. J Eur Acad Dermatol Venereol. 2019;33(4):718–24.
54. Abeck D, Schmidt T, Fesq H, Strom K, Mempel M, Brockow K, et al. Long-term efficacy of medium-dose UVA1 phototherapy in atopic dermatitis. J Am Acad Dermatol. 2000;42(2):254–7.
55. Bogaczewicz J, Malinowska K, Sysa-Jedrzejowska A, Wozniacka A. Medium-dose ultraviolet A1 phototherapy improves SCORAD index and increases mRNA expression of interleukin-4 without direct effect on human beta defensin-1, interleukin-10, and interleukin-31. Int J Dermatol. 2016;55(7):E380–E5.
56. Mavilia L, Mori M, Rossi R, Campolmi P, Puglisi Guerra A, Lotti T. 308 nm monochromatic excimer light in dermatology: personal experience and review of the literature. G Ital Dermatol Venereol. 2008;143(5):329–37.
57. Wollenschlager I, Hermann J, Ockenfels HM. Targeted UVB-308 nm (NUVB) therapy with excimer laser in the treatment of atopic dermatitis and other inflammatory dermatoses. Hautarzt. 2009;60(11):898–906.
58. Oh CT, Kwon TR, Seok J, Choi EJ, Kim SR, Jang YJ, et al. Effect of a 308-nm excimer laser on atopic dermatitis-like skin lesions in NC/Nga mice. Laser Surg Med. 2016;48(6):629–37.
59. Kurosaki Y, Tsurumachi M, Kamata Y, Tominaga M, Suga Y, Takamori K. Effects of 308 nm excimer light treatment on the skin microbiome of atopic dermatitis patients. Photodermatol Photoimmunol Photomed. 2019;36(3):185–91.
60. Choi SY, Oh CT, Kwon TR, Kwon HJ, Choi EJ, Jang YJ, et al. Gain-switched 311-nm Ti:Sapphire laser might be a potential treatment modality for atopic dermatitis. Laser Med Sci. 2016;31(7):1437–45.
61. Soliman A, Nofal E, Nofal A, El Desouky F, Asal M. Combination therapy of methotrexate plus NBUVB phototherapy is more effective than methotrexate monotherapy in the treatment of chronic plaque psoriasis. J Dermatol Treat. 2015;26(6):528–34.

Allergen Immunotherapy for Atopic Dermatitis

Dong-Ho Nahm, Kwang Hoon Lee, and Chang Ook Park

Introduction

Atopic dermatitis (AD) is a common chronic inflammatory skin disease characterized by itching, dry skin, eczema, and frequent association with a personal or familial history of atopic diseases [1]. Hypersensitivity reaction (allergic reaction) to environmental agents has been suggested as an important pathogenetic mechanism responsible for the development and maintenance of chronic skin inflammation in AD [1]. However, the pathogenetic mechanism of AD seems to be more complexly associated with genetic predisposition, environmental triggering factor, immune dysfunction, hypersensitivity reaction, chronic skin inflammation, and skin barrier defect [2].

Current standard medical therapy for AD using topical corticosteroids or topical calcineurin inhibitors is mainly focused on transient symptomatic relief, and its clinical efficacy is often disappointing to both patients and physicians [2]. Although a significant number of patients with moderate-to-severe AD can be improved by a systemic treatment with corticosteroid, cyclosporine, or methotrexate, there is a possibility of systemic toxicity from long-term treatment with these compounds [1]. Recent randomized clinical trials showed that significant clinical improvements could be induced by the treatment with monoclonal antibody to interleukin (IL)-4 receptor alpha (Dupilumab) or monoclonal antibody to IL-13 in patients with moderate-to-severe AD [3–6]. These results suggest that hypersensitivity reaction (allergic reaction characterized by activation of Th2 immune pathway) plays a key role in pathogenesis of AD and could be a useful therapeutic target for AD [2]. Because clinical efficacies of currently available pharmacological therapies for AD are transient and incomplete, further development of a new therapeutic modality is required to improve the long-term clinical course of AD [2].

Allergen immunotherapy (also named as allergen-specific immunotherapy or allergy immunotherapy, AIT) is a treatment method of administering increasing doses of a clinically relevant allergen to a patient with allergic disease [7–10]. Methodologically, AIT can be performed by subcutaneous injection (subcutaneous immunotherapy: SCIT) or sublingual administration (sublingual immunotherapy: SLIT) [8, 9]. AIT can decrease

D.-H. Nahm (✉)
Department of Allergy and Clinical Immunology, Ajou University School of Medicine, Suwon, Korea (Republic of)
email: dhnahm@gmail.com

K. H. Lee · C. O. Park
Department of Dermatology, Cutaneous Biology Research Institute, Yonsei University College of Medicine, Seoul, Korea (Republic of)

K. H. Lee et al. (eds.), *Practical Insights into Atopic Dermatitis*,
https://doi.org/10.1007/978-981-15-8159-5_18

a hypersensitivity reaction to allergen, reduce the clinical symptoms induced by exposure to allergen, prevent sensitization to a new allergen, and produce a sustained clinical improvement even after discontinuation of treatment [7–10]. The clinical efficacy of AIT has been proven for the treatment of allergic rhinitis, allergic asthma, and bee venom hypersensitivity by systematic reviews analyzing multiple randomized, double-blind, placebo-controlled clinical trials (strong evidence) [11–13]. The disease-modifying effects of AIT have been proven for allergic asthma and allergic rhinitis [14–16]. A meta-analysis of randomized clinical trials on AIT in patients with AD provided a moderate-level evidence of the clinical efficacy for AD [14]. However, the clinical usefulness of AIT for AD is still controversial [13]. This controversy is mainly due to limited numbers of well-designed randomized controlled clinical trials evaluating the clinical efficacy of AIT in patients with AD. Other disadvantages of clinical application of AIT for AD are lack of knowledge on the degree of clinical efficacy, no available clinical or biological marker to predict a favorable clinical response, and risk of systemic allergic reaction including anaphylaxis.

AIT has an important advantage as a treatment for AD compared to other pharmacological therapies because AIT has a potential as a disease-modifying therapy for AD that can change a long-term clinical course of AD [2, 17]. There have been several reports on the long-term clinical improvement (clinical remission) after AIT in patients with AD [18, 19]. However, a further well-designed clinical trial is needed to confirm the long-term disease-modifying clinical efficacy of AIT in patients with AD.

History of AIT for AD

Historically, SCIT was firstly implemented by Noon in England in 1911 for patients with seasonal allergic rhinitis and allergic conjunctivitis sensitized to grass pollen [20].

In 1953, Diamond HE firstly reported the eight patients with respiratory allergic and concomitant AD who experienced a clinical improvement of AD after SCIT with inhalant allergens for the treatment of respiratory allergic diseases [21].

In 1960, Tuft L reported the results of SCIT with inhalant allergens in 101 patients with AD and a favorable clinical response was observed after SCIT in 77.2% of the patients. In this report, clinical exacerbation of AD was observed in the 5 of 101 patients and it was developed at 12–48 h after SCIT and 4 of the 5 patients discontinued the SCIT due to this "delayed adverse reaction" [22].

In 1974, Kauffman HS and Roth HL reported the results of the first randomized placebo-controlled clinical trial on the efficacy of AIT in 52 children and adult patients with AD [23].

In 2013, Bae JM et al. reported the results of the first meta-analysis on AIT for AD and confirmed a significant therapeutic benefit for patients with AD by analyzing eight randomized placebo-controlled clinical trials sensitized to inhalant allergens (moderate-level evidence) (Fig. 1) [13]. However, this findings is based on an analysis of a small

Study or Subgroup	log[Odds Ratio]	SE	Treatment Total	Placebo Total	Weight	Odds Ratio IV, Random, 95% CI	Year
Kaufman et al.	1.7047	0.6703	26	26	13.5%	5.50 [1.48, 20.46]	1974
Warner et al.	2.2336	1.0494	9	11	10.9%	9.33 [1.19, 72.99]	1978
Glover et al.	-0.3409	0.8283	13	13	12.4%	0.71 [0.14, 3.61]	1992
Leroy et al.	2.6847	0.87	12	11	12.1%	14.65 [2.66, 80.63]	1993
Galli et al.	0.0588	0.7074	16	18	13.2%	1.06 [0.27, 4.24]	1994
Silny et al.	3.5835	1.3176	10	10	9.2%	36.00 [2.72, 476.25]	2006
Pajno et al.	4.1359	0.6849	26	22	13.4%	62.55 [16.34, 239.43]	2007
Novak et al.	0.1995	0.3332	107	55	15.3%	1.22 [0.64, 2.35]	2012
Total (95% CI)			**219**	**166**	**100.0%**	**5.35 [1.61, 17.77]**	

Heterogeneity: Tau² = 2.34; Chi² = 41.00, df = 7 (P <.00001); I^2 = 83%
Test for overall effect: Z = 2.74 (P =.006)

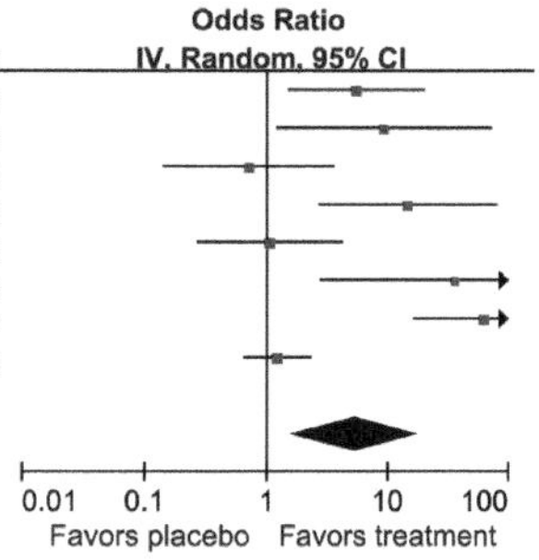

Fig. 1 Meta-analysis of eight randomized controlled trials of allergen immunotherapy in patients with atopic dermatitis. A random-effects model was used to produce data. Allergen immunotherapy has a significant positive effect on atopic dermatitis (odds ratio [OR], 5.35; 95% CI, 1.61–17.77; number needed to treat, 3; 95% CI, 2–9) [13]

number of randomized controlled trials with considerable heterogeneity among trials [13].

In 2013, Gendelman SR et al. reported a systematic review using the Grading of Recommendations Assessment, Development, and Evaluation (GRADE) system to evaluate clinical efficacy of AIT for AD by analyzing seven randomized placebo-controlled trials [24]. Although all seven randomized placebo-controlled trials reported a significant improvement of clinical symptoms, the authors concluded the strength of recommendation for use of AIT in patients with AD as weak because of a small number of randomized controlled trials and methodological shortcomings in the study designs of these trials. They suggested a need for an additional high-quality evidence to evaluate the clinical efficacy of AIT in AD [24].

In 2016, Tam HH et al. reported a Cochrane systematic review on the clinical efficacy of AIT for the treatment of AD by analyzing 12 eligible randomized controlled trials. The evidence regarding efficacy of AIT for AD was marked by inconsistency in study findings and the low grade of evidence. This systematic review concludes that there is no consistent evidence that AIT is effective for treating AD due to low quality of evidence and further large, rigorously conducted randomized controlled trials using modern high-quality allergens are needed [25].

Scientific Rationale of AIT for AD: Importance of Allergic Mechanism in the Pathogenesis of AD

The AD seems to be a multifactorial complex disorder caused and maintained by multiple pathogenetic elements including genetic predisposition, environmental triggering factor, immune dysfunction, hypersensitivity reaction, chronic skin inflammation, and skin barrier defect [2]. However, the precise interactions among the multiple pathogenetic elements involved in the development and maintenance of AD are not completely understood yet.

Hypersensitivity reaction (allergic reaction) to environmental allergen plays a critical role in the development and maintenance of AD based on the multiple evidences (Table 1) [2]. These evidences provide scientific a rationale supporting allergen-specific therapies including avoidance of a clinically relevant sensitized allergen and AIT in patients with AD.

Table 1 Evidences supporting a key role of allergic mechanism in the pathogenesis of atopic dermatitis

1. Exposure to a sensitized allergen (skin contact, inhalation, etc.) aggravates pre-existing eczematous skin lesion or induces new eczematous skin lesion in patients with atopic dermatitis.
2. Avoidance of a sensitized allergen induces clinical improvement in patients with atopic dermatitis.
3. Allergen immunotherapy that administering increasing doses of a clinical relevant sensitized allergen to induce an allergen-specific immune tolerance provides in clinical improvement in patients with atopic dermatitis sensitized to inhalant allergens.
4. Allergic sensitization to common inhalant or food allergen is present in the majorities of patients with atopic dermatitis (80–90%).
5. Serum IgE levels are increased in majorities of patients with atopic dermatitis
6. Patients with atopic dermatitis are frequently affected by coexisting other allergic diseases (allergic rhinitis, allergic keratoconjunctivitis, and asthma).
7. Children with atopic dermatitis frequently outgrow the atopic dermatitis before the puberty and progress to asthma and allergic rhinitis ("allergic march").
8. Significant clinical improvement of atopic dermatitis can be induced by monoclonal antibody to IL-4 receptor alpha blocking the biological effects of both IL-4 and IL-13 (main cytokines from Th2 cells).
9. Immunoadsorption selectively removing IgE antibodies from plasma using an anti-IgE antibody column induced significant clinical improvements in patients with severe atopic dermatitis.
10. Passive transfer of atopic dermatitis in recipient following bone marrow transplantation from a donor with atopic dermatitis.

Method of AIT

Subcutaneous Allergen Immunotherapy and Sublingual Allergen Immunotherapy

Subcutaneous injection of allergen extract (SCIT) has been the predominant method for AIT since 1911 when the Noon reported the first successful implementation of AIT with grass pollen extract in patients with seasonal allergic rhinoconjunctivitis [20].

However, clinical application of sublingual administration of the allergen extract (SLIT) has been increased and is now a dominant method of AIT in European countries since 1986 when the Scadding GK and Brostoff J reported the first successful trial of sublingual administration of house dust mite extract in liquid form in patients with allergic rhinitis [26]. SLIT can be self-administered by patient or caregiver at home and allergen extract (either liquid or tablet form) is placed under the tongue for at least 1–2 min and then is swallowed. Recently, clinical efficacy and safety of SLIT for respiratory allergic diseases including allergic rhinitis and allergic asthma have been clearly demonstrated by randomized controlled studies [27, 28]. Systemic allergic reaction is very rare with SLIT [27].

The indication of SLIT is basically the same as SCIT. However, SLIT is clinically useful for the patient who experienced severe allergic reaction during SCIT, or the patient dislikes or fears injection therapy (especially in children), or patient with difficulty for regular hospital visits due to their occupation (company employee or student), or patient who live in the distant location from the hospital (Table 2).

Although there are only small numbers of studies comparing the clinical efficacy of SCIT and SLIT, clinical efficacy of SCIT seems to be higher than the SLIT (Table 2) [29].

Table 2 Comparison of subcutaneous allergen immunotherapy and sublingual allergen immunotherapy

	Subcutaneous allergen immunotherapy	Sublingual allergen immunotherapy
History	From 1911	From 1986
Treatment method	Subcutaneous injection at the hospital	Sublingual self-administration at home
Safety	Rarely, severe systemic allergic reaction (anaphylaxis) can occur (mostly within 30 min after injection)	Very low risk of a severe systemic allergic reaction
A useful indication	Patients who can regularly visit hospital for 3–5 years	Patients who cannot regularly visit hospitals due to variable reasons (occupation or distant location)
Therapeutic efficacy	High	Moderate to high
Advantage	High therapeutic efficacy	High safety and easiness for patients

The Schedules of AIT

In a traditional schedule of SCIT, weekly subcutaneous injections of increasing doses of allergen extract are required for 12–16 weeks during the initial buildup phase, and it is followed by maintenance phase of administering the same maximum maintenance dose at every 4–6 weeks [8, 9].

The duration of initial buildup phase can be shortened by applying cluster, rush, and ultra-rush schedules. In a cluster schedule, multiple injections of allergen extract (usually 2–3 times at each visit with 30 min intervals) are performed on nonconsecutive days. On the other hand, multiple injections of allergen extract can be performed to reach a maximum maintenance dose within 1–3 days (rush schedule) or only 1 day (ultra-rush schedule) [30–33]. No significant increase in incidence of systemic allergic reaction and more rapid clinical improvement has been observed by the cluster schedule compared to the conventional schedule [34]. A rush schedule or ultra-rush schedule is frequently associated with increased incidence of systemic allergic reaction but this risk can be reduced by the premedication with oral antihistamine and using a low-to-medium potency allergen extract for AIT. Systemic reactions can be properly managed by timely administration of systemic rescue medications (systemic antihistamines, corticosteroids, and/or epinephrine) during proper monitoring of development of patients on AIT [30–33]. In patients with AD, rush or ultra-rush schedules of AIT were well tolerated and could be a useful method to start an AIT [31, 33].

Shorter buildup phase with fewer injections and reduced risk of systemic reaction is possible for AIT in patients with AD using the modified allergen extracts (allergoids such as depigmented, glutaraldehyde-treated, polymerized, and aluminum hydroxide-adsorbed allergen extract) or allergen extract adsorbed to adjuvant particles (aluminum hydroxide or tyrosine) designed to decrease a systemic absorption of allergen [32, 33].

For SLIT, the period of buildup phase is very short or frequently is not needed [8].

Total Duration of AIT

The duration of AIT is usually 3–5 years [8]. Prospective studies on the duration and effect of SCIT with grass pollen extract for allergic rhinitis and SCIT with house dust mite extract for allergic asthma suggested that 3 years of AIT can produce a prolonged clinical improvement after discontinuation of AIT [15, 35]. A prospective study on SLIT with house dust mite extract in patients with allergic rhinitis reported improvement of clinical symptoms lasting for more than 7 years after 3 years of SLIT [36]. SLIT for 4 years was associated with longer duration of clinical improvement compared to SLIT for 3 years in patient with allergic rhinitis [36]. Unfortunately, there are few clinical studies on the optimal duration of AIT in patients with AD.

Selection of Allergen for AIT

Method to Select a Clinically Relevant Allergen for AIT

In patients with respiratory allergic diseases (allergic rhinitis, allergic asthma, and allergic conjunctivitis), allergens with proven clinical efficacy for AIT by randomized, double-blind, placebo-controlled studies are pollens (grass pollens, tree pollens, and weed pollens), house dust mites, fungi (*Alternaria* and *Cladosporium*), and animal allergens (dog and cat) [8, 9].

The majority of patients with allergic diseases in the real clinical practice are sensitized to multiple different allergens (polysensitization). Not all of these sensitized allergens are clinically relevant. Moreover, AIT with the most relevant single allergen is equally effective in both monosensitized and polysensitized patients [37]. In general, the clinical efficacy and immunomodulatory effect of AIT for allergic diseases are limited to the allergen included in the allergen extract used for AIT [9]. Majorities of the published randomized controlled studies on the clinical efficacy of AIT have been performed with a single allergen extract [8]. When selecting an allergen for AIT, it is desirable to include a single allergen or as few as possible numbers of allergens (less than 2 or 3 allergens) [38].

It is important to select a clinically relevant allergen for AIT to obtain a favorable clinical efficacy. When selecting an allergen to be included for AIT, there should be an objective evidence supporting the presence of a strong allergic reaction to the allergen (strong positive results in allergy skin prick test (≥3+) and/or serum allergen-specific IgE antibody test (≥3.5 kU/L) in the patient. The allergen should be frequently exposed in real life of the patients and there should be a clear evidence of the cause–result association between exposure to allergen and the development of the clinical symptom by careful medical history or allergen challenge test (atopy patch test, nasal challenge test, or bronchial challenge test).

An allergen that has been proven to be effective for AIT in patients with AD by double-blind controlled studies is the house dust mite [13]. House dust mite is the most common clinically relevant allergen associated with AD in the majority of developed countries [39]. AIT with house dust mite extract should be considered as a treatment option for patients with AD having strong allergy to house dust mite confirmed by allergy skin test and/or serum allergen-specific IgE antibody test [39]. However, uncontrolled observational studies suggested that AIT with other inhalant allergens including pollens (birch, tree) and animal danders (cat and dog) was also clinically useful in patients with AD [40–42].

Type of Commercial Allergen Preparations for AIT

Commercial allergen preparations for SCIT include an unmodified aqueous allergen extract (Hollister-Stier Inc., USA), an allergen extract adsorbed to aluminum hydroxide (Allergopharma, Germany; ALK, Denmark) or tyrosine (Allergy Therapeutics, UK), and a modified allergen (allergoid) such as depigmented glutaraldehyde-treated, polymerized, and aluminum hydroxide-adsorbed allergen extract (LETI Pharma, Spain).

Preparations for SCIT containing allergen extract adsorbed to aluminum hydroxide or tyrosine have high safety with low risk of systemic allergic reaction including anaphylaxis compared to the aqueous allergen extract [31, 33, 43].

Commercial allergen preparations for SLIT are either in forms of the aqueous allergen extract, dried tablet containing unmodified allergen extract (Stallergenes, France; ALK-Abelló, Denmark), or dried tablet containing modified allergen extract (Lofarma, Italy).

There is an important technical limitation of currently available commercial allergen preparations for AIT. There is no standardization on the total amount of allergenic protein, the major allergen concentration, and the biological activity of allergen extracts to compare the allergenic potencies of allergen preparations from different manufacturers. These limitations result in difficulty for physicians who select an optimal preparation for AIT in each patients with allergic diseases by physicians.

Patient Selection

Clinical Indication of AIT in Patients with AD

AIT can be performed in patients with AD when a sensitization to inhalant allergen (house dust mite, pollen, animal dander, etc.) is confirmed by allergy tests (allergy skin test and/or serum allergen-specific IgE antibody test). When there is a clear association between exposure to allergen and development of allergic symptom (either by careful medical history or allergen challenge test), when adequate avoidance of the allergen is difficult, and when clinical symptom of allergic diseases is not adequately controlled by medical treatments, AIT can be attempted (Table 3) [7, 8].

Table 3 Clinical indication of allergen immunotherapy in patients with atopic dermatitis

Presence of IgE-mediated sensitization (skin prick test and/or serum-allergen specific IgE test).
Presence of a clear association between the allergen exposure and the development of clinical symptoms.
Difficult to avoid allergen exposure.
Difficult to control clinical symptoms by medical treatments.
Availability of a standardized high-quality allergen extract preparation for allergen immunotherapy.
Presence of evidences for safety and efficacy of the allergen extract preparation for allergen immunotherapy.

Contraindication of AIT in Patients with AD

AIT is not generally performed in patients with uncontrolled severe bronchial asthma, patients with autoimmune disease, severe immune deficiency or malignant disease, patients with uncontrolled severe cardiovascular diseases who cannot receive epinephrine injection to treat anaphylaxis that can be occurred during AIT, and patients on current treatment with beta-blocker (due to inefficacy of epinephrine treatment). SCIT is contraindicated for infants under 5 years of age. On the other hand, SLIT is known to be safe for children over 3-years old. Initiation of AIT in pregnant women is contraindicated. However, pregnant women who are already undergoing AIT can continue the therapy during pregnancy (Table 4).

Mechanism of AIT

The mechanism of AIT has not yet been fully understood. In the past, it has been speculated that increased serum allergen-specific IgG (especially particularly IgG4) antibodies (also called blocking antibodies) after immunotherapy block the binding between allergen and IgE antibodies and suppress allergic reaction and improve clinical symptom [44].

Table 4 Contraindications for allergen immunotherapy in patients with atopic dermatitis

Uncontrolled severe bronchial asthma.
Uncontrolled severe cardiovascular disease.
Current treatment with beta-blocker.
Severe immunodeficiency.
Autoimmune diseases.
Malignant diseases.
Children of less than 5 years of age (less than 3 years of age for sublingual immunotherapy).
Initiation of allergen immunotherapy during pregnancy.

Recent studies on AIT suggest that allergen administered subcutaneously or sublingually for AIT stimulates dendritic cells (antigen-presenting cells) to activate regulatory T cells (Treg cells) to secrete IL-10 and transforming growth factor-β (TGF-β). The IL-10 and TGF-β inhibit type 2 helper T cells (Th2 cells) and decrease the production of allergen-specific IgE antibodies from B cell. The IL-10 and TGF-β also activate the type 1 helper T cells (Th1 cells) to produce interferon-gamma (IFN-γ) and stimulate the production of allergen-specific IgG4 antibodies from B cells and these suppress allergic inflammation of target tissue and induce clinical improvement in patients with allergic diseases [45] (Fig. 2).

In patients with AD, AIT significantly decreased serum levels of allergen-specific IgE antibodies, increased serum levels of allergen-specific IgG4 antibodies, and increased serum IL-10 and IFN-γ levels [46, 47].

Clinical Efficacy of AIT

Evaluation of Clinical Efficacy of AIT in Patients with AD

To evaluate the therapeutic effect of AIT objectively, the changes in the clinical severity score, degree of improvement of clinical symptom, and requirement of topical and systemic medication should be assessed and recorded before and after AIT. It is also clinically useful to record the extent of involvement of AD by photographs of the same lesion before and after treatment. To assess the clinical severity in patients with AD, Eczema Area and Severity Index (EASI), SCORAD (SCORing Atopic Dermatitis) score, and Investigator's Global Assessment (IGA), visual analogue scale (VAS), Patient-oriented Eczema Measure (POEM), and Dermatology Life Quality Index (DLQI) are useful [48].

Clinical Efficacy of AIT in Patients with AD

In 2006, Werfel T et al. reported a multicenter randomized study evaluating clinical efficacy of SCIT in 89 adult patients with severe AD (SCORAD score ≥ 40) sensitized to house dust mite. This study demonstrated that SCIT significantly reduced the clinical severity of AD measured by SCORAD score and decreased topical corticosteroid use in patient group treated with high-dose of house dust mite extract compared to the patient group treated with lower dose of house dust mite extract [49]. In 2012, Novak N et al. reported a randomized, double-blind, placebo-controlled study evaluating clinical efficacy of SCIT with house dust mite extract in 168 adult patients with AD. This study showed no significant difference in changes of clinical severity score (SCORAD score) for 18 months between treatment group and placebo group. However, a subgroup analysis showed that SCIT with house dust mite significantly reduced the clinical severity score (SCORAD score) compared to placebo in patients with severe AD (SCORAD > 50) [47].

In 2007, Pajno GB et al. reported a randomized, double-blind, placebo-controlled study evaluating the clinical efficacy of SLIT in 56 children with AD sensitized to house dust mite. This study showed that SLIT with house dust mite extract significantly reduced the clinical severity of AD measured by SCORAD score and patient-rated subjective overall severity score measured by visual analogue scale in children with mild-to-moderate AD (SCORAD score ≤ 40) compared to the placebo treatment. In this study, SLIT was not effective in children with severe AD (SCORAD score > 40) [50]. In

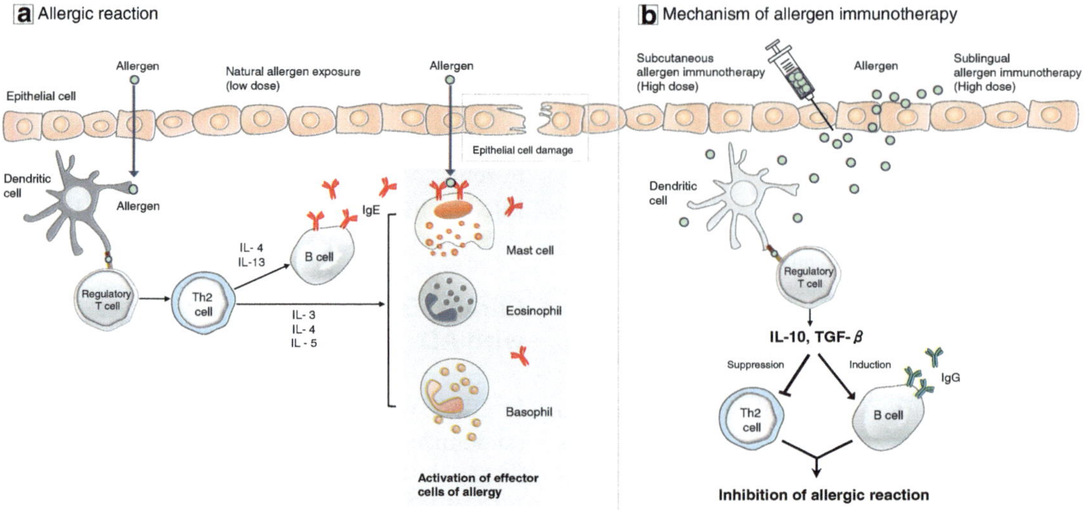

Fig. 2 Mechanism of allergen immunotherapy. Allergens administered subcutaneously or sublingually stimulate dendritic cells (DCs) and DCs activates regulatory T cells (Treg cells) to secrete IL-10 and TGF-β. IL-10 and TGF-β inhibit Th2 cells, stimulate activation of Th1 cells, and promote the production allergen-specific IgG4 antibodies to allergen (blocking antibodies) (**b**). These suppress allergic inflammation of target tissue (**a**) and induce clinical improvement in patients with allergic diseases

Table 5 Clinical efficacy of allergen immunotherapy in patients with atopic dermatitis

Allergen immunotherapy is clinically beneficial in patients with atopic dermatitis sensitized to house dust mite.
Subcutaneous allergen immunotherapy can improve clinical severity score and reduce requirement of topical corticosteroid in adult patients with severe atopic dermatitis sensitized to house dust mite.
Sublingual allergen immunotherapy can improve clinical severity score and patient-rated overall severity score in children and adult patients with mild-to-moderate atopic dermatitis sensitized to house dust mite.

2014, Qin Y et al. reported a randomized controlled study evaluating clinical efficacy of SLIT in 107 adult patients with AD sensitized house dust mite. This study showed that SLIT with house dust mite extract provided significant improvements in the clinical severity score (SCORAD), medication requirement, and patients-rated subjective overall severity in treatment group compared to the control group [51].

Overall, AIT is clinically beneficial in patients with AD sensitized to house dust mite (Table 5).

Characteristics of Patients with AD Who Experienced a Favorable Clinical Response After AIT

AIT can be clinically effective in patients with AD sensitized to inhalant allergens (house dust mite and pollens). However, there has been yet no validated clinical or biological marker to predict a favorable clinical response of AIT in patients with AD. However, previous observational studies suggest that patients showing a favorable clinical response to AIT with AD have the following characteristics; high serum levels of allergen-specific IgE antibodies for house dust mite (>3.5 kU/L), severe AD (SCORAD score > 50), children or adolescent (<12 years), and short disease duration (≤10 years) at the timing of initiation of AIT (Table 6) [19, 47, 52].

Long-Term Clinical Efficacy of AIT in Patients with AD

In patients with respiratory allergic diseases including allergic asthma and allergic rhinitis, AIT can improve clinical symptom, reduce

Table 6 Characteristics of patients with atopic dermatitis with a favorable clinical response to allergen immunotherapy

Sensitization to house dust mite
High serum levels of allergen-specific IgE antibody (>3.5 kU/L)
Severe atopic dermatitis (SCORAD > 50)
Children or adolescent (age < 12 years)
Short disease duration (≤10 years)

requirement of medication, decrease the degree of allergic reaction to the specific allergen, decrease nonspecific hyperreactivity of the respiratory tract, and decrease the serum allergen-specific IgE antibody level [45]. A certain proportion of patients with respiratory allergic diseases who have undergone AIT for a sufficient period (3–5 years) can experience a long-term clinical improvement even after discontinuing AIT [15, 35, 36]. AIT also can prevent sensitization to a new allergen and prevent the development of asthma in children with allergic rhinitis [16, 53]. AIT is regarded as a disease-modifying therapy for respiratory allergic diseases [8].

Unfortunately, there are only a few reports on the long-term clinical efficacy of AIT in patients with AD. In 1985, Chait I and Allkins V reported a patient with life-long severe AD who experienced a clinical remission lasting for more than 4 years after 1 year of SCIT with house dust mite extract [18]. In 2016, Lee J et al. reported a retrospective analysis on the 217 patients with AD who received SCIT with house dust mite extract for more than 3 years and this study showed that 45% of patients experienced a complete or near complete remission of clinical symptoms after AIT for more than 3 years [19]. These results suggest that AIT has a potential to be a disease-modifying therapy for AD. However, further well-designed clinical studies on a long-term clinical efficacy of AIT for AD are needed to confirm this possibility.

Safety of AIT

Side effects of AIT include local and systemic allergic reactions caused by the administration of allergen extract. It is important to educate patients on the risk, nature of side effects, and how to deal with the side effects before the initiation of AIT (Table 7).

Table 7 Precautions for subcutaneous allergen immunotherapy

1. Observe the patient for at least 30 min in the hospital after subcutaneous injection of allergen extract to monitor a possible development of systemic allergic reaction (anaphylaxis, etc.).
2. Postpone an injection of allergen extract when a patient has a fever or an acute asthmatic attack.
3. If the injection interval is significantly delayed from regular schedule, the injection dose of allergen extract should be reduced and then increased in the next regular visit.
4. If severe local or systemic allergic reactions occur in the previous allergen injection, the injection dose of allergen extract should be reduced in the next schedule.
5. Patients should be advised to take a second-generation oral antihistamine as a premedication at least 2 h before subcutaneous injection of allergen extract to reduce the risk of development of systemic allergic reaction.

A local injection site reaction can occur after SCIT. Injection site can be itchy and swollen at several hours after subcutaneous injection of allergen. If severe local edema occurs and the diameter of the injection site reaction is too large, there is a risk of development of systemic allergic reaction in the next allergen injection and allergen dose for SCIT should be reduced at the next schedule. The systemic allergic reactions include the occurrence of generalized urticaria, dyspnea due to bronchoconstriction, or acute systemic allergic reactions (anaphylaxis) which can be a critical condition manifested by severe breathing difficulties due to edema of upper airway (laryngeal edema), a hypotension, and loss of consciousness [54].

Since most of these severe systemic allergic reactions occur within 30 min after subcutaneous injection of allergen extract, patients should be observed for at least 30 min at the hospital after SCIT and possible development of any side effects should be assessed before leaving hospital. In the event of a systemic allergic reaction, systemic antihistamine, systemic corticosteroid, inhalant bronchodilator, and intramuscular epinephrine should be administered according to the severity of symptoms. If systemic allergic reaction (anaphylaxis) or severe exacerbation of clinical symptoms of atopic dermatitis was occurred in the previous injection, or the intended injection schedule was significantly delayed more than 6 weeks, next administration dose of allergen for AIT should be reduced to prevent a possible development of systemic allergic reaction. To reduce the risk of development of systemic allergic reaction, patients should be advised to take a second-generation oral antihistamine as a premedication at least 2 h before subcutaneous injection of allergen extract for AIT (Table 7).

In addition, delayed side reaction manifested by temporal exacerbation of existing AD lesions developing at 12–72 h after SCIT was reported in a few (less than 5%) patients with AD [21, 22]. If delayed side reaction is suspected in patients with AD, the allergen dose for AIT should be reduced in next visit, and gradually increased again to prevent development of the delayed side reaction. However, if the symptoms continue even after the administration of reduced allergen doses, discontinuation of SCIT or switch to SLIT should be considered in the patients. The SLIT is more safer than SCIT. Common side reaction of SLIT is a local irritation in the oral cavity (pruritus or edema) or gastrointestinal side effect (nausea, vomiting, diarrhea, abdominal pain, etc.), but development of severe systemic allergic reaction (anaphylaxis) is very rare during SLIT [8, 29].

Limitations of Current form of AIT

Various attempts have been made to improve the efficacy and safety of AIT in allergic diseases. However, there are several important limitations of AIT (Table 8). To solve these limitations, the development of a new therapeutic product for AIT is needed. However, high cost and risk to perform well-designed large multicenter randomized, double-blind, placebo-controlled clinical trials are major obstacles for the development of new products for AIT [8].

Table 8 Limitations (unmet needs) of allergen immunotherapy

- Absence of clinical or biological markers to predict the effectiveness of allergen immunotherapy.
- Difficulty in selecting optimal commercial allergen extracts for allergen immunotherapy due to lack of standardized information of an allergenic potency and major allergen content of commercial allergen extracts.
- Difficulty in selecting the route of allergen immunotherapy due to lack of studies comparing efficacy and safety of subcutaneous allergen immunotherapy and sublingual allergen immunotherapy.
- Decreased patient long-term compliance for allergen immunotherapy need of 3–5 years of maintenance treatment duration.
- Risk of severe systemic allergic reaction (anaphylaxis) during subcutaneous allergen immunotherapy.

Comparison of AIT and Monoclonal Antibody Therapy for the Treatment of AD

Monoclonal antibody to IL-4 receptor alpha (Dupilumab) can provide a rapid-onset clinical improvement within 1 week after the initiation of the treatment and long-term clinical improvement by a regular maintenance treatment [3–5]. AIT provides a significant clinical improvement from 1 to 9 months after the initiation of treatment in patients with AD, but it's clinical efficacy is long-term lasting even after discontinuation of the treatment [49, 50, 55]. These two treatment methods have a common disadvantage of incomplete clinical efficacy in certain proportions of patients with AD. Therefore, a combination therapy with AIT with monoclonal antibody to IL-4 receptor alpha (Dupilumab) might provide a rapid-onset long-term clinical improvement in patients with AD.

Recent Trials and Future Directions for the Development of AIT

There have been trials to minimize the risk of side effects and maximize the clinical efficacy of AIT. Current attempts to develop AIT include:

(1) a modification of allergen (allergen peptides, recombinant allergen, and chemically modified allergen), (2) addition of a new adjuvant (cytosine–phosphate–guanine toll-like receptor agonist, etc.), (3) changes in the routes of allergen administration (intralymphatic injection, epicutaneous route, microneedle patches, etc.), and (4) monoclonal antibody to major allergen of cat [54–60].

In the future, various combination therapies including AIT, monoclonal antibody therapy, and immunomodulatory drugs (including methotrexate or Janus kinase inhibitors) might improve clinical outcomes in patients with AD [3–6, 61–63].

Conclusion

AIT has the potential to improve a long-term clinical course of AD. There have been trials for development of new immunomodulatory therapy for AD. Many new drugs for AD including monoclonal antibodies (target antigens) and new immunomodulatory small molecule compounds (Janus kinase inhibitors, etc.) are on the clinical trials. Therefore, a personalized immunomodulatory therapy combining AIT with other immunomodulatory modalities (monoclonal antibodies and/or small molecule compounds) might improve long-term clinical outcomes of AD in the future (Table 9).

Table 9 Present and future of immunomodulatory therapy for atopic dermatitis

Present	Future
Transient symptomatic treatment Nonspecific transient immune suppression with pharmacological therapy Monoclonal antibody inhibiting specific immune pathway	Long-term treatment-free of clinical remission Correction of immune dysfunction and hypersensitivity by induction of immune tolerance Combinations of multiple antigen-specific and nonspecific immunomodulatory modalities

Key Points

- Allergen immunotherapy is clinically effective in patients with atopic dermatitis sensitized to house dust mite.
- Allergen immunotherapy can be conducted by either subcutaneous route or sublingual route.
- Subcutaneous immunotherapy is effective in patients with severe atopic dermatitis, children or adolescents with atopic dermatitis, and patients with short disease duration.
- Sublingual immunotherapy is effective in patients with mild-to-moderate atopic dermatitis.
- Allergen immunotherapy for more than 3–5 years is required to produce long-term clinical improvement.
- Patients should be monitored at a hospital for more than 30 min after subcutaneous injection of allergen extract to monitor risk of development of systemic allergic reaction including anaphylaxis.

References

1. Akdis CA, Akdis M, Bieber T, Bindslev-Jensen C, Boguniewicz M, Eigenmann P, et al. Diagnosis and treatment of atopic dermatitis in children and adults: European Academy of Allergology and Clinical Immunology/American Academy of Allergy, Asthma and Immunology/PRACTALL Consensus Report. J Allergy Clin Immunol. 2006;118:152–69. https://doi.org/10.1016/j.jaci.2006.03.045.
2. Nahm DH. Personalized immunomodulatory therapy for atopic dermatitis: an allergist's view. Ann Dermatol. 2015;27:355–63. https://doi.org/10.5021/ad.2015.27.4.355.
3. Thaci D, Simpson EL, Beck LA, Bieber T, Blauvelt A, Papp K, et al. Efficacy and safety of dupilumab in adults with moderate-to-severe atopic dermatitis inadequately controlled by topical treatments: a randomised, placebo-controlled, dose-ranging phase 2b trial. Lancet. 2016;387(10013):40–52. https://doi.org/10.1016/S0140-6736(15)00388-8.
4. Simpson EL, Bieber T, Guttman-Yassky E, et al. Two Phase 3 trials of dupilumab versus placebo in atopic

dermatitis. N Engl J Med. 2016;375:2335–48. https://doi.org/10.1056/NEJMoa1610020.

5. Blauvelt A, de Bruin-Weller M, Gooderham M, Cather JC, Weisman J, Pariser D, et al. Long-term management of moderate-to-severe atopic dermatitis with dupilumab and concomitant topical corticosteroids (LIBERTY AD CHRONOS): a 1-year, randomised, double-blinded, placebo-controlled, phase 3 trial. Lancet. 2017;389(10086):2287–303. https://doi.org/10.1016/S0140-6736(17)31191-1.
6. Simpson EL, Flohr C, Eichenfield LF, Bieber T, Sofen H, Taieb A, et al. Efficacy and safety of lebrikizumab (an anti-IL-13 monoclonal antibody) in adults with moderate-to-severe atopic dermatitis inadequately controlled by topical corticosteroids: a randomized, placebo-controlled phase II trial (TREBLE). J Am Acad Dermatol. 2018;78:863–71 e11. https://doi.org/10.1016/j.jaad.2018.01.017.
7. Bousquet J, Lockey R, Malling HJ. Allergen immunotherapy: therapeutic vaccines for allergic diseases. A WHO position paper. J Allergy Clin Immunol. 1998;102:558–62. https://doi.org/10.1016/s0091-6749(98)70271-4.
8. Jutel M, Agache I, Bonini S, Burks AW, Calderon M, Canonica W, et al. International consensus on allergy immunotherapy. J Allergy Clin Immunol. 2015;136:556–68. https://doi.org/10.1016/j.jaci.2015.04.047.
9. Joint Task Force on Practice Parameters, American Academy of Allergy, Asthma and Immunology, American College of Allergy, Asthma and Immunology, Joint Council of Allergy, Asthma and Immunology. Allergen immunotherapy: a practice parameter second update. J Allergy Clin Immunol. 2007;120(3 Suppl):S25–85. https://doi.org/10.1016/j.jaci.2007.06.019.
10. Burks AW, Calderon MA, Casale T, Cox L, Demoly P, Jutel M, et al. Update on allergy immunotherapy: American Academy of Allergy, Asthma & Immunology/European Academy of Allergy and Clinical Immunology/PRACTALL consensus report. J Allergy Clin Immunol. 2013;131:1288–96 e3. https://doi.org/10.1016/j.jaci.2013.01.049.
11. Pipet A, Botturi K, Pinot D, Vervloet D, Magnan A. Allergen-specific immunotherapy in allergic rhinitis and asthma. Mechanisms and proof of efficacy. Respir Med. 2009;103:800–12. https://doi.org/10.1016/j.rmed.2009.01.008.
12. Boyle RJ, Elremeli M, Hockenhull J, Cherry MG, Bulsara MK, Daniels M, et al. Venom immunotherapy for preventing allergic reactions to insect stings. Cochrane Database Syst Rev. 2012;10:CD008838. https://doi.org/10.1002/14651858.CD008838.pub2.
13. Bae JM, Choi YY, Park CO, Chung KY, Lee KH. Efficacy of allergen-specific immunotherapy for atopic dermatitis: a systematic review and meta-analysis of randomized controlled trials. J Allergy Clin Immunol. 2013;132:110–7. https://doi.org/10.1016/j.jaci.2013.02.044.
14. Jacobsen L, Niggemann B, Dreborg S, Ferdousi HA, Halken S, Host A, et al. Specific immunotherapy has long-term preventive effect of seasonal and perennial asthma: 10-year follow-up on the PAT study. Allergy. 2007;62:943–8. https://doi.org/10.1111/j.1398-9995.2007.01451.x.
15. Durham SR, Walker SM, Varga EM, Jacobson MR, O'Brien F, Noble W, et al. Long-term clinical efficacy of grass-pollen immunotherapy. N Engl J Med. 1999;341:468–75. https://doi.org/10.1056/NEJM199908123410702.
16. Des Roches A, Paradis L, Menardo JL, Bouges S, Daures JP, Bousquet J. Immunotherapy with a standardized Dermatophagoides pteronyssinus extract. VI. Specific immunotherapy prevents the onset of new sensitizations in children. J Allergy Clin Immunol. 1997;99:450–3. https://doi.org/10.1016/s0091-6749(97)70069-1.
17. Lee J, Park CO, Lee KH. Specific immunotherapy in atopic dermatitis. Allergy Asthma Immunol Res. 2015;7(3):221–9. https://doi.org/10.4168/aair.2015.7.3.221.
18. Chait I, Allkins V. Remission of life-long atopic dermatitis after hyposensitisation to house dust mite. Practitioner. 1985;229:609, 612.
19. Lee J, Lee H, Noh S, Bae BG, Shin JU, Park CO, et al. Retrospective analysis on the effects of house dust mite specific immunotherapy for more than 3 years in atopic dermatitis. Yonsei Med J. 2016;57:393–8. https://doi.org/10.3349/ymj.2016.57.2.393.
20. Noon L. Prophylactic inoculation against hay fever. Lancet. 1911;177:1572–3.
21. Diamond HE. Atopic dermatitis caused by inhalant antigens and its immunologic therapy. Ann Allergy. 1953;11:146–56.
22. Tuft L. Studies in atopic dermatitis. V. Problems in inhalant hyposensitization and results of treatment. J Allergy. 1960;31:1–11. https://doi.org/10.1016/0021-8707(60)90019-8.
23. Kaufman HS, Roth HL. Hyposensitization with alum precipitated extracts in atopic dermatitis: a placebo-controlled study. Ann Allergy. 1974;32:321–30.
24. Gendelman SR, Lang DM. Specific immunotherapy in the treatment of atopic dermatitis: a systematic review using the GRADE system. Ann Allergy Asthma Immunol. 2013;111:555–61. https://doi.org/10.1016/j.anai.2013.08.020.
25. Tam HH, Calderon MA, Manikam L, Nankervis H, Nunez IG, Williams HC, et al. Specific allergen immunotherapy for the treatment of atopic eczema: a Cochrane systematic review. Allergy. 2016;71:1345–56. https://doi.org/10.1111/all.12932.
26. Scadding GK, Brostoff J. Low dose sublingual therapy in patients with allergic rhinitis due to house dust mite. Clin Allergy. 1986;16:483–91. https://doi.org/10.1111/j.1365-2222.1986.tb01983.x.
27. Frew AJ. Sublingual immunotherapy. N Engl J Med. 2008;358:2259–64. https://doi.org/10.1056/NEJMct0708337.

28. Virchow JC, Backer V, Kuna P, Prieto L, Nolte H, Villesen HH, et al. Efficacy of a house dust mite sublingual allergen immunotherapy tablet in adults with allergic asthma: a randomized clinical trial. JAMA. 2016;315:1715–25. https://doi.org/10.1001/jama.2016.3964.
29. Nelson HS, Makatsori M, Calderon MA. Subcutaneous immunotherapy and sublingual immunotherapy: comparative efficacy, current and potential indications, and warnings—United States versus Europe. Immunol Allergy Clin North Am. 2016;36:13–24. https://doi.org/10.1016/j.iac.2015.08.005.
30. Cox L. Accelerated immunotherapy schedules: review of efficacy and safety. Ann Allergy Asthma Immunol. 2006;97:126–37. https://doi.org/10.1016/S1081-1206(10)60003-8.
31. Kim ME, Kim JE, Sung JM, Lee JW, Choi GS, Nahm DH. Safety of accelerated schedules of subcutaneous allergen immunotherapy with house dust mite extract in patients with atopic dermatitis. J Korean Med Sci. 2011;26:1159–64. https://doi.org/10.3346/jkms.2011.26.9.1159.
32. Casanovas M, Martín R, Jiménez C, Caballero R, Fernández-Caldas E. Safety of an ultra-rush immunotherapy build-up schedule with therapeutic vaccines containing depigmented and polymerized allergen extracts. Int Arch Allergy Immunol. 2006;139:153–8. https://doi.org/10.1159/000090392.
33. Lee SH, Kim ME, Shin YS, Ye YM, Park HS, Nahm DH. Safety of ultra-rush schedule of subcutaneous allergen immunotherapy with house dust mite extract conducted in an outpatient clinic in patients with atopic dermatitis and allergic rhinitis. Allergy Asthma Immunol Res. 2019;11:846–55. https://doi.org/10.4168/aair.2019.11.6.846.
34. Tabar AI, Echechipia S, Garcia BE, Olaquibel JM, Lizaso MT, Gomez B, et al. Double-blind comparative study of cluster and conventional immunotherapy schedules with Dermatophagoides pteronyssinus. J Allergy Clin Immunol. 2005;116:109–18. https://doi.org/10.1016/j.jaci.2005.05.005.
35. Des Roches A, Paradis L, Knani J, Hejjaoui A, Dhivert H, Chanez P, et al. Immunotherapy with a standardized Dermatophagoides pteronyssinus extract V Duration of the efficacy of immunotherapy after its cessation. Allergy. 1996;51:430–3. https://doi.org/10.1111/j.1398-9995.1996.tb04643.x.
36. Marogna M, Spadolini I, Massolo A, Canonica GW, Passalacqua G. Long-lasting effects of sublingual immunotherapy according to its duration: a 15-year prospective study. J Allergy Clin Immunol. 2010;126:969–75. https://doi.org/10.1016/j.jaci.2010.08.030.
37. Calderon MA, Cox L, Casale TB, Moingeon P, Demoly P. Multiple-allergen and single-allergen immunotherapy strategies in polysensitized patients: looking at the published evidence. J Allergy Clin Immunol. 2012;129:929–34. https://doi.org/10.1016/j.jaci.2011.11.019.
38. Calderon MA, Cox LS. Monoallergen sublingual immunotherapy versus multiallergen subcutaneous immunotherapy for allergic respiratory diseases: a debate during the AAAAI 2013 Annual Meeting in San Antonio, Texas. J Allergy Clin Immunol Pract. 2014;2:136–43. https://doi.org/10.1016/j.jaip.2013.12.008.
39. Thomas WR. House dust allergy and immunotherapy. Hum Vaccin Immunother. 2012;8:1469–78. https://doi.org/10.4161/hv.20812.
40. Novak N, Thaci D, Hoffmann M, Folster-Holst R, Biedermann T, Homey B, et al. Subcutaneous immunotherapy with a depigmented polymerized birch pollen extract—a new therapeutic option for patients with atopic dermatitis. Int Arch Allergy Immunol. 2011;155:252–6. https://doi.org/10.1159/000320058.
41. Chu H, Park KH, Kim SM, Lee JH, Park JW, Lee KH, et al. Allergen-specific immunotherapy for patients with atopic dermatitis sensitized to animal dander. Immun Inflamm Dis. 2020;8:165–9. https://doi.org/10.1002/iid3.291.
42. Silny W, Czarnecka-Operacz M. Specific immunotherapy in the treatment of patients with atopic dermatitis—results of double blind placebo controlled study. Pol Merkur Lekarski. 2006;21:558–65.
43. Müller UR. Venom immunotherapy: aqueous vs. aluminium hydroxide adsorbed extracts. Allergy. 2004;59:577–8. https://doi.org/10.1111/j.1398-9995.2004.00494.x.
44. Ring J, Gutermuth J. 100 years of hyposensitization: history of allergen-specific immunotherapy (ASIT). Allergy. 2011;66:713–24. https://doi.org/10.1111/j.1398-9995.2010.02541.x.
45. Jutel M, Agache I, Bonini S, Burks AW, Calderon M, Canonica W, et al. International consensus on allergen immunotherapy II: mechanisms, standardization, and pharmacoeconomics. J Allergy Clin Immunol. 2016;137:358–68. https://doi.org/10.1016/j.jaci.2015.12.1300.
46. Zhong H, Deng X, Song Z, Darsow U, Chen W, Chen S, et al. Immunological changes after ASIT in AD allergen-specific immunotherapy and their potential correlation with clinical response in patients with atopic dermatitis patients sensitized to house dust mite. J Eur Acad Dermatol Venereol. 2015;29:1318–24. https://doi.org/10.1111/jdv.12813.
47. Novak N, Bieber T, Hoffmann M, Folster-Holst R, Homey B, Werfel T, et al. Efficacy and safety of subcutaneous allergen-specific immunotherapy with depigmented polymerized mite extract in atopic dermatitis. J Allergy Clin Immunol. 2012;130:925–31 e4. https://doi.org/10.1016/j.jaci.2012.08.004.
48. Chopra R, Vakharia PP, Simpson EL, Paller AS, Silverberg JI. Severity assessments used for inclusion criteria and baseline severity evaluation in atopic dermatitis clinical trials: a systematic review. J Eur Acad Dermatol Venereol. 2017;31:1890–9. https://doi.org/10.1111/jdv.14483.
49. Werfel T, Breuer K, Rueff F, Przybilla B, Worm M, Grewe M, et al. Usefulness of specific immunotherapy in patients with atopic dermatitis and allergic sensitization to house dust mites: a multi-centre, random-

ized, dose-response study. Allergy. 2006;61:202–5. https://doi.org/10.1111/j.1398-9995.2006.00974.x.
50. Pajno GB, Caminiti L, Vita D, Barberio G, Salzano G, Lombardo F, et al. Sublingual immunotherapy in mite-sensitized children with atopic dermatitis: a randomized, double-blind, placebo-controlled study. J Allergy Clin Immunol. 2007;120:164–70. https://doi.org/10.1016/j.jaci.2007.04.008.
51. Nahm DH, Kim ME, Kwon B, Cho SM, Ahn A. Clinical efficacy of subcutaneous allergen immunotherapy in patients with atopic dermatitis. Yonsei Med J. 2016;57:1420–6. https://doi.org/10.3349/ymj.2016.57.6.1420.
52. Qin YE, Mao JR, Sang YC, Li WX. Clinical efficacy and compliance of sublingual immunotherapy with Dermatophagoides farinae drops in patients with atopic dermatitis. Int J Dermatol. 2014;53:650–5. https://doi.org/10.1111/ijd.12302.
53. Purello-D'Ambrosio F, Gangemi S, Merendino RA, Isola S, Puccinelli P, Parmiani S, et al. Prevention of new sensitizations in monosensitized subjects submitted to specific immunotherapy or not. A retrospective study. Clin Exp Allergy. 2001;31:1295–302. https://doi.org/10.1046/j.1365-2222.2001.01027.x.
54. Cox L, Larenas-Linnemann D, Lockey RF, Passalacqua G. Speaking the same language: the World Allergy Organization subcutaneous immunotherapy systemic reaction grading system. J Allergy Clin Immunol. 2010;125:569–74, 574.e1-574.e7. https://doi.org/10.1016/j.jaci.2009.10.060.
55. Bussmann C, Maintz L, Hart J, Allam JP, Vrtala S, Chen KW, et al. Clinical improvement and immunological changes in atopic dermatitis patients undergoing subcutaneous immunotherapy with a house dust mite allergoid: a pilot study. Clin Exp Allergy. 2007;37:1277–85. https://doi.org/10.1111/j.1365-2222.2007.02783.x.
56. Rajakulendran M, Tham EH, Soh JY, Van Bever HP. Novel strategies in immunotherapy for allergic diseases. Asia Pac Allergy. 2018;8:e14. https://doi.org/10.5415/apallergy.2018.8.e14.
57. Casale TB, Stokes JR. Future forms of immunotherapy. J Allergy Clin Immunol. 2011;127:8–15. https://doi.org/10.1016/j.jaci.2010.10.034.
58. Orengo JM, Radin AR, Kamat V, Badithe A, Ben LH, Bennett BL, et al. Treating cat allergy with monoclonal IgG antibodies that bind allergen and prevent IgE engagement. Nat Commun. 2018;9:1421. https://doi.org/10.1038/s41467-018-03636-8.
59. Wollenberg A, Barbarot S, Bieber T, Christen-Zaech S, Deleuran M, Fink-Wagner A, et al. Consensus-based European guidelines for treatment of atopic eczema (atopic dermatitis) in adults and children: part II. J Eur Acad Dermatol Venereol. 2018;32:850–78. https://doi.org/10.1111/jdv.14888.
60. Kim JH, Shin JU, Kim SH, Noh JY, Kim HR, Lee J, et al. Successful transdermal allergen delivery and allergen-specific immunotherapy using biodegradable microneedle patches. Biomaterials. 2018;150:38–48. https://doi.org/10.1016/j.biomaterials.2017.10.013.
61. Leroy BP, Boden G, Lachapelle JM, Jacquemin MG, Saint-Remy JM. A novel therapy for atopic dermatitis with allergen-antibody complexes: a double-blind, placebo-controlled study. J Am Acad Dermatol. 1993;28(2 Pt 1):232–9. https://doi.org/10.1016/0190-9622(93)70033-p.
62. Nahm DH, Lee ES, Park HJ, Kim HA, Choi GS, Jeon SY. Treatment of atopic dermatitis with a combination of allergen-specific immunotherapy and a histamine-immunoglobulin complex. Int Arch Allergy Immunol. 2008;146:235–40. https://doi.org/10.1159/000115892.
63. Baris S, Kiykim A, Ozen A, Tulunay A, Karakoc-Aydiner E, Barlan IB. Vitamin D as an adjunct to subcutaneous allergen immunotherapy in asthmatic children sensitized to house dust mite. Allergy. 2014;69:246–53. https://doi.org/10.1111/all.12278.

Treatment Algorithms

Ji Hyun Lee and Joo Young Roh

Introduction

Atopic dermatitis (AD) is a pruritic inflammatory cutaneous disorder, with an estimated prevalence of up to 20% of children and 10% of adults [1–6]. AD is a diagnosis based on clinical features [7]. Disease-specific genetic factors, immunologic factors, and environmental factors contribute to the development of AD. AD patients' symptoms improve and worsen by various factors.

Treatment of AD is divided into basic management including education, topical and systemic treatment, and phototherapy (Fig. 1). Basic treatment of AD includes a basic skin care through moisturizer and the avoidance of triggering factor to avoid causative allergens and irritants. In recent years, the importance of education has emerged, with the emphasis on patient compliance with treatment. The main pharmacological treatment of AD is topical and systemic therapeutics. The potency of topical steroids and topical calcineurin inhibitor is selected according to the patients' age, lesion, and severity. Systemic therapy is used for active treatment of AD. Biologics have recently been challenged in addition to conventional immumomodulators such as short-term corticosteroid and cyclosporine. Depending on the patient, phototherapy is added.

Firstly, the patient's severity through history taking as well as scoring should be identified. AD is treated according to its severity (Fig. 2). Korean Atopic Dermatitis Association (KADA) defined the severity of AD according to Eczema Area and Severity index (EASI) score and SCOring Atopic Dermatitis (SCORAD) index. Mild AD, EASI < 16, SCORAD < 25; moderate AD, $16 \leq$ EASI < 23, $25 \leq$ SCORAD < 50; and severe AD, EASI score ≥ 23, SCORAD ≥ 50. Correlation between EASI score and SCORAD index has been validated [8, 9].

Expert consensus also emphasized that the grade should be increased if pruritus numerical rating scale is higher than 7 ($\geq$7) or dermatology life quality index (DLQI) score exceeds 10.

Mild AD is sufficient for basic treatment. In some cases, topical steroids or topical calcineurin inhibitors may be added. In addition to basic treatment, moderate-to-severe AD is controlled by systemic immunomodulators and biologics such as dupilumab. Depending on the patient's symptoms, phototherapy can be applicable. In patients with mild-to-severe AD, proactive treatment may be given according to the lesion.

J. H. Lee
Department of Dermatology, Seoul St. Mary's Hospital, College of Medicine, The Catholic University of Korea, Seoul, Korea (Republic of)

J. Y. Roh (✉)
Department of Dermatology, Gil Medical Center, Gachon University College of Medicine, Incheon, Korea (Republic of)
e-mail: jyroh1@gilhospital.com

K. H. Lee et al. (eds.), *Practical Insights into Atopic Dermatitis*,
https://doi.org/10.1007/978-981-15-8159-5_19

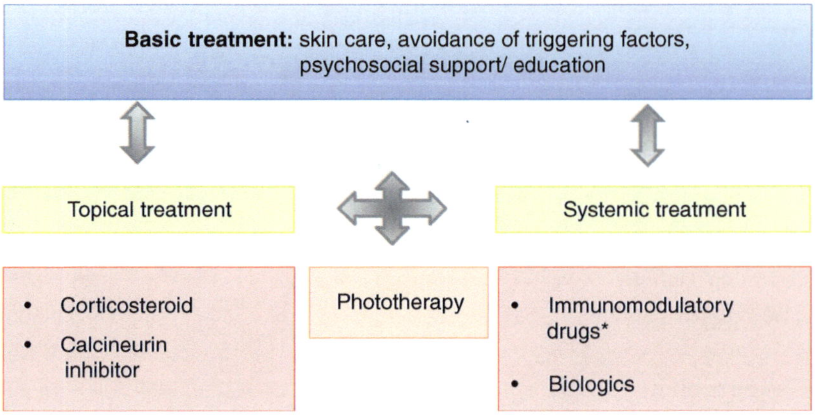

Fig. 1 Current therapy for patients with atopic dermatitis. *Immunomodulatory drugs: corticosteroid, cyclosporine, methotrexate, azathioprine, and mycophenolate mofetil

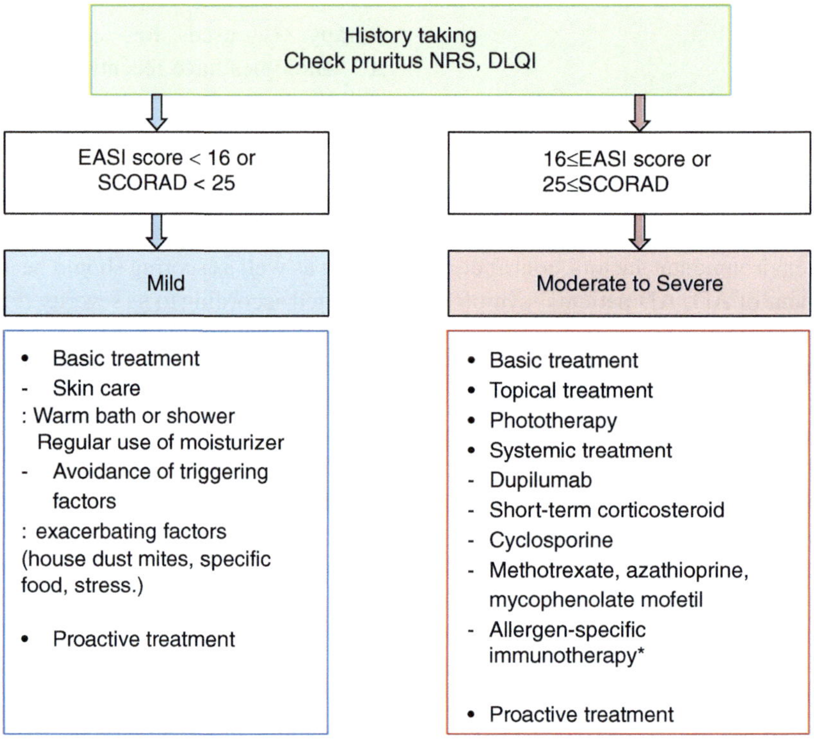

Fig. 2 Treatment for atopic dermatitis according to the severity. *SCORAD*: SCOring Atopic Dermatitis, *EASI*: eczema area and severity index, *AD*: atopic dermatitis, *NRS*: numerical rating scale, DLQI: dermatology life quality index. Even mild atopic dermatitis with an EASI score of <16 is defined as moderate atopic dermatitis if the day or nighttime NRS is ≥7 through history taking. Even mild atopic dermatitis with an EASI score of <16 is defined as moderate atopic dermatitis if DLQI is >10 through history taking. *Allergen-specific immunotherapy (ASIT) is considered in moderate to severe AD patients who are resistant to other treatments, however, it could also be considered in mild cases

I. Basic Treatment

Application of moisturizer improves barrier dysfunctions [10]. It is also important to control the environmental factors through avoidance of the triggering allergens and irritants (house dust mites, specific food, stress, etc.). Patient-specific structural educational program with psychological support is important in its long-term management and treatment adherence [11]. Education through in-depth individual interviews with patients is the main factor in the success of treatment.

II. Topical Treatment

In the case of AD that is not controlled by basic treatment, first consider topical treatment. Topical treatment should be selected and maintained based on the patient's risk-benefits.

1. Topical Corticosteroids

Topical corticosteroids are first-line topical therapeutics for controlling AD and relieving pruritus [12]. These improve AD lesions. Especially, topical corticosteroids have been used for proactive treatment (once or twice weekly application) and have been known to reduce acute flares but have no side effects [13–15].

2. Topical Calcineurin Inhibitors

Topical calcineurin inhibitors, pimecrolimus cream, and tacrolimus ointment, have a short-term as well as a long-term without skin atrophy and improve AD [7, 16]. These are also used for proactive treatment [17, 18].

3. Small Molecules

Crisaborole, a phosphodiesterase 4 (PDE4) inhibitor, is approved by the Food and Drug Administration (FDA) for atopic dermatitis (AD) in 2016.

III. Phototherapy

Phototherapy can be used for managing AD through anti-inflammatory and immunosuppressive effects. Phototherapy includes UVB (mostly narrowband (NB-UVB) of 311 nm and less frequently broadband (BB-UVB)), UVA (especially UVA1 of 340–400 nm), and photochemotherapy. There is evidence for the use of NB-UVB and UV-A1 phototherapy in moderate-to-severe atopic dermatitis. NB-UVB has been indicated for chronic moderate-to-severe AD, while UVA1 is used for acute phase AD [19, 20].

IV. Systemic Treatment

The following systemic treatment should be considered in moderate-to-severe recalcitrant AD.

1. Systemic Corticosteroid

Although systemic steroid improves AD, most studies recommend short-term use of systemic steroids in patients with AD, taking into account side effects [15, 21–25]. Adverse effects of long-term use of systemic steroids include impaired glucose tolerance, diabetes, hypertension, hyperlipidemia, gastritis, peptic ulcer, weight gain, osteoporosis, hypothalamic–pituitary–adrenal axis suppression, emotional changes, fluid retention, and opportunistic infections [24, 25].

2. Systemic Immunomodulators

Systemic immunosuppressants include cyclosporine, methotrexate, azathioprine, and mycophenolate mofetil. They are used in severe and difficult to treat AD patients. Cyclosporine is administered as the first drug, but other immune modulators can be considered if AD treatment of cyclosporine is insufficient or intolerant.

1) Cyclosporine

Cyclosporine is recommended as a first-line drug for moderate-to-severe AD [15]. After withdrawal of the drug, attention is needed, as the symptoms of atopic dermatitis may worsen.

2) Methotrexate

Compared with cyclosporine, a similar improvement rate was observed at 16 weeks with a low frequency of adverse events [26].

3) Azathioprine

Compared to methotrexate, azathioprine has been reported to be effective and safe, but side effects such as bone marrow suppression remain [15, 27–30].

4) Mycophenolate Mofetil

A meta-analysis showed a 38.3% improvement in severity after mycophenolate mofetil [31].

5) Biologics

Biologics are emerging as important treatment options in patients with moderate-to-severe AD. Dupilumab, a fully human IL-4Rα monoclonal antibody inhibits both IL-4 and IL-13 signaling, has shown its efficacy and safety in patients with moderate-to-severe AD [32–34]. First, two phase 3 trials of identical design (SOLO 1 and SOLO 2) [32] showed the efficacy and safety of dupilumab monotherapy. Based on the results of this trial, dupilumab was approved by the US Food and Drug Administration in 2017 for adult patients with moderate to severe AD. In a long-term clinical trial (LIBERTY AD CHRONOS) [33] of dupilumab for 52 weeks in combination with concomitant low- or medium-potency topical corticosteroids, dupilumab also showed efficacy and safety in treatment of AD. Lebrikizumab and tralokinumab, monoclonal antibodies, can be considered in moderate to severe AD [35, 36]. Nemolizumab, an anti-IL-31 receptor A monoclonal antibody, improved pruritus, dermatitis, and sleep disturbance in AD patients [36]. Small molecules such as apremilast, a PDE 4 inhibitor [37–42], Janus kinase (JAK) inhibitors [43, 44], and histamine receptor antagonists [45, 46] also being studied in the treatment of AD.

3. Allergen-Specific Immunotherapy

Allergen-specific immunotherapy (ASIT) is considered in moderate-to-severe AD patients who are resistant to other treatments, however, it could also be considered in mild cases. ASIT is recommended for AD patients who have hypersensitivity to house dust mites, pollen, mold, fungi, hymenoptera, and animal allergens [23]. Because of potentially serious side effects such as systemic allergic reaction and anaphylaxis, close monitoring is recommended [47].

Discussion

AD is a chronic, relapsing inflammatory disorder. Therefore, appropriate treatment should be given to the AD severity following relapsing or flare-up. In patients with mild symptoms, it is essential to have skin care and avoid triggering factors. Psychological support with education is helpful for controlling AD. In some cases, topical treatments are used.

In addition to basic treatment, depending on the severity, active treatment with topical and systemic modalities is required. In addition, even if AD lesions improve, proactive treatment is needed to maintain the therapy.

References

1. Bieber T. Atopic dermatitis. N Engl J Med. 2008;358(14):1483–94.
2. Odhiambo JA, Williams HC, Clayton TO, Robertson CF, Asher MI, Group IPTS. Global variations in prevalence of eczema symptoms in children from ISAAC Phase Three. J Allergy Clin Immunol. 2009;124(6):1251–8.e23.
3. Lee JH, Han KD, Kim KM, Park YG, Lee JY, Park YM. Prevalence of atopic dermatitis in Korean children based on data from the 2008–2011 Korean National Health and Nutrition Examination Survey. Allergy Asthma Immunol Res. 2016;8(1):79–83.
4. Lee JH, Son SW, Cho SH. A comprehensive review of the treatment of atopic eczema. Allergy Asthma Immunol Res. 2016;8(3):181–90.
5. Silverberg JI, Hanifin JM. Adult eczema prevalence and associations with asthma and other health and demographic factors: a US population-based study. J Allergy Clin Immunol. 2013;132(5):1132–8.
6. Shaw TE, Currie GP, Koudelka CW, Simpson EL. Eczema prevalence in the United States: data from the 2003 National Survey of Children's Health. J Invest Dermatol. 2011;131(1):67–73.
7. Ashcroft DM, Dimmock P, Garside R, Stein K, Williams HC. Efficacy and tolerability of topical pimecrolimus and tacrolimus in the treatment of atopic dermatitis: meta-analysis of randomised controlled trials. BMJ. 2005;330(7490):516.
8. Kim JESM, Park GH, Lee UH, Lee JH, Han TY, Koh HC, Jang YH, Kim HO, Na CH, Lew BL, Ahn JY,

Park CO, Seo YJ, Lee YW, Sohn SW, Park YL. 2019 consensus Korean diagnostic guidelines to define severity classification and treatment refractoriness for atopic dermatitis: objective and subjective assessment of severity. Ann Dermatol. 2019;31(6):654–61.
9. Oranje AP, Glazenburg EJ, Wolkerstorfer A, de Waard-van der Spek FB. Practical issues on interpretation of scoring atopic dermatitis: the SCORAD index, objective SCORAD and the three-item severity score. Br J Dermatol. 2007;157(4):645–8.
10. Czarnowicki T, Malajian D, Khattri S, Correa da Rosa J, Dutt R, Finney R, et al. Petrolatum: barrier repair and antimicrobial responses underlying this "inert" moisturizer. J Allergy Clin Immunol. 2016;137(4):1091–102.e7.
11. Weber MB, Fontes Neto Pde T, Prati C, Soirefman M, Mazzotti NG, Barzenski B, et al. Improvement of pruritus and quality of life of children with atopic dermatitis and their families after joining support groups. J Eur Acad Dermatol Venereol. 2008;22(8):992–7.
12. Sher LG, Chang J, Patel IB, Balkrishnan R, Fleischer AB Jr. Relieving the pruritus of atopic dermatitis: a meta-analysis. Acta Derm Venereol. 2012;92(5):455–61.
13. Berth-Jones J, Damstra RJ, Golsch S, Livden JK, Van Hooteghem O, Allegra F, et al. Twice weekly fluticasone propionate added to emollient maintenance treatment to reduce risk of relapse in atopic dermatitis: randomised, double blind, parallel group study. BMJ. 2003;326(7403):1367.
14. Hanifin J, Gupta AK, Rajagopalan R. Intermittent dosing of fluticasone propionate cream for reducing the risk of relapse in atopic dermatitis patients. Br J Dermatol. 2002;147(3):528–37.
15. Roekevisch E, Spuls PI, Kuester D, Limpens J, Schmitt J. Efficacy and safety of systemic treatments for moderate-to-severe atopic dermatitis: a systematic review. J Allergy Clin Immunol. 2014;133(2):429–38.
16. Queille-Roussel C, Paul C, Duteil L, Lefebvre MC, Rapatz G, Zagula M, et al. The new topical ascomycin derivative SDZ ASM 981 does not induce skin atrophy when applied to normal skin for 4 weeks: a randomized, double-blind controlled study. Br J Dermatol. 2001;144(3):507–13.
17. Wollenberg A, Reitamo S, Girolomoni G, Lahfa M, Ruzicka T, Healy E, et al. Proactive treatment of atopic dermatitis in adults with 0.1% tacrolimus ointment. Allergy. 2008;63(7):742–50.
18. Gollnick H, Kaufmann R, Stough D, Heikkila H, Andriano K, Grinienko A, et al. Pimecrolimus cream 1% in the long-term management of adult atopic dermatitis: prevention of flare progression. A randomized controlled trial. Br J Dermatol. 2008;158(5):1083–93.
19. Garritsen FM, Brouwer MW, Limpens J, Spuls PI. Photo(chemo)therapy in the management of atopic dermatitis: an updated systematic review with implications for practice and research. Br J Dermatol. 2014;170(3):501–13.
20. Meduri NB, Vandergriff T, Rasmussen H, Jacobe H. Phototherapy in the management of atopic dermatitis: a systematic review. Photodermatol Photoimmunol Photomed. 2007;23(4):106–12.
21. Calzavara Pinton P, Cristaudo A, Foti C, Canonica GW, Balato N, Costanzo A, et al. Diagnosis and management of moderate to severe adult atopic dermatitis: a Consensus by the Italian Society of Dermatology and Venereology (SIDeMaST), the Italian Association of Hospital Dermatologists (ADOI), the Italian Society of Allergy, Asthma and Clinical Immunology (SIAAIC), and the Italian Society of Allergological, Environmental and Occupational Dermatology (SIDAPA). G Ital Dermatol Venereol. 2018;153(2):133–45.
22. Drucker AM, Eyerich K, de Bruin-Weller MS, Thyssen JP, Spuls PI, Irvine AD, et al. Use of systemic corticosteroids for atopic dermatitis: International Eczema Council consensus statement. Br J Dermatol. 2018;178(3):768–75.
23. Kim JE, Kim HJ, Lew BL, Lee KH, Hong SP, Jang YH, et al. Consensus guidelines for the treatment of atopic dermatitis in Korea (part II): systemic treatment. Ann Dermatol. 2015;27(5):578–92.
24. Sidbury R, Davis DM, Cohen DE, Cordoro KM, Berger TG, Bergman JN, et al. Guidelines of care for the management of atopic dermatitis: section 3. Management and treatment with phototherapy and systemic agents. J Am Acad Dermatol. 2014;71(2):327–49.
25. Yu SH, Drucker AM, Lebwohl M, Silverberg JI. A systematic review of the safety and efficacy of systemic corticosteroids in atopic dermatitis. J Am Acad Dermatol. 2018;78(4):733–40.e11.
26. Goujon C, Viguier M, Staumont-Salle D, Bernier C, Guillet G, Lahfa M, et al. Methotrexate versus cyclosporine in adults with moderate-to-severe atopic dermatitis: a phase III randomized noninferiority trial. J Allergy Clin Immunol Pract. 2018;6(2):562–9.e3.
27. Schram ME, Roekevisch E, Leeflang MM, Bos JD, Schmitt J, Spuls PI. A randomized trial of methotrexate versus azathioprine for severe atopic eczema. J Allergy Clin Immunol. 2011;128(2):353–9.
28. Gerbens LAA, Hamann SAS, Brouwer MWD, Roekevisch E, Leeflang MMG, Spuls PI. Methotrexate and azathioprine for severe atopic dermatitis: a 5-year follow-up study of a randomized controlled trial. Br J Dermatol. 2018;178(6):1288–96.
29. Wollenberg A, Barbarot S, Bieber T, Christen-Zaech S, Deleuran M, Fink-Wagner A, et al. Consensus-based European guidelines for treatment of atopic eczema (atopic dermatitis) in adults and children: part II. J Eur Acad Dermatol Venereol. 2018;32(6):850–78.
30. Rajagopalan M, De A, Godse K, Krupa Shankar DS, Zawar V, Sharma N, et al. guidelines on management of atopic dermatitis in India: an evidence-based review and an expert consensus. Indian J Dermatol. 2019;64(3):166–81.
31. Phan K, Smith SD. Mycophenolate mofetil and atopic dermatitis: systematic review and meta-analysis. J Dermatolog Treat. 2019:1–18. https://doi.org/10.1080/09546634.2019.1642996.

32. Simpson EL, Bieber T, Guttman-Yassky E, Beck LA, Blauvelt A, Cork MJ, et al. Two phase 3 trials of dupilumab versus placebo in atopic dermatitis. N Engl J Med. 2016;375(24):2335–48.
33. Blauvelt A, de Bruin-Weller M, Gooderham M, Cather JC, Weisman J, Pariser D, et al. Long-term management of moderate-to-severe atopic dermatitis with dupilumab and concomitant topical corticosteroids (LIBERTY AD CHRONOS): a 1-year, randomised, double-blinded, placebo-controlled, phase 3 trial. Lancet. 2017;389(10086):2287–303.
34. de Bruin-Weller M, Thaci D, Smith CH, Reich K, Cork MJ, Radin A, et al. Dupilumab with concomitant topical corticosteroid treatment in adults with atopic dermatitis with an inadequate response or intolerance to ciclosporin A or when this treatment is medically inadvisable: a placebo-controlled, randomized phase III clinical trial (LIBERTY AD CAFE). Br J Dermatol. 2018;178(5):1083–101.
35. Simpson EL, Flohr C, Eichenfield LF, Bieber T, Sofen H, Taieb A, et al. Efficacy and safety of lebrikizumab (an anti-IL-13 monoclonal antibody) in adults with moderate-to-severe atopic dermatitis inadequately controlled by topical corticosteroids: a randomized, placebo-controlled phase II trial (TREBLE). J Am Acad Dermatol. 2018;78(5):863–71.e11.
36. Wollenberg A, Howell MD, Guttman-Yassky E, Silverberg JI, Kell C, Ranade K, et al. Treatment of atopic dermatitis with tralokinumab, an anti-IL-13 mAb. J Allergy Clin Immunol. 2019;143(1):135–41.
37. Abrouk M, Farahnik B, Zhu TH, Nakamura M, Singh R, Lee K, et al. Apremilast treatment of atopic dermatitis and other chronic eczematous dermatoses. J Am Acad Dermatol. 2017;77(1):177–80.
38. Farahnik B, Beroukhim K, Nakamura M, Abrouk M, Zhu TH, Singh R, et al. Use of an oral phosphodiesterase-4 inhibitor (apremilast) for the treatment of chronic, severe atopic dermatitis: a case report. Dermatol Online J. 2017;23:5.
39. Samrao A, Berry TM, Goreshi R, Simpson EL. A pilot study of an oral phosphodiesterase inhibitor (apremilast) for atopic dermatitis in adults. Arch Dermatol. 2012;148(8):890–7.
40. Saporito RC, Cohen DJ. Apremilast use for moderate-to-severe atopic dermatitis in pediatric patients. Case Rep Dermatol. 2016;8(2):179–84.
41. Simpson EL, Imafuku S, Poulin Y, Ungar B, Zhou L, Malik K, et al. A phase 2 randomized trial of apremilast in patients with atopic dermatitis. J Invest Dermatol. 2019;139(5):1063–72.
42. Volf EM, Au SC, Dumont N, Scheinman P, Gottlieb AB. A phase 2, open-label, investigator-initiated study to evaluate the safety and efficacy of apremilast in subjects with recalcitrant allergic contact or atopic dermatitis. J Drugs Dermatol. 2012;11(3):341–6.
43. Guttman-Yassky E, Silverberg JI, Nemoto O, Forman SB, Wilke A, Prescilla R, et al. Baricitinib in adult patients with moderate-to-severe atopic dermatitis: a phase 2 parallel, double-blinded, randomized placebo-controlled multiple-dose study. J Am Acad Dermatol. 2019;80(4):913–21.e9.
44. Levy LL, Urban J, King BA. Treatment of recalcitrant atopic dermatitis with the oral Janus kinase inhibitor tofacitinib citrate. J Am Acad Dermatol. 2015;73(3):395–9.
45. Murata Y, Song M, Kikuchi H, Hisamichi K, Xu XL, Greenspan A, et al. Phase 2a, randomized, double-blind, placebo-controlled, multicenter, parallel-group study of a H4 R-antagonist (JNJ-39758979) in Japanese adults with moderate atopic dermatitis. J Dermatol. 2015;42(2):129–39.
46. Werfel T, Layton G, Yeadon M, Whitlock L, Osterloh I, Jimenez P, et al. Efficacy and safety of the histamine H4 receptor antagonist ZPL-3893787 in patients with atopic dermatitis. J Allergy Clin Immunol. 2019;143(5):1830–7.e4.
47. Pajno GB, Caminiti L, Vita D, Barberio G, Salzano G, Lombardo F, et al. Sublingual immunotherapy in mite-sensitized children with atopic dermatitis: a randomized, double-blind, placebo-controlled study. J Allergy Clin Immunol. 2007;120(1):164–70.

Part VII

Prevention

Prevention of Atopic Dermatitis

Eung Ho Choi

Introduction

Atopic dermatitis (AD) develops during the first 6 months of life in 45% of affected subjects and by 5 years of age in 85% of them [1]. AD generally begins in infancy, accompanied by food allergy, followed by the occurrence of asthma and allergic rhinitis at school age, which is the so-called atopic march. AD is chronic in nature because only half of children with AD have disease resolution in adulthood [2, 3].

Skin barrier dysfunction has been suggested to play an essential role in initiation of early AD. Antigen penetration through a compromised barrier likely leads to increased innate immune responses, antigen-presenting cell stimulation, and priming of distinct eczema [4–6]. In a T_H2-promoting environment, T-cell/B-cell interactions in regional draining lymph nodes lead to excessive IgE production. Simultaneous redistribution of memory T cells into the circulation exacerbates AD through cutaneous T-cell infiltration, and then spreads beyond the skin to include food allergy, asthma, and allergic rhinitis [7].

Stratum corneum (SC) intercellular lipids are important for the development of AD. The extracellular matrix in the SC is rich in ceramides, cholesterol, and free fatty acids, which are maintained at an optimal ratio [8]. Disruption of the lipid composition is documented in both lesional and nonlesional AD skin [9]. Additionally, the *TMEM79* gene, which is involved in secretion of lamellar bodies (LBs), was shown to be associated with AD [10]. These alterations increase transepidermal water loss (TEWL), reduce skin hydration, and impair skin barrier function [9]. A transcriptomic analysis of pediatric AD skin showed abnormalities in lipid metabolism genes despite the lack of *FLG* mutation [11]. This suggests that lipid abnormalities contribute independently to skin barrier dysfunction. A meta-analysis of the AD transcriptome presented significant negative correlations between key epidermal lipids and T_H2 activation [12].

In addition, restoring SC lipids is beneficial for patients with AD. Ceramide-dominant moisturizers have been shown to restore skin barrier integrity [13, 14]. Epidermal lipid synthesis and metabolism are regulated by nuclear hormone receptors (NHRs) and, in turn, epidermal lipid metabolites can serve as ligands for NHRs. Liver X receptor (LXR) is a transcription factor that can be activated by a number of small-molecule agonists. In animal models LXR agonists were shown to have beneficial effects on the skin, including increasing lamellar lipid levels and keratinocyte differentiation and decreasing

E. H. Choi (✉)
Department of Dermatology, Yonsei University Wonju College of Medicine, Wonju, Korea (Republic of)
e-mail: choieh@yonsei.ac.kr

K. H. Lee et al. (eds.), *Practical Insights into Atopic Dermatitis*,
https://doi.org/10.1007/978-981-15-8159-5_20

inflammation [15]. A topical LXR agonist is being tested in patients with AD.

Because AD and the atopic march mostly present in early infancy, primary prevention should be attempted as early as possible. Excessive T- and B-cell activation in the blood and skin occurs subsequently to promote the development of other allergic symptoms. Therefore, various strategies have to be taken into account to avoid the first stage of this march.

Moisturizers

Moisturizers were shown to improve skin barrier function and reduce inflammation [16, 17]. Moisturizers used in premature newborns decrease TEWL, dermatitis severity, and bacterial colonization [18, 19]. The compromised skin barrier of neonates predisposes them to development of AD at an early age. Skin barrier dysfunction, measured as increased TEWL, determined at birth and at 2 months of age, was significantly predictive of AD at 12 months in a large birth cohort study [20]. These changes were seen in both high- and low-risk infants and were independent of *FLG* mutations. Accordingly, a lowest-quartile TEWL at birth was protective against AD. The implication was that skin barrier dysfunction could facilitate allergen entry and allergic response priming. Thus, possible primary interventions to prevent AD are focusing on improving skin barrier integrity, including supplementing barrier function with moisturizers.

Some interventional studies have shown some promise in AD prevention in specific settings. A pilot study in 2010 showed that emollient therapy in 22 infants aged 3 weeks to 6 months at high risk of AD was useful and safe as a prevention strategy. Infants treated with a petrolatum-based cream showed a 50% reduction in the cumulative incidence of AD in comparison with controls [21]. Another pilot study of 56 infants with xerosis reported that regular moisturizing with oil baths over 6 months resulted in significantly less AD in the treatment group compared to the control [22]. In 2014, two prospective randomized controlled studies were reported. One randomized controlled trial in British and American neonates enrolled 124 high-risk neonates. They were treated with at least once-daily application of full-body emollients from 3 weeks of life for 6 months. The primary outcome of the cumulative incidence of AD at 6 months showed a 50% relative risk reduction in the treated group [23]. Another concomitant randomized controlled trial study from Japan reported a 32% reduction in AD diagnosis at age 32 weeks in 118 high-risk infants who received daily moisturizing from birth. IgE sensitization to egg white, skin hydration, and *S. aureus* colonization were also assessed at week 32. No differences were observed in IgE sensitization and *S. aureus* colonization between the intervention and the control groups, whereas the intervention group had significantly higher SC hydration [24]. The strategy of daily application of moisturizer to prevent AD in infants at high risk is reasonable but may not offer lifetime prevention.

According to Korea Health Insurance Corporation data from 2010 to 2015, the prevalence of AD continues to decrease in children between the ages of 0 and 9 years. We guessed the following reasons. More than 70% of Korean mothers have higher education than college graduation, so they fully understood the importance of moisturizers and start applying them as soon as the baby is born.

Probiotics

Early in pregnancy, limited microbial exposure and changes in the growth and composition of intestinal microbiota such as antibiotics, dietary habits, and other lifestyle influences could contribute to increased incidence and severity of allergic disorders [25]. In utero exposure to bacterial patterns primes the immune system and/or the epithelium to respond appropriately to pathogens and commensals after birth. A meta-analysis reported that antibiotic exposure during the last two trimesters of pregnancy increases the risk of wheeze/asthma at 3 years [26].

In infancy, microbiome alteration is an important risk factor for allergic diseases. Evidence suggests that the microbial environment plays a significant role in the pathogenesis of allergic diseases [27]. Changes in the resident microbiome, with production of protective metabolites, such as short-chain fatty acids, tryptophan, or zwitterionic polysaccharides, can have defensive effects against allergic diseases and may occur through the diet or exposure to siblings, daycare, dogs, or farming environments.

Possible strategies to prevent allergic diseases are correction of dysbiosis and increased exposure to beneficial microbes [28]. From this point of view, probiotics, acting as promoters of an adequate balance in the gut microbiota [29], have been suggested as an intervention to prevent allergic diseases [30]. Prenatal and postnatal (maternal and child) supplementation of *Lactobacillus rhamnosus* showed promise in prevention [31]. Conversely, early experiments showed that probiotics (e.g., *Lactobacillus reuteri*) given prenatally in pregnant women and postnatally in infants did not reduce the occurrence of AD but possibly reduced IgE-associated AD [32]. In a double-blind, placebo-controlled trial, *L. rhamnosus* GG alone reduced AD by half in high-risk infants [33]. A successful trial involved the randomization of 415 pregnant women to receive interventions from 36 weeks' gestation until 3 months postpartum [34]. The intervention was a randomized comparison of milk without probiotics versus a blend of probiotic milk containing *L. rhamnosus* GG, *Lactobacillus acidophilus* La-5, and *Bifidobacterium animalis* subsp. *lactis* Bb-12. At 6 years of age, the children whose mothers had received probiotics had a significantly lower prevalence of AD. However, other allergic diseases were not prevented in this study [34].

A meta-analysis of 17 randomized controlled trials found a significantly lower risk ratio for AD in infants treated pre- and postnatally with probiotics (relative risk [RR] 0.78 [95% confidence interval (CI) 0.69–0.89], $P = 0.0003$) [35]. Several other systematic reviews and/or meta-analyses have confirmed similar findings [36]. Most studies started probiotics in the last 2–4 weeks of gestation, with one randomized controlled trial starting them 2 months before delivery with the intention to influence postnatal gut colonization [37]. A subgroup meta-analysis found a significant effect of giving both pre- and postnatal probiotics, as opposed to giving postnatal supplementation alone [35]. Although one meta-analysis reported that treatment with *Lactobacillus* alone or in combination with *Bifidobacterium* was protective [35], others found the most significant reduction in eczema when a mixture of strains was used [38]. *Lactobacillus rhamnosus* is one specific strain shown to have a protective effect and was used either alone or as part of a mixture in the two largest cohort studies [39–42]. Daily use of *L. rhamnosus* HN001 in pregnant women from 35 weeks gestation until 6 months after delivery if breastfeeding and in infants from birth until 2 years showed a 50% reduction in AD prevalence when the children were 2, 4, and 6 years of age. Subgroup meta-analyses revealed that probiotics prevented AD for the first 2 years of life, but then there was a relative loss of efficacy [38].

Diet

Possible benefits of exclusive breastfeeding and/or supplementation with hydrolyzed formula in high-risk children were discussed. Elimination diets for mothers were not recommended. A beneficial role of supplements including vitamin D, selenium, fish oil, borage oil, and zinc sulfate was not found [43]. A National Institute of Allergy and Infectious Diseases consensus group made the following recommendations. A restricted maternal diet during pregnancy or lactation in high-risk mothers was not recommended. Breastfeeding exclusively for the first 4–6 months was recommended. Hydrolyzed formulas were suggested as a possible preventive strategy in high-risk infants as a breastfeeding alternative [44].

It was hypothesized that early sensitization to food allergens might be due to their ingestion through breast milk, which explains the reactions to foods never consumed before [45]. A microarray with antibodies against ten major food allergens was performed with breast milk from 14 Spanish women. All allergens including the most potent peanut allergen (Ara h 2) were detected with a wide variation in protein concentrations in breast milk [46]. Therefore, breastfeeding could be a gateway of IgE sensitization to food allergens dissolved in maternal milk. The first allergenic contact may be important because it might lead in the future to an allergic state in the child regarding both sensitization and tolerance. However, avoidance of cow's milk and egg during lactation did not prevent food sensitization in infants [47].

Common food allergens cross the placenta because they were detected in amniotic fluid from pregnant women at 15–20 weeks of gestation and from 20 women after delivery [48]. In addition, 9 of 37 newborns with positive IgE responses to ovalbumin in cord blood developed an egg allergy or AD by 14 months of age [49]. However, avoiding allergenic foods in pregnancy does not reduce the risk of atopy in intervention studies [50]. Observational studies reported that low consumption of peanuts, tree nuts, or cow's milk in pregnancy, particularly among nonallergic women, may possibly increase the risk of allergy to peanuts, tree nuts, and cow's milk, respectively. In addition, maternal wheat intake is low, making it a risk factor for AD [51, 52].

Whether allergy is prevented by reducing or increasing exposure to food allergens or delaying or advancing weaning is still being debated. Current evidence does not show that AD incidence is lower in breastfed infants [53]. Yet, breastfeeding remains the cornerstone of infants' nutrition program because of its benefits for growth and immune maturation. Thus, it is recommended for at least 6 months. Moreover, early weaning is beneficial to prevent AD occurrence in children [54]. Delay in the intake of solid food above the recommended minimum age did not show a preventive effect on allergy in infants at high or normal risk [55]. However, early intake of six allergenic foods such as peanuts, cooked egg, cow's milk, sesame, whitefish, and wheat from 3 months of age did not prevent allergic diseases at 1 and 3 years of age in the general population [56]. A protective effect against the development of peanut allergy has been shown by introduction of peanuts between 4 and 11 months of age among high-risk children [57].

Evidence showing that n-3 long-chain polyunsaturated fatty acid (LCPUFA) supplementation during pregnancy and/or lactation prevents allergy was limited in a systematic review [58]. Few differences in childhood allergic diseases were seen between women who were supplemented with n-3 LCPUFAs and those who were not. On the other hand, a prospective study reported that n-3 LCPUFA supplementation during infancy may reduce the risk of skin and respiratory allergic diseases in childhood [59].

Therefore, diet-related strategies to prevent AD have focused on early introduction of complementary foods and dietary supplementation with probiotics and unsaturated fatty acids.

Other Factors

The role of other factors including vaccinations, allergen avoidance, and breastfeeding in preventing AD is still arguable [60, 61].

Other risk factors for AD, obesity, or low vitamin D levels in pregnancy have been discussed. Accelerated growth and a relative increase in abdominal circumference between the first and the second trimesters of pregnancy were associated with a higher risk of AD [62]. It could be maternal obesity that represents a key factor for the regulation of neonatal immune system development [63]. In a Taiwanese pediatric study, low maternal 25-hydroxyvitamin D levels were linked to an increased risk of allergic sensitization, early childhood AD, and asthma [64]. Conversely, the levels of 25-hydroxyvitamin D in mid gestation and at birth were not associated with the risk of AD among children within the first 4 years of life [65]. In a meta-analysis, a moderate association was found between low maternal vitamin D levels and increased risk of childhood AD in the offspring [66].

Delivery by cesarean section (CS) may predispose toward development of a food allergy in early childhood. A birth cohort study from Greece showed that children born by CS had a threefold probability of developing a food allergy in the first 3 years of life, especially those with an allergic predisposition [67]. However, in agreement with a previous report, no effect on the risk of AD was shown [62].

In a Danish nationwide cohort study, seasons influenced the risk of AD, with the highest risk in children born during fall and the lowest risk in those born during spring [68]. This result could be explained by transcutaneous allergen exposure and dry skin in the winter season. In this cohort study, neonatal jaundice also was a weak but significant risk factor for childhood AD. In a population-based study, neonatal jaundice was associated with the development of allergic diseases, mostly allergic rhinitis and AD [69]. Moreover, this risk was linked with high bilirubin levels requiring phototherapy [70].

Pollutants associated with climate factors may differentially impact AD prevalence and severity, some with apparent harmful effects [71]. On the other hand, lower UVB exposure could contribute to the increased AD incidence among industrialized countries [72]. This result could be partially explained by reduced exposure to solar irradiation in children living in urban areas.

The association between the exposure to pets (especially cats and dogs) and the prevalence of allergic diseases is inconsistent. Early exposure to dogs or cats and the prevalence of allergic diseases among school-aged children was analyzed. After multivariate analyses, only exposure to dogs, both indoors and outdoors, was significantly associated with a decrease in the prevalence of AD (odds ratios [ORs] 0.40 [95% CI 0.20–0.79] and 0.38 [95% CI 0.18–0.83], respectively). Therefore, exposure to dogs, whether indoor or outdoor pets, is associated with a decreased prevalence of AD [73].

Conclusions

Although AD is largely genetic in nature, low-risk prevention strategies have been attempted to reduce the likelihood of a first onset of AD in pre disposed individuals. Moisturizer application from early infancy, use of probiotics during pregnancy and lactation in mother and neonate, and early complementary food intake are some possible methods recommended for primary prevention of AD. Eventually AD prevention needs to select who could be candidates for testing the most effective prevention strategies in practice. So far, decisions on high-risk groups have been based solely on parental memory. Therefore, recently developed methods that can easily and quickly detect predictive biomarkers for AD onset, including gene mutations, have to be used, and they will increase the effects of methods aimed at preventing AD development.

References

1. Kay J, Gawkrodger DJ, Mortimer MJ, Jaron AG. The prevalence of childhood atopic eczema in a general population. J Am Acad Dermatol. 1994;30(1):35–9.
2. Spergel JM, Paller AS. Atopic dermatitis and the atopic march. J Allergy Clin Immunol. 2003;112(6 Suppl):S118–S27.
3. Spergel JM. From atopic dermatitis to asthma: the atopic march. Ann Allergy Asthma Immunol. 2010;105(2):99–117.
4. Chamlin SL, Kao J, Frieden IJ, Sheu MY, Fowler AJ, Fluhr JW, et al. Ceramide-dominant barrier repair lipids alleviate childhood atopic dermatitis: changes in barrier function provide a sensitive indicator of disease activity. J Am Acad Dermatol. 2002;47(2):198–208.
5. Elias PM, Hatano Y, Williams ML. Basis for the barrier abnormality in atopic dermatitis: outside-inside-outside pathogenic mechanisms. J Allergy Clin Immunol. 2008;121(6):1337–43.
6. Nickoloff BJ, Naidu Y. Perturbation of epidermal barrier function correlates with initiation of cytokine cascade in human skin. J Am Acad Dermatol. 1994;30(4):535–46.
7. Czarnowicki T, Krueger JG, Guttman-Yassky E. Novel concepts of prevention and treatment of atopic dermatitis through barrier and immune manipulations with implications for the atopic march. J Allergy Clin Immunol. 2017;139(6):1723–34.
8. Elias PM, Crumrine D, Rassner U, Hachem J-P, Menon GK, Man W, et al. Basis for abnormal desquamation and permeability barrier dysfunction in RXLI. J Invest Dermatol. 2004;122(2):314–9.
9. Jungersted JM, Scheer H, Mempel M, Baurecht H, Cifuentes L, Høgh JK, et al. Stratum corneum lipids, skin barrier function and filaggrin mutations in patients with atopic eczema. Allergy. 2010;65(7):911–8.
10. Saunders SP, Goh CSM, Brown SJ, Palmer CNA, Porter RM, Cole C, et al. Tmem79/Matt is the matted mouse gene and is a predisposing gene for atopic dermatitis in human subjects. J Allergy Clin Immunol. 2013;132(5):1121–9.

11. Cole C, Kroboth K, Schurch NJ, Sandilands A, Sherstnev A, O'Regan GM, et al. Filaggrin-stratified transcriptomic analysis of pediatric skin identifies mechanistic pathways in patients with atopic dermatitis. J Allergy Clin Immunol. 2014;134(1):82–91.
12. Ewald DA, Malajian D, Krueger JG, Workman CT, Wang T, Tian S, et al. Meta-analysis derived atopic dermatitis (MADAD) transcriptome defines a robust AD signature highlighting the involvement of atherosclerosis and lipid metabolism pathways. BMC Med Genet. 2015;8:60.
13. Kim M, Jung M, Hong S-P, Jeon H, Kim M-J, Cho M-Y, et al. Topical calcineurin inhibitors compromise stratum corneum integrity, epidermal permeability and antimicrobial barrier function. Exp Dermatol. 2010;19(6):501–10.
14. Sajić D, Asiniwasis R, Skotnicki-Grant S. A look at epidermal barrier function in atopic dermatitis: physiologic lipid replacement and the role of ceramides. Skin Therapy Lett. 2012;17(7):6–9.
15. Schmuth M, Moosbrugger-Martinz V, Blunder S, Dubrac S. Role of PPAR, LXR, and PXR in epidermal homeostasis and inflammation. Biochim Biophys Acta. 2014;1841(3):463–73.
16. Czarnowicki T, Malajian D, Khattri S, Correa da Rosa J, Dutt R, Finney R, et al. Petrolatum: barrier repair and antimicrobial responses underlying this "inert" moisturizer. J Allergy Clin Immunol. 2016;137(4):1091–102.e7.
17. Giam YC, Hebert AA, Dizon MV, Van Bever H, Tiongco-Recto M, Kim K-H, et al. A review on the role of moisturizers for atopic dermatitis. Asia Pac Allergy. 2016;6(2):120–8.
18. Pabst RC, Starr KP, Qaiyumi S, Schwalbe RS, Gewolb IH. The effect of application of aquaphor on skin condition, fluid requirements, and bacterial colonization in very low birth weight infants. J Perinatol. 1999;19(4):278–83.
19. Nopper AJ, Horii KA, Sookdeo-Drost S, Wang TH, Mancini AJ, Lane AT. Topical ointment therapy benefits premature infants. J Pediatr. 1996;128(5 Pt 1):660–9.
20. Kelleher M, Dunn-Galvin A, Hourihane JOB, Murray D, Campbell LE, McLean WHI, et al. Skin barrier dysfunction measured by transepidermal water loss at 2 days and 2 months predates and predicts atopic dermatitis at 1 year. J Allergy Clin Immunol. 2015;135(4):930–5.e1.
21. Simpson EL, Berry TM, Brown PA, Hanifin JM. A pilot study of emollient therapy for the primary prevention of atopic dermatitis. J Am Acad Dermatol. 2010;63(4):587–93.
22. Kvenshagen BK, Carlsen KH, Mowinckel P, Berents TL, Carlsen KCL. Can early skin care normalise dry skin and possibly prevent atopic eczema? A pilot study in young infants. Allergol Immunopathol (Madr). 2014;42(6):539–43.
23. Simpson EL, Chalmers JR, Hanifin JM, Thomas KS, Cork MJ, McLean WHI, et al. Emollient enhancement of the skin barrier from birth offers effective atopic dermatitis prevention. J Allergy Clin Immunol. 2014;134(4):818–23.
24. Horimukai K, Morita K, Narita M, Kondo M, Kitazawa H, Nozaki M, et al. Application of moisturizer to neonates prevents development of atopic dermatitis. J Allergy Clin Immunol. 2014;134(4):824–30.e6.
25. Abrahamsson TR, Wu RY, Jenmalm MC. Gut microbiota and allergy: the importance of the pregnancy period. Pediatr Res. 2015;77(1-2):214–9.
26. Zhao D, Su H, Cheng J, Wang X, Xie M, Li K, et al. Prenatal antibiotic use and risk of childhood wheeze/asthma: a meta-analysis. Pediatr Allergy Immunol. 2015;26(8):756–64.
27. von Mutius E. The microbial environment and its influence on asthma prevention in early life. J Allergy Clin Immunol. 2016;137(3):680–9.
28. Blattner CM, Crosby MS, Goedken M, Murase JE. Update: do probiotics prevent or treat pediatric atopic dermatitis? Pediatr Allergy Immunol. 2016;27(4):425–8.
29. Caffarelli C, Cardinale F, Povesi-Dascola C, Dodi I, Mastrorilli V, Ricci G. Use of probiotics in pediatric infectious diseases. Expert Rev Anti-Infect Ther. 2015;13(12):1517–35.
30. Lundelin K, Poussa T, Salminen S, Isolauri E. Long-term safety and efficacy of perinatal probiotic intervention: evidence from a follow-up study of four randomized, double-blind, placebo-controlled trials. Pediatr Allergy Immunol. 2017;28(2):170–5.
31. Foolad N, Brezinski EA, Chase EP, Armstrong AW. Effect of nutrient supplementation on atopic dermatitis in children: a systematic review of probiotics, prebiotics, formula, and fatty acids. JAMA Dermatol. 2013;149(3):350–5.
32. Abrahamsson TR, Jakobsson T, Böttcher MF, Fredrikson M, Jenmalm MC, Björkstén B, et al. Probiotics in prevention of IgE-associated eczema: a double-blind, randomized, placebo-controlled trial. J Allergy Clin Immunol. 2007;119(5):1174–80.
33. Kalliomäki M, Salminen S, Arvilommi H, Kero P, Koskinen P, Isolauri E. Probiotics in primary prevention of atopic disease: a randomised placebo-controlled trial. Lancet. 2001;357(9262):1076–9.
34. Simpson MR, Dotterud CK, Storrø O, Johnsen R, Øien T. Perinatal probiotic supplementation in the prevention of allergy related disease: 6 year follow up of a randomised controlled trial. BMC Dermatol. 2015;15:13.
35. Panduru M, Panduru NM, Sălăvăstru CM, Tiplica GS. Probiotics and primary prevention of atopic dermatitis: a meta-analysis of randomized controlled studies. J Eur Acad Dermatol Venereol. 2015;29(2):232–42.
36. Boulos S, Yan AC. Current concepts in the prevention of atopic dermatitis. Clin Dermatol. 2018;36(5):668–71.
37. Rautava S, Kainonen E, Salminen S, Isolauri E. Maternal probiotic supplementation during pregnancy and breast-feeding reduces the risk of

eczema in the infant. J Allergy Clin Immunol. 2012;130(6):1355–60.
38. Zuccotti G, Meneghin F, Aceti A, Barone G, Callegari ML, Di Mauro A, et al. Probiotics for prevention of atopic diseases in infants: systematic review and meta-analysis. Allergy. 2015;70(11):1356–71.
39. Kukkonen K, Savilahti E, Haahtela T, Juntunen-Backman K, Korpela R, Poussa T, et al. Probiotics and prebiotic galacto-oligosaccharides in the prevention of allergic diseases: a randomized, double-blind, placebo-controlled trial. J Allergy Clin Immunol. 2007;119(1):192–8.
40. Wickens K, Black PN, Stanley TV, Mitchell E, Fitzharris P, Tannock GW, et al. A differential effect of 2 probiotics in the prevention of eczema and atopy: a double-blind, randomized, placebo-controlled trial. J Allergy Clin Immunol. 2008;122(4):788–94.
41. Wickens K, Black P, Stanley TV, Mitchell E, Barthow C, Fitzharris P, et al. A protective effect of Lactobacillus rhamnosus HN001 against eczema in the first 2 years of life persists to age 4 years. Clin Exp Allergy. 2012;42(7):1071–9.
42. Wickens K, Stanley TV, Mitchell EA, Barthow C, Fitzharris P, Purdie G, et al. Early supplementation with Lactobacillus rhamnosus HN001 reduces eczema prevalence to 6 years: does it also reduce atopic sensitization? Clin Exp Allergy. 2013;43(9):1048–57.
43. Bronsnick T, Murzaku EC, Rao BK. Diet in dermatology: part I. Atopic dermatitis, acne, and nonmelanoma skin cancer. J Am Acad Dermatol. 2014;71(6):1039.e1–e12.
44. Boyce JA, Assa'ad A, Burks AW, Jones SM, Sampson HA, Wood RA, et al. Guidelines for the diagnosis and management of food allergy in the United States: summary of the NIAID-sponsored expert panel report. Nutr Res. 2011;31(1):61–75.
45. Pastor-Vargas C, Maroto AS, Díaz-Perales A, Villaba M, Casillas Diaz N, Vivanco F, et al. Sensitive detection of major food allergens in breast milk: first gateway for allergenic contact during breastfeeding. Allergy. 2015;70(8):1024–7.
46. Schocker F, Baumert J, Kull S, Petersen A, Becker W-M, Jappe U. Prospective investigation on the transfer of Ara h 2, the most potent peanut allergen, in human breast milk. Pediatr Allergy Immunol. 2016;27(4):348–55.
47. Kramer MS, Kakuma R. Maternal dietary antigen avoidance during pregnancy or lactation, or both, for preventing or treating atopic disease in the child. Cochrane Database Syst Rev. 2012;2012(9):CD000133-CD.
48. Pastor-Vargas C, Maroto AS, Díaz-Perales A, Villalba M, Esteban V, Ruiz-Ramos M, et al. Detection of major food allergens in amniotic fluid: initial allergenic encounter during pregnancy. Pediatr Allergy Immunol. 2016;27(7):716–20.
49. Kamemura N, Kawamoto N, Nakamura R, Teshima R, Fukao T, Kido H. Low-affinity allergen-specific IgE in cord blood and affinity maturation after birth. J Allergy Clin Immunol. 2014;133(3):904–5.e6.
50. Kramer MS, Kakuma R. Maternal dietary antigen avoidance during pregnancy or lactation, or both, for preventing or treating atopic disease in the child. Evid Based Child Health. 2014;9(2):447–83.
51. Bunyavanich S, Rifas-Shiman SL, Platts-Mills TA, Workman L, Sordillo JE, Camargo CA Jr, et al. Peanut, milk, and wheat intake during pregnancy is associated with reduced allergy and asthma in children. J Allergy Clin Immunol. 2014;133(5):1373–82.
52. Tuokkola J, Luukkainen P, Tapanainen H, Kaila M, Vaarala O, Kenward MG, et al. Maternal diet during pregnancy and lactation and cow's milk allergy in offspring. Eur J Clin Nutr. 2016;70(5):554–9.
53. Tan H-TT, Ellis JA, Koplin JJ, Matheson MC, Gurrin LC, Lowe AJ, et al. Filaggrin loss-of-function mutations do not predict food allergy over and above the risk of food sensitization among infants. J Allergy Clin Immunol. 2012;130(5):1211–3.e3.
54. Turati F, Bertuccio P, Galeone C, Pelucchi C, Naldi L, Bach JF, et al. Early weaning is beneficial to prevent atopic dermatitis occurrence in young children. Allergy. 2016;71(6):878–88.
55. Ricci G, Cipriani F. Which advises for primary food allergy prevention in normal or high-risk infant? Pediatr Allergy Immunol. 2016;27(8):774–8.
56. Perkin MR, Logan K, Tseng A, Raji B, Ayis S, Peacock J, et al. Randomized trial of introduction of allergenic foods in breast-fed infants. N Engl J Med. 2016;374(18):1733–43.
57. Du Toit G, Roberts G, Sayre PH, Bahnson HT, Radulovic S, Santos AF, et al. Randomized trial of peanut consumption in infants at risk for peanut allergy. N Engl J Med. 2015;372(9):803–13.
58. Gunaratne AW, Makrides M, Collins CT. Maternal prenatal and/or postnatal n-3 long chain polyunsaturated fatty acids (LCPUFA) supplementation for preventing allergies in early childhood. Cochrane Database Syst Rev. 2015;2015(7):CD010085-CD.
59. Foiles AM, Kerling EH, Wick JA, Scalabrin DMF, Colombo J, Carlson SE. Formula with long-chain polyunsaturated fatty acids reduces incidence of allergy in early childhood. Pediatr Allergy Immunol. 2016;27(2):156–61.
60. Oszukowska M, Michalak I, Gutfreund K, Bienias W, Matych M, Szewczyk A, et al. Role of primary and secondary prevention in atopic dermatitis. Postepy Dermatol Alergol. 2015;32(6):409–20.
61. Williams HC, Chalmers JR, Simpson EL. Prevention of atopic dermatitis. F1000 Med Rep. 2012;4:24.
62. Parazzini F, Cipriani S, Zinetti C, Chatenoud L, Frigerio L, Amuso G, et al. Perinatal factors and the risk of atopic dermatitis: a cohort study. Pediatr Allergy Immunol. 2014;25(1):43–50.
63. Wilson RM, Marshall NE, Jeske DR, Purnell JQ, Thornburg K, Messaoudi I. Maternal obesity alters immune cell frequencies and responses in umbilical cord blood samples. Pediatr Allergy Immunol. 2015;26(4):344–51.

64. Chiu C-Y, Huang S-Y, Peng Y-C, Tsai M-H, Hua M-C, Yao T-C, et al. Maternal vitamin D levels are inversely related to allergic sensitization and atopic diseases in early childhood. Pediatr Allergy Immunol. 2015;26(4):337–43.
65. Gazibara T, Elbert NJ, den Dekker HT, de Jongste JC, Reiss I, McGrath JJ, et al. Associations of maternal and fetal 25-hydroxyvitamin D levels with childhood eczema: the Generation R Study. Pediatr Allergy Immunol. 2016;27(3):283–9.
66. Wei Z, Zhang J, Yu X. Maternal vitamin D status and childhood asthma, wheeze, and eczema: a systematic review and meta-analysis. Pediatr Allergy Immunol. 2016;27(6):612–9.
67. Papathoma E, Triga M, Fouzas S, Dimitriou G. Cesarean section delivery and development of food allergy and atopic dermatitis in early childhood. Pediatr Allergy Immunol. 2016;27(4):419–24.
68. Egeberg A, Andersen YMF, Gislason G, Skov L, Thyssen JP. Neonatal risk factors of atopic dermatitis in Denmark—results from a nationwide register-based study. Pediatr Allergy Immunol. 2016;27(4):368–74.
69. Wei C-C, Lin C-L, Shen T-C, Kao C-H. Neonatal jaundice and risks of childhood allergic diseases: a population-based cohort study. Pediatr Res. 2015;78(2):223–30.
70. Das RR, Naik SS. Neonatal hyperbilirubinemia and childhood allergic diseases: a systematic review. Pediatr Allergy Immunol. 2015;26(1):2–11.
71. Kathuria P, Silverberg JI. Association of pollution and climate with atopic eczema in US children. Pediatr Allergy Immunol. 2016;27(5):478–85.
72. Thyssen JP, Zirwas MJ, Elias PM. Potential role of reduced environmental UV exposure as a driver of the current epidemic of atopic dermatitis. J Allergy Clin Immunol. 2015;136(5):1163–9.
73. Bedolla-Barajas M, Morales-Romero J, Bedolla-Pulido TI, Bedolla-Pulido TR, Meza-López C, Pulido-Guillén NA. Exposure to dogs but not cats is associated to a decrease in the prevalence in atopic dermatitis amongst school-children. Allergol Immunopathol (Madr). 2018;46(5):431–7.

GPSR Compliance

The European Union's (EU) General Product Safety Regulation (GPSR) is a set of rules that requires consumer products to be safe and our obligations to ensure this.

If you have any concerns about our products, you can contact us on ProductSafety@springernature.com

In case Publisher is established outside the EU, the EU authorized representative is:

Springer Nature Customer Service Center GmbH
Europaplatz 3
69115 Heidelberg, Germany

Batch number: 10731385

Printed by Printforce, the Netherlands